Other monographs in the series, *Major Problems in Clinical Pediatrics:*

Bell and McCormick: *Increased Intracranial Pressure in Children* — published in July 1972

Cornblath and Schwartz: *Disorders of Carbohydrate Metabolism in Infancy* — published in February 1966

Oski and Naiman: *Hematologic Problems in the Newborn* — Second Edition published in March 1972

Rowe and Mehrizi: *The Neonate with Congenital Heart Disease* — published in June 1968

Brewer: *Juvenile Rheumatoid Arthritis* — published in January 1970

Smith: *Recognizable Patterns of Human Malformation* — published in February 1970

Solomon and Esterly: *Neonatal Dematology* — published in January 1973

Scriver and Rosenberg: *Amino Acid Metabolism and Its Disorders* — published in October 1973

THE LUNG AND ITS DISORDERS IN THE NEWBORN INFANT

Third Edition

By

Mary Ellen Avery, A.B., M.D.

Professor and Chairman, Department of Pediatrics,
Faculty of Medicine, McGill University;
Physician-in Chief, Montreal Children's Hospital;
Formerly physician-in-charge, Newborn Nurseries,
Johns Hopkins Hospital, Baltimore, Maryland

and

Barry D. Fletcher, B.A., M.D., C.M.

Assistant Professor, Department of Diagnostic Radiology,
Lecturer in Pediatrics, Faculty of Medicine,
McGill University; Radiologist, Montreal Children's Hospital

Volume I in the Series
MAJOR PROBLEMS IN CLINICAL PEDIATRICS

ALEXANDER J. SCHAFFER
Consulting Editor

W. B. Saunders Company, Philadelphia, London, Toronto 1974

W. B. Saunders Company: West Washington Square
Philadelphia, Pa. 19105

12 Dyott Street
London, WCIA 1DB

833 Oxford Street
Toronto, Ontario M8Z 5T9

The Lung and its Disorders in the Newborn Infant   ISBN 0-7216-1467-1

Print No.   9   8   7   6   5   4   3   2   1

Foreword

Everyone who has any interest in neonatology is acquainted with Dr. Mary Ellen Avery's *The Lung and Its Disorders in the Newborn Infant*. This was the original volume in our series entitled *Major Problems in Clinical Pediatrics*. Published in 1964, its excellence was of a quality all our subsequent contributors have tried hard to attain. By 1968 Dr. Avery deemed it outdated, so rapidly had new knowledge in the field accrued, and her second edition became available. Now, five years later, she feels constrained to update it and revise it once more, for the same good reasons.

This time she has enlisted the help of Dr. Barry D. Fletcher. Dr. Fletcher is an Assistant Professor of Radiology at McGill University and Radiologist at the Montreal Children's Hospital. He received his earlier training in the Radiology Department of the Johns Hopkins Hospital, focusing his interest largely upon infants and children. With his expert assistance, the radiographic illustrations, so very important a part of a work of this nature, have been augmented in number, selected with even greater care, and reproduced with more precision.

Again the authors have come up with "the last word" on this subject.

ALEXANDER J. SCHAFFER, M.D.

Preface to the Third Edition

Why a third edition? The answer is that observations made on infants and laboratory studies in the past five years are of such significance that they deserve to be collected in one place; the student who confines his reading to the second edition would be lacking some very important information, particularly in the area of artificial respiration; and finally, I enjoy the opportunity to read critically and try to understand events in a rapidly moving specialty.

This edition allows me to introduce a new author, Dr. Barry Fletcher. In both previous editions I relied heavily on the advice of first Dr. Olga Baghdassarian, and later Dr. John Dorst, radiologists at the Johns Hopkins Hospital. Dr. Fletcher, radiologist at the Montreal Children's Hospital now brings to these pages increased emphasis on the important role of radiographic studies in both investigation and diagnosis.

A new setting, Montreal, has provided new opportunities to study respiratory problems in the fetus and newborn. The neonatal intensive care unit at the Montreal Children's Hospital under Dr. Leo Stern, the respiratory function laboratory under Dr. Pierre Beaudry, and the nurseries of the Royal Victoria Hospital under Dr. Robert Usher all provide clinical stimulation; the physiology department of McGill University, under Dr. David Bates, has been a superb setting in which to pursue animal studies, and the cooperation of Dr. Thurlbeck and Dr. Wang of the department of pathology has been invaluable. The research fellows since 1968, Drs. John Knelson, Robert Kotas, and H. William Taeusch, have been largely responsible for the studies from our laboratory, some of which have made it clear that the third edition is due.

I remain indebted to former fellows who contributed so much to the earlier editions, they are Drs. George Brumley, Sue Buckingham, Shirley Borkowf, Victor Chernick, Robert deLemos, Axel Fenner, W. Alan Hodson, Richard Nachman, Colin Normand, Hooshang Shaibani, and Jack Wolfsdorf.

Many of our colleagues have contributed helpful criticism and suggestions to this edition. Dr. Robert L. Williams extensively revised the chapter on perinatal circulation, and Dr. Ronald Shapera reviewed the section on infections. To them, and to all those who have participated in "newborn rounds" in recent years, this volume is our way of saying, "Thank you."

MARY ELLEN AVERY

Preface to the
First Edition

A monograph devoted to one organ at one time of life can be written only if innumerable investigators at the bedside and in the laboratory have directed their attention to the problem over many years. This work is a compilation of the experience in many parts of the world. It follows the publication of textbooks devoted to the newborn infant and his illnesses, upon which I have relied in great measure to provide the background and perspective needed to focus upon the lung. Three books in particular, Clement Smith's *Physiology of the Newborn Infant* (Thomas), William Silverman's *Dunham's Premature Infants* (Hoeber), and Alexander Schaffer's *Diseases of the Newborn* (Saunders), have provided much useful information about newborn infants. Potter's *Pathology of the Fetus and Infant* (Year Book) and Spencer's *Pathology of the Lung* (Macmillan) also furnished a wealth of information and references.

But interest in a subject and desire to assemble information about it could never have come from textbooks alone. Much came from opportunities for clinical and laboratory experience at the Johns Hopkins and Boston Lying-In Hospitals, and in the Department of Physiology, Harvard School of Public Health. But even more came from the stimulation of my teachers. I cannot possibly acknowledge everyone who has helped make this work possible. I cite for special mention Dr. George Anderson, who reminded me that the newborn infant has special and puzzling problems; Drs. Harry Gordon, Alexander Schaffer, and Janet Hardy, who by their stimulating rounds in the nurseries of The Johns Hopkins Hospital interested me in devoting special attention to newborn infants; Drs. Jere Mead, James Whittenberger, and Charles D. Cook at Harvard, who communicated much of their enthusiasm and knowledge about the physiology of the lung; and especially Dr. Clement Smith, whose own great interest in, and knowledge of, the newborn infant was shared through both his writings and his teaching to me as his research fellow for two years at the Boston Lying-In Hospital, and more recently in the preparation of this work. I gratefully acknowledge the encouragement of my present chief, Dr. Robert Cooke, Professor of Pediatrics at Johns Hopkins, who has turned me loose in the newborn nurseries at Hopkins, and Drs. Richard Riley and Richard Shepard, who provide constant stimulation and advice on respiratory physiology. What is useful in this book is in large measure due to the observations and teachings of these people. What is missing or erroneous is in no measure their responsibility. I have tried to put together the pieces of a puzzle. Portions of a picture emerge. Probably some pieces are wrong, others are missing. If this work serves to stimulate others to help complete the picture, I shall be justly rewarded.

It is appropriate to acknowledge as well the changing status of medical investigation in this country. My predecessors for the most part accumulated their experience and wrote their works in the midst of the pressures of pediatric practice or large routine laboratory and teaching responsibilities. I have been relatively free to pursue investigations as they seemed appropriate, and to read at length, with only as many clinical and teaching responsibilities as were important to stimulate the investigative ones. This has been possible in large measure because of the generosity of the National Institutes of Health. A special traineeship provided support for the first three years after a pediatric residency, and subsequently research grants have made possible much of the work that is presented in this book. I am also indebted to The Maryland Heart Association and The American Thoracic Society for financial support, and to The John and Mary R. Markle Foundation for its great generosity in encouraging me to devote the largest portion of my time to teaching and research.

I am indebted to my many colleagues at The Johns Hopkins Hospital and elsewhere who endured endless questioning about some of the conditions discussed in these pages, and especially Dr. Alexander Schaffer, who reviewed the entire text. Dr. Olga Baghdassarian of the Department of Radiology not only collected most of the films, but wrote some of the descriptions of them, and wrote the section on "Roentgenographic Evaluation of the Chest."

The text could not have appeared in its present form without the assistance of Miss Carol Hoffman, who helped with the drawings and literature survey, Mrs. Joan Holthaus, who typed the manuscript, and Mrs. Dorothy Lyne, who assisted with the manuscript.

I wish to thank Dr. Robert R. Wright and Mr. Charles Stuart of The University of California Medical Center for their courtesy in allowing me to reproduce on the end sheets their beautiful photomicrographs of lung tissue which were originally published in Science, Vol. 137, August 24, 1962.

And finally I wish to acknowledge the great assistance and advice of the staff of W. B. Saunders Company.

MARY ELLEN AVERY

Contents

xi

PART II   DISORDERS OF RESPIRATION IN THE NEWBORN PERIOD

Chapter Eight

NORMAL AND ABNORMAL AIRWAYS

Chapter Thirteen

Normal Development and Physiology of the Fetal and Neonatal Lung

Chapter One

LUNG DEVELOPMENT

The pediatrician has a special interest in the problem of lung growth since he is called upon to care for immature infants. Organ maturation must evolve to a degree capable of function before extrauterine life is possible; not infrequently it appears that viability of the prematurely born infant is limited by the lung. It is not until the 28th week of gestation that the potential airway and capillary proliferation around the airway are sufficient for gas exchange.

DEVELOPMENT OF THE AIRWAYS

Before the period of viability, the lung is essentially a glandular organ, with closed air spaces. In a 24-day embryo, there is an outpouching of the gut; at 26 to 28 days, two primary branches appear, which are the major bronchi; for the next three months, growth consists of branching of the endodermal tube into the surrounding mesenchyme. The mesenchyme itself is of two types, a relatively cellular one, which surrounds the endodermal tree, and a less cellular one, which fills the remaining space. Ham and Baldwin (1941) suggest that the more cellular mesenchyme is the source of the nonepithelial elements in the alveolar walls, and the noncellular type gives rise to pleura, subpleural connective tissue, interlobular septa, and cartilage of the bronchial tree.

Cartilage deposition begins at about 10 weeks. By 16 weeks, antenatal formation of new bronchi is nearly complete, but cartilage continues to appear until the 24th week, when it reaches the same extent as is found at term (Fig. 1–1).

3

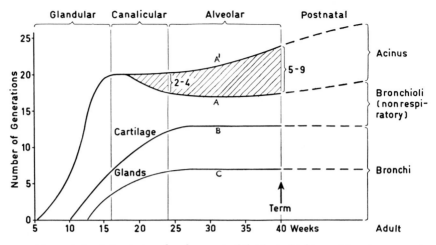

Figure 1–1. Intrauterine development of the bronchial tree. Line A represents the number of bronchial generations, and A¹ the respiratory bronchioles and alveolar ducts. B is the extension of cartilage along the bronchial tree, and C the extension of mucous glands. (From Bucher, U., and Reid, L.: Thorax *16:*207, 1961.)

By 12 weeks the lobes of the lung are well demarcated. Elastic fiber bundles are present in the walls of the trachea and main bronchi, as well as the pulmonary artery and pleura (Loosli and Potter, 1959). Septa can first be recognized between the 18th and 20th weeks of fetal life. They consist of sheets of areolar tissue which pass for varying distances from their pleural attachments into the lung. They have the same distribution in the fetus as in the adult, most numerous at the sharp edges of the lung and sparse over the lateral aspects (Reid and Rubino, 1959).

It has long been known that the respiratory epithelium is rich in glycogen in embryonic life (Bernard, 1859). It is most abundant in regions of the lung where cell division is most rapid, and disappears from mature cells when citric acid cycle activity increases (Sorokin et al., 1959). Sorokin suggested that glycogen is required to support epidermal mitosis in embryonic tissues. He established this dependence on glycolysis by means of tissue explants; growth and differentiation proceeded in like fashion whether the fetal lungs were raised on standard media or media with added malonate or cyanide, or in the absence of air. Only the explants given fluoride, which inhibits glycolysis, failed to differentiate (Sorokin, 1961).

During rapid lung growth, the epithelial mass increases relative to mesenchyme (Fauré-Fremiet and Dragoiu, 1923). Mitotic counts show two epithelial divisions per stromal division during early and late organogeny, and a higher ratio in mid-development (Sorokin et al., 1959). With unequal cell division, it would be expected that the more rapidly dividing tissues would branch (Fig. 1–2). Cannulization of the airways occurs at approximately 20 weeks, with the appearance of a cuboidal cell lining (Laumonier, 1952).

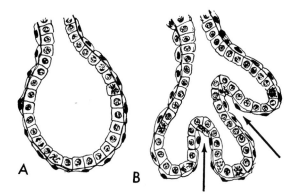

Figure 1-2. Schematic illustration of the role of cell division in branching of the developing lung. (From Sorokin et al.: Developmental Biology 1:125, 1959.)

Terminal airsacs or alveoli appear as outpouchings of the bronchioles, and after 28 weeks these alveoli increase in number to form multiple pouches of a common chamber known as an alveolar duct. The time of appearance of alveoli in the human lung is not constant, but may begin at 28 weeks and progress to term, since frequently some terminal airspaces are lined by cuboidal epithelium near term. This observation has led to confusion about the role of air breathing in "flattening" cuboidal epithelium. Farber and Wilson (1933), and later Whitehead et al. (1942), felt that epithelium was flattened as a result of the introduction of air at birth. The excised lungs of stillborn infants, after artificial respiration, showed less cuboidal epithelium than did the control lung. Potter (1953) based exception to this suggestion on extensive observations indicating that the histologic structure of the lungs is essentially the same after birth as before birth. Parmentier (1962) confirmed these findings in human and rat lungs. He saw progressive differentiation of lung structures in utero with attenuation of alveolar epithelium. The strongest evidence that attenuation of epithelium can occur in the absence of air breathing is that of Sorokin (1961), who demonstrated the formation of thin-walled alveoli in tissue explants of embryonic lung. Electron micrographs of fetal lungs likewise show an abrupt attenuation of cuboidal cell cytoplasm extending over adjacent capillaries (Low and Sampaio, 1957).

A most significant milestone in lung development appears to occur at about 26 to 28 weeks when the fetus weighs about 1 kg. At this time the capillary network, which arose about the 20th week from vascular structures in the mesenchyme, proliferates close to the developing airway (Potter, 1953). Extrauterine existence is not possible until there is a sufficiently extensive surface area of the lung for gas exchange (Fig. 1-3).

Extensive studies of lung growth in tissue culture have clarified a number of questions: for example, it is evident that the lung in organ culture is capable of being a self-developing entity; since being

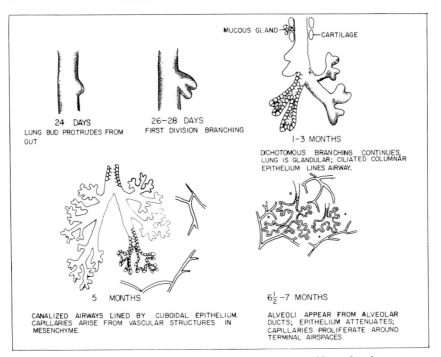

Figure 1–3. Diagrammatic representation of the stages of lung development.

separated from the embryo and the mother, rudiments of the lung can develop *in vitro*. The older the fetal lung fragments are at the time of initiation of culture, the better the prospects of obtaining a differentiated organ. *In vitro* blood vessels do not develop to the extent that they do *in vivo*.

Evidence of an inductive capacity of the investing mesenchyme comes from the studies of Rudnick with the chick lung and Sampaolo and Sampaolo with the rabbit lung. The removal of the mesenchyme from the lung bud interrupts the process of epithelial branching. Once the mesenchyme is regenerated, the growth of the epithelium proceeds. The epithelium alone isolated *in vitro* is incapable of morphogenesis. Alescio and Cassini have reported that the substitution of bronchial mesenchyme for tracheal mesenchyme promotes the development of a supernumerary bud at the grafting site. These studies indicate that the pulmonary epithelium is capable of budding in a given region for some time after it would normally stop doing so.

DEVELOPMENT OF GLANDS AND CILIA

By eight weeks, long after the trachea is lined by the pulmonary endoderm, a secondary invagination of its epithelium occurs to form the paratracheal mucous glands (Sorokin, 1960). Cilia are evident in the trachea and main bronchi at 10 weeks, and in the peripheral airways by 13 weeks (Bucher and Reid, 1961). Goblet cells with PAS positive material appear in the bronchial epithelium at 13 to 14 weeks. Glands appear first as solid buds from the basal layers of the surface epithelium, at about the 14th to 16th weeks of gestation, and later as tubules which branch and form mucus-containing acini (Thurlbeck et al., 1961; Sorokin, 1960; Bucher and Reid, 1961). Granular acini can be identified by 26 weeks. From their staining characteristics, it appears that the fetal acini contain some acid mucopolysaccharide, which may contribute to the acid pH of tracheal fluid (Reid, 1967).

THE ALVEOLAR CELLS AND THEIR LINING LAYER

It is now well established that the terminal airspaces, or alveoli, which appear about the 26th to 28th weeks of gestation are lined by epithelium. However, until the era of the electron microscope, anatomists did not agree on this point, and indeed the controversy raged whether the airspaces were a type of functional interstitial emphysema or were actually lined by cells (Macklin, 1936; Bertalanffy and LeBlond, 1955). Alveolar cells normally indistinguishable by the light microscope could be seen in some pathologic conditions in which edema raised them from the underlying tissue (Miller, 1950). In 1953, Low published electron micrographs that demonstrated a continuous squamous epithelium with long thin cells and an attenuated cytoplasm. Bertalanffy and LeBlond (1955) pointed out that the alveolar cells, although a rather complex group, could be divided into two chief types, on the basis of orth-fixed preparations stained with Masson's trichrome. One type consisted of vacuolated alveolar cells with some lipoidal material (type II cells), while the other cells were nonvacuolated and looked like connective tissue (type I cells). A number of desquamated macrophages were apparent in the airspaces.

Extensive studies of the morphology of the alveolar cells have emphasized the presence of numerous cytoplasmic inclusions, endoplasmic reticulum, and mitochondria. Only recently have nerve fibers been found intimately associated with the alveolar lining cells. Hung et al. (1972) described two types of unmyelinated fibers adjacent to alveolar cells and suggested that both afferent and efferent innervation is present.

Bertalanffy and LeBlond (1953) showed further that in the lung of the rat there was a constant loss of alveolar cells which was balanced by rapid mitotic proliferation of other cells; the vacuolated cells were renewed about once a month, the nonvacuolated cells about every eight days.

Peculiar osmiophilic inclusions in the vacuolated cells were noted by Karrer (1956) in the mouse lung and were subsequently identified in all mammalian lungs studied (Schulz, 1959) (Fig. 1–4).

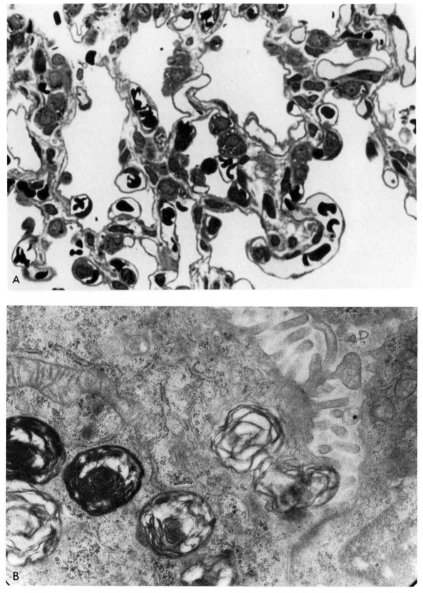

Figure 1–4. A, Normal lung of a term, 40-hour-old infant. Note the inclusion-containing vacuolated large alveolar cells in this Epon-embedded 1 μ section of lung. × 640. B, Electron micrograph of inclusion-containing alveolar cell of the human. Note that one appears to be entering the lumen. × 36,600. Lead acetate stain. (A and B from Balis et al.: Lab. Invest. *15:*530, 1966.)

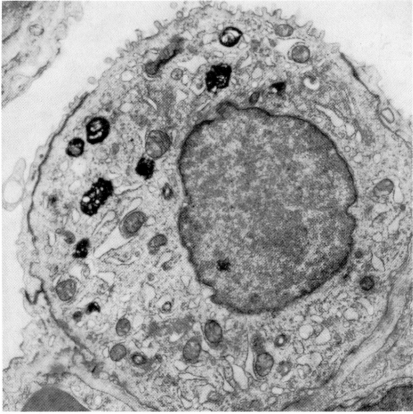

C

Figure 1–4 Continued. C, A great alveolar cell, or granular pneumonocyte. Note the many mitochondria, osmiophilic inclusion bodies, extensive endoplasmic reticulum, Golgi apparatus, and multivesicular bodies. This particular cell is from an adult opossum; similar cells are seen in all mammalian lungs. × 14,200. (*C* from Sorokin, S.: J. Histochem. Cytochem. *14:*890, 1967.)

They appear late in the developing mouse, or at about 18 days of a 19- to 20-day gestation (Woodside and Dalton, 1958). The time of appearance in the human fetal lung is variable, having been noted in the lung of an infant of 840 gm. (Campiche et al., 1962). In a more extensive survey, Spear et al. described them in some lungs of 310-, 600-, and 710-gm. fetuses, although they were not regularly seen before 900 gm. (1969). Lauweryns mentions typical lamellar bodies and multivesicular bodies in the cylindrical cells of an infant of 240 gm. (20 weeks) (1970). They are first seen in the lamb at 120 days of a 147- day gestation (Kikkawa et al., 1965). The identity and function of these inclusions are not definitely established. Buckingham and Avery (1962) suggested that the inclusions could be the source of a material which lowers surface tension at the alveolar-air interface. Klaus et al. (1962) added significant support to this suggestion from three lines of evidence. First, they correlated the presence of osmiophilic inclusions with surface activity in lung extracts in dog, cat, rat, mouse, rabbit, and man. Second, both osmiophilic inclusions and surface activity were decreased in vagotomized guinea pigs. And third, surface activity was present in the isolated mitochondrial fraction of homogenized and ultracentrifuged lung tissue, which also contained the inclusions. Still additional evidence for the association of osmiophilic inclusions and surface activity came from studies of guinea pigs exposed to 15 per cent carbon dioxide for more than 24 hours. Both osmiophilic inclusions and surface activity were deficient in these animals during the phase of uncompensated respiratory acidosis, but both reappeared with compensation of the acidosis (Schaefer et al., 1963). Consistent with its being a lysosome rather than a transformed mitochondrion, the limiting membrane of the inclusion stains with alkaline phosphatase. Although the role of the inclusions is not established, the association with the surfactant suggests that it is a storage site.

The possibility that the large alveolar cells were secretory was suggested by Macklin (1954) and supported by electron micrographs which show osmiophilic inclusions in the process of entering the airspaces (Bensch et al., 1964; Balis and Conen, 1964; Hatasa and Nakamura, 1965). Improvements in the techniques of lung fixation permitted Gil and Weibel to demonstrate a duplex alveolar lining layer. Occasionally osmiophilic lamellae of tubular myelin figures were noted in continuity with the surface film (Fig. 1–5). These findings support the theory that the osmiophilic material in the inclusions is secreted to the alveolar surface and accumulates there. Its removal is presumably by ingestion by macrophages, although further studies on this topic are in order.

The large or vacuolated alveolar cell may also be the site of the synthesis of phospholipids, presumably an important component of the surfactant. Isotopically tagged glucose or acetate is converted to palmitate and incorporated into lecithin by lung slices or even the mitochondrial fraction of lung (Felts, 1965; Tombropoulos, 1964). Autoradiographic studies suggest that the accumulation of the tagged H^3 acetate or palmitate injected into the living rabbit only occurs in the cytoplasm of the large alveolar cell (Buckingham et al., 1966). Morphologic and cytochemical studies show that the large alveolar cell contains an extensive Golgi apparatus, multivesicular bodies, and granular endoplasmic reticulum, all characteristics of cells having synthetic activity. They are active for NADP diaphorase and glucose-6-phosphate dehydrogenase, distinguishing them from alveolar phagocytes (Sorokin, 1967).

The function of the alveolar lining layer in stabilizing airspaces was not appreciated until the mid-1950's. Pattle (1958) investigated foam expressed from lung parenchyma and noted the long survival of small bubbles suspended in saline. He deduced that surface tension

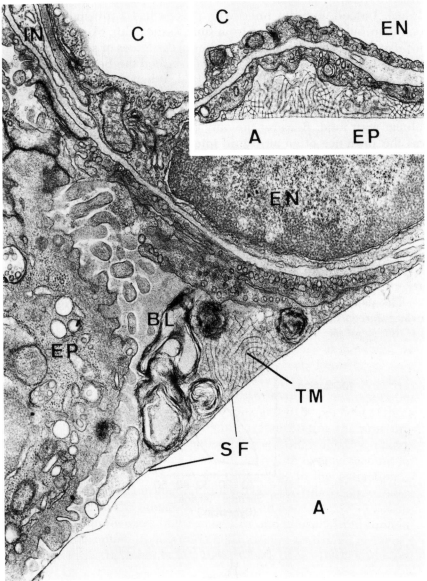

Figure 1–5.   Thin section of lung tissue fixed by sequential vascular perfusion of glutaraldehyde, osmium tetroxide, and uranyl acetate. Tubular myelin figures accumulate in the depression in the epithelial surface (magnified 26,400 ×). A = alveolus, C = capillary, TM = tubular myelin figures, SF = surface film, BL = base layer, EP = alveolar epithelium, and EN = capillary endothelium. (Courtesy of Prof. Ewald Weibel, Anatomisches Institut, Bern, Switzerland.)

Induction of Surfactant

Against the background of the descriptive studies of the ontogeny of the surfactant, and as an incidental observation made during studies on the initiation of parturition in the lamb, Liggins noted that lambs born after cortisol infusion of the ewe were viable at an earlier age than expected (1969). Learning of Liggins's initial observation by way of a personal communication at a combined meeting of the New Zealand Obstetrical and Pediatric Societies in 1968, Avery and others pursued the possibility that accelerated appearance of the pulmonary surfactant could be achieved by induction of the capacity of type II cells to synthesize it by steroids. The first suggestion of such a possibility was made by Buckingham in 1968 by analogy with changes demonstrated in the intestinal epithelium a number of years before by Moog (1953). The demonstration of accelerated lung maturation was reported by deLemos et al. (1969, 1970). They infused hydrocortisone into one lamb from each of the seven sets of twins and used the other as a control. In each cortisol-treated twin the lung was "more mature" than in the control. A saline-treated fetus showed no effect. Further evidence of acceleration of surfactant protection by glucocorticoids in the lamb was reported by Platzker et al. (1972). Surfactant production could be detected in dexamethasone-treated lambs as early as 108 days of gestation. At 126 days' gestation the tracheal flux of surface-active material increased 370 per cent after two days of treatment.

In order to see if the ability to accelerate synthesis of the surfactant was unique to the lamb, or if it might occur in other species, Kotas and Avery conducted systematic studies on 228 fetal rabbits from 24 days of gestation to term (31 days) (1971). The trends in time were for a greater distensibility of the lung when inflated with air post-mortem, and greater stability on deflation, indicative of the presence of the surfactant. One fetus in each of 15 litters was given a single dose of a long-acting glucocorticoid, 9α-fluoroprednisolone on day 24. After sacrifice on day 26 or 27, the lungs of the treated fetuses resembled those of a 29- to 30-day fetus. Wang et al. (1971) studied these same lungs morphologically and demonstrated an increase in attenuation of the alveolar cells with more osmiophilic inclusions per cell in the steroid-treated rabbits. Motoyama et al. (1971) confirmed these findings with the injection of 0.5 to 1 mg. of hydrocortisone sodium succinate into the fetal rabbit and further noted that the injected fetuses on delivery were more active and breathed better than their littermate controls. The enhanced survival of prematurely delivered rabbits after cortisol injection 48 hours earlier was further studied by Taeusch et al. (1972). They noted that the survival correlated with the degree of maturity of the lung and that it was significantly increased after cortisol. An effect on the fetus adjacent to the treated one was also evident, as if some cortisol could diffuse to the neighbor. The longest survival was after direct injection, next longest among the neighbors, and shortest among the more distant littermates, suggesting a dose-response relationship (Fig. 1–4). Farrell and Zachman (1972) repeated the studies of Kotas and Avery (1971) with 9α-fluoroprednisolone acetate injected into fetal rabbits at 23 to 24 days and measured the lecithin content of the lung parenchyma a few days later. The treated group had 96 mg./gm. dry weight of lung, compared to 70 mg./gm. in the controls. They also examined four enzymes in the two major biosynthetic pathways. The only significant change was in the level of phosphorylcholine-glyceride transferase, which was elevated 45 per cent in the steroid-treated group, suggesting acceleration of the choline incorporation pathway.

Further evidence for the role of the intact pituitary-adrenal axis for the maturation of the fetal lung comes from experimental ablation of the hypophysis or adrenals. Fetal hypophysectomy in goats led to a delay in lung maturation (DeLemos et al., 1971) and in decapitated fetal rats a similar observation was reported by Blackburn et al. (1972). They found enlarged lungs with more immature cells in the rats decapitated on the 16th day of gestation. Lung lecithin at term was decreased in the decapitated fetuses.

The mechanism by which cortisol accelerates lung maturation is not established. However, recently it has been suggested that steroid hormones require specific receptor molecules in their target tissue in order for steroids to affect it. Ballard and Ballard (1972) examined fetal rabbit tissues for the presence of glucocorticoid receptors using H_3 dexamethasone. Receptor activity was found in the soluble cytoplasmic fraction from all fetal tissues studied but was in highest concentration in the lung. The concentration was constant during the last 12 days of gestation. Nuclear binding sites for tritiated cortisol were demonstrated in fetal lung by Giannopoulos et al. (1972). They further showed the specifity of the sites for compounds with glucocorticoid activity and the failure to bind progesterone or testosterone. The uptake of tritiated cortisol increased from day 20 and reached a maximum at 28 to 30 days of gestation. The uptake was somewhat lower in newborn rabbits. Thus, cortisol-binding sites are present in both nuclei and cytoplasm of fetal lung cells, suggesting that this compound, rather than one of its metabolites, plays a role in induction of enzymes necessary for surfactant synthesis.

The possibility that alterations in surfactant production can be achieved with other compounds as well is suggested by the evidence that thyroid administration or withdrawal in the rat profoundly affects the numbers of osmiophilic inclusions in the type II cells of the alveoli. Both storage and production of surfactant were augmented by thyroid, according to Redding et al. (1972). Acceleration of lung maturation in the fetal rabbit was achieved with thyroid injected into the fetuses by Wu et al. (1971).

DEVELOPMENT OF THE PULMONARY VESSELS AND LYMPHATICS

An understanding of the development of the pulmonary vessels elucidates a number of malformations of the vessels and associated malformations of the lung (Ferencz, 1961; Spencer, 1962; Neill, 1956).

The lung bud, which arises from the primitive gut, receives its blood supply initially from a series of paired segmental arteries that arise from the dorsal aorta caudal to the aortic arches. The vessels end in a plexus of capillaries in the growing lung.

The anlage of the pulmonary artery first appears in the 7.0-mm. embryo as a projection from the ventral end of the fourth aortic arch. The dorsal portion of that projection, which is the sixth aortic arch, joins the dorsal aorta and supplies the developing lung. Another protrusion extends caudally from the ventral portion of the sixth arch and fuses with the dorsal portion. This ventrocaudal portion of the sixth arch also joins the pulmonary capillary plexus and eventually becomes the pulmonary artery, while the dorsal portion forms the ductus arteriosus. The pulmonary capillaries lose their original connections with the segmental dorsal aortic arches, except for the first pair, which persist as bronchial arteries. The pattern of branching of the pulmonary arteries follows that of the airways, with the addition of many "supernumerary" arteries. These side branches extend only short distances before they break into a capillary bed which crosses the boundaries of respiratory units (Elliott and Reid, 1965).

The bronchial arterial circulation in the human fetus and the newborn has some features that are less common in later life. Direct anastomotic connections between bronchial and pulmonary arteries have been demonstrated by serial sectioning (Wagenvoort, 1967) and by microangiographic studies (Robertson, 1967) (Fig. 1–7). In some infants who died during the first year of life, the anastomoses were observed to be fibrotic, suggesting that they gradually disappear. Lungs of premature infants showed branches of the bronchial arteries ending in pulmonary alveolar capillaries; similar vessels were not found in children over six weeks of age. The functional significance of the anastomoses in fetal lungs is not known; however, bronchopulmonary blood flow in the fetal lamb has been measured as less than 5 per cent of the total flow. When the pulmonary artery was occluded, pressure in the peripheral end dropped from 60 mm. Hg to 2 to 4 mm. Hg, suggesting a very small functional contribution by bronchial vessels (Campbell et al., 1967).

The primitive pulmonary vein first appears as an evagination of the superior wall of the left atrium in the 4.0-mm. embryo and in the 6- to 7-mm. embryo unites with the capillary plexus (Neill, 1956). Before this union, blood from the capillary plexus drains into the cardinal

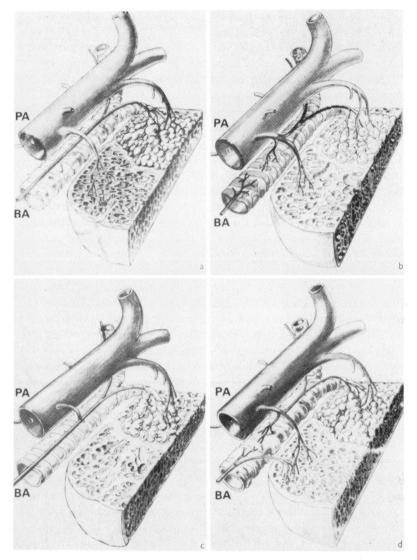

Figure 1–7. Schematic representation of vascular patterns in the lung. *a,* The usual pattern of pulmonary and bronchial artery distribution in the lung. *b,* One pattern of branching of the pulmonary artery to supply a bronchus. *c,* A bronchopulmonary anastomosis. *d,* The bronchial artery supplying the lung parenchyma. (From Robertson, B.: Acta Paediat. Scand. 56:261, 1967.)

and vitello-umbilical veins, especially the anterior cardinal vein. When the veins regroup in the 7.0-mm. embryo (28 to 30 days) blood from both lungs drains into the evagination of the left atrium, which is close to the sinus venosus. Subsequently, the common trunk is absorbed into the wall of the sinus until its four component veins enter the future atrium as four separate veins.

The bronchial veins develop from the splanchnic system and empty into the pulmonary veins, except for those that continue to drain into the azygos vein deriving from the persistent cardinal and portal veins.

The lymphatics appear in the 26-mm. embryo (60 days) in the hilar region, and are present in the lung by 70 days (Tobin, 1957). At about 100 days' gestation valves are visible in the pericardial lymphatic plexus (Kampmeier, 1928). The lymphatic system in the newborn lung surrounds the bronchi, pulmonary arteries, and veins, and can be traced distally to the alveolar ducts. Flow is centripetal except immediately under the pleura, where the lymph flows along superficial lymphatic channels before returning to the hilum.

Progressive changes in the histology of the pulmonary vessels take place during fetal life, but the changes are most marked in association with respiration after birth. Histologic development is complete first in the lobar arteries, then in the smaller segmented and subsegmental vessels. Arteries at all levels pass through a stage of having a very narrow lumen of 2 to 8 μ, or less than the size of red blood cells. In the seven-week fetus the lobar arteries are narrow; by eight to 10 weeks these arteries are expanded but the subsegmental ones are narrow. The terminal and respiratory arteries remain narrow until 34 to 38 weeks; but the respiratory arterioles are the only vessels with a narrow lumen at term (Kaufman, 1964). Gradually the lumina of both arteries and arterioles enlarge, and the amount of smooth muscle increases during the latter half of gestation (O'Neal et al., 1957). For the first four days after birth very few changes are noted, but at 10 days of extrauterine life the lumina are much wider, regardless of the time of birth. An increase in lumen size after birth has been noted in a premature infant of five months' gestation who survived for 10 days (Larroche et al., 1959).

The functional corollary of these anatomical observations has been investigated in lambs of differing gestational ages (Dawes, 1958). Isolated, perfused lungs of immature fetal lambs before and after ventilation showed very little increase in flow, with increase in pulmonary arterial perfusion pressure. The vascular bed of the mature fetus permitted a modest increase in flow, with increase in pressure. No significant increase in flow was measured in the immature animal after ventilation, whereas nearly a 10-fold increase in flow was achieved with high perfusion pressures in the animal at term.

The possibility of abnormal thickening of neonatal pulmonary arterial walls was suggested by Goldberg et al. on the basis of studies in rats (1971). They exposed pregnant rats to 13 per cent oxygen throughout gestation, and compared the histology of the pulmonary vessels of the fetuses to those of control fetal and neonatal rats. Medial hypertrophy was prominent in the small arteries of the hypoxic group but decreased in the first weeks after birth.

POSTNATAL GROWTH OF THE LUNG

No sudden structural or histochemical events in the cells lining the airspaces herald or accompany birth. Sorokin and coworkers (1959) found that the time of appearance of glycogen, mucoproteins, muco-polysaccharides, alkaline and acid phosphatase activity, and succinic dehydrogenase was predictable in rats and guinea pigs, although it was different in the two animals. The chemical maturation of the lung was not accelerated by birth, but rather proceeded in a uniform manner whether the fetus was in utero or prematurely delivered (Table 1–1). (See page 14.)

The terminal airsacs are shallow and wide-mouthed in the newborn infant, and not until several months after birth do they assume a cup-shaped configuration. Before birth the terminal respiratory bronchioles are smooth; after several months new alveoli appear proximal to the terminal airspace by transformation of preexisting respiratory bronchioles (Boyden and Tompsett, 1965). If the functional unit is the terminal saccule, as suggested by Boyden and Tompsett, the larger radius would not only tend to prevent atelectasis in the first months of life, but also limit the surface area available for gas exchange.

Lung growth proceeds with respect to an increase in the number of bronchiolar divisions, alveoli, alveolar diameters, and surface area for gas exchange. The studies of Dunnill (1962) are of special interest in this regard, since the lungs studied were all fixed with formalin vapor at a volume as near as possible to that of the thorax of the cadaver. Statistical methods were used to estimate mean alveolar dimensions (Weibel and Gomez, 1962) (Table 1–2). Angus and Thurlbeck (1972) point out the large variation in the numbers of alveoli between individuals of a given age. The mean value for adults was 375×10^6 with a range of 212 to 605×10^6. The total number of alveoli was significantly related to body length. Conversely the number of conducting airways tended to be constant regardless of body size. Given the wide range of variability in alveolar number, it is not possible from studies published to date to conclude at what age further generation of alveoli stops. They may form as long as body length increases.

The dimensional relationships of the lung at different ages permit some interesting inferences about function. Note that the numbers of alveoli and airways increase about 10-fold from infancy to adulthood. Lung surface area, on the other hand, increases some 20-fold, or about the same as the increase in body weight. At first this would appear to be a reasonable relationship, since the area for gas exchange should bear some relationship to the mass of cells undergoing metabolism. However, the metabolism of the infant is nearly double that of the adult when it is expressed per kilogram body weight. Thus, the infant

Table 1-1. Some Histochemical Events in Developing Human Lungs*

Age Months	Glycogen				Mucus	Elastic Tissue	Succinic Dehydrogenase	Alk. Phos.	Acid Phos.	Esterase
	Col. Ep.	Buds	Stroma	Vess.						
1	+ 2	+ 2	low	0	0	membranes	+ uniform	+ ep. / + pul. artery / + col. ep. / 0 buds	low all	low all
2		+ 3	+	+ 2						
3			+ 2			< membranes col. ep.	< proximal ep.	trachea not uniform, low pul. artery / + bronch. vess. / 0 large vess.	< ep. / 0 buds	<trachea and bronchi
4	+				+ glands / low goblet / + 2 glands	+ 2 vess. / + bronchi	+ 2 col. ep. / + buds / + vascular musc.			+ 2 cil. ep. / + prox. musc. / + small bronchi
5	low	+	+ 3		+ goblet				+ 2 ep.	
6	low	+		+	+ 3 glands / + 2 goblet	+ 3 vess. / + 2 trachea / low cub. ep.	+ bronchial musc.			
7	0	low	+ 4	0	+ 4 glands / + 3 goblet / low alveolar cell	+ alveoli and small vess.		+ glands and goblet cells / low septal cells and leukocytes / low col. ep.	+ 2 glands	+ 2 bronchioles
8		0	low	0	+ alveolar cell	+ 2 alveoli well defined in lung		low col. ep.		+ cub. ep.
9		0	0		glands and goblet to bronchioles					

Only changes in histochemical reactivity, together with the approximate dates of their incidence, are recorded. Rough quantitation is given by the arbitrary scale, low to + 4.

acid phos. = acid phosphatase col. ep. = columnar epithelium musc. = smooth muscle vess. = blood vessels
alk. phos. = alkaline phosphatase cub. ep. = cuboidal epithelium prox. = proximal < = increase
cil. ep. = ciliated epithelium goblet = goblet cells pul. = pulmonary

*From Sorokin, S.: Acta Anatomica 40:105, 1960. Reproduced courtesy of the author and S. Karger, Basel/New York.

Table 1–2. Effect of Age on Lung Size*

Age	Numbers of Alveoli ($X\ 10^6$)	Number of Airways ($X\ 10^6$)	Air-Tissue Interface (m^2)	Body Surface Area (m^2)
Birth	24	1.5	2.8	0.21
3 months	77	2.5	7.2	0.29
7 months	112	3.7	8.4	0.38
13 months	129	4.5	12.2	0.45
4 years	257	7.9	22.2	0.67
8 years	280	14.0	32.0	0.92
Adult	296	14.0	75.0	1.90
Approximate fold-increase birth to adult	10	10	21	9

* Data of Dunnill, M. S.: Thorax 77:329, 1962.

would appear to have less reserve lung surface area for added metabolism than the adult.

An important relationship between the conductance of the peripheral and central airways, as it is affected by age, was described by Hogg et al. (1970). Using a retrograde catheter technique on excised human lungs, they found little change with age in the conductance of the airways central to the 12th to the 15th generation; conductance of the more peripheral airways increased sharply at about age five years. They speculate that the seriousness in infants of lower airway obstructive disease, such as cystic fibrosis and bronchiolitis, relates to the dimensions of the airways.

Chapter Two

THE FETAL LUNG

PHYSICAL PROPERTIES

The physical properties of the lung of the fetus bear on the problems associated with the first inflation of the lung at birth. Are the airspaces empty in the sense of alveolar wall touching alveolar wall, or are they slightly distended with fluid? If fluid is present, what is its source, and what is the pleural pressure in the fetus? These questions have interested investigators for many years, at least since 1879 when Hermann measured pleural pressure and found it to be atmospheric. Addison and How (1913) found fluid in the lungs of fetal sheep and dogs; however, Krogh in 1936 assumed that the lung was at minimal volume but that the thoracic cavity was filled with fluid. Recent studies directed to these questions have clarified, although not yet fully answered, them (Agostoni et al., 1958; Avery, 1962).

Observations of respiratory movements in fetal animals (p. 27) and the finding of amniotic sac contents in the lungs of some infants who died from nonpulmonary causes in the neonatal period suggested that some ebb and flow of amniotic fluid may occur in the fetus (Farber and Sweet, 1931; Ahvenainen, 1948; Camerer, 1938).

The volume of fluid that may be present just before birth has not been measured in the human infant. The possibility that the lungs are not at minimal volume was supported by roentgenographic studies in which oxygen was placed in the stomach before the first breath. The position of the diaphragm and the shape of the thorax were about the same after aeration of the lungs as they were before (Lind et al., 1966).

In fetal goats, it also appears that the lungs are partly fluid-filled. This observation is based on three lines of evidence obtained from goats delivered by cesarean section and sacrificed before the first breath with magnesium sulfate given intravenously to stop the circula-

22

tion and by clamping of the trachea to prevent lung volume change. First, the fetal lungs weighed two to three times as much as lungs of newborn goats of the same size; second, the specific gravity of the fetal lung was 1.011 to 1.019, compared to 1.052 and 1.050 in newborn goats, suggesting the presence of a fluid of low specific gravity. And third, pleural pressure in the fetal goat was atmospheric. This last observation suggests that fluid is present in the lung. If it were not, and the lung were at minimal volume, the thorax would be at less than its resting volume, and, to the extent determined by its pressure-volume characteristics, would tend to become larger. Such an outward recoil of the thorax would lower pleural pressure. If the lungs were partly distended with fluid, the thorax would be nearer its relaxation volume and pleural pressure could be atmospheric (Avery and Cook, 1961). Karlberg (1960) found no appreciable negative intraesophageal pressures in normal infants before the first breath, although a water-filled catheter in the esophagus would not permit detection of slightly subatmospheric pressures, since the baseline would be uncertain. The volume of liquid in the lungs of the fetal lamb, measured by dilution techniques, was about 50 ml. in a 3.5-kg. animal, or approximately equal to the functional residual capacity, that is, the volume of air in the lung at the end of a quiet expiration (Howatt et al., 1965).

The rate of postnatal disappearance of fluid in the lung was estimated from lung weight/body weight ratios of littermates of puppies (Avery, 1961) (Fig. 2–1). The decrease in lung weight over the first hours of life was variable. In lambs too, the water content was slightly

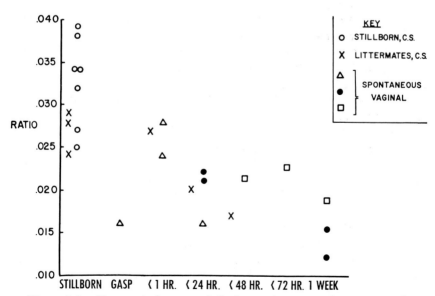

Figure 2–1. Changes in lung weight/body weight ratio with time in newborn puppies. (From Fomon, S. J., (ed.): *Normal and Abnormal Respiration in Children,* Ross Laboratories, 37th Ross Conference on Pediatric Research, Columbus, 1961.)

below the fetal range by one hour of age and well below it by two to three hours of age (Orzalesi et al., 1965). Many more observations are needed for an understanding of this phenomenon; but it is probable that great variation will be found, since in newborn infants rales, presumably associated with this fluid, may linger, or may vanish with one good cry.

AMNIOTIC FLUID AND LUNG SECRETIONS

The potential airways of the fetus are in contact with the amniotic fluid if the glottis is open. It is germane to consider the nature of amniotic fluid and the fluid that comes from the trachea, since they provide the internal environment of the fetal lung. It is both disconcerting and challenging to consider the state of our knowledge on this subject, recently reviewed by Ann Reynolds (1972).

As early as 1902, Jacque measured in animals the osmolarity of amniotic fluid and fetal and maternal blood (cited by Needham, 1931) and found that the osmolarity of the amniotic fluid decreased until, at term, it was hypo-osmolar with respect to the fetal blood. In the human, Battaglia et al. (1959) showed the changes throughout pregnancy to be from 289 mOsm./kg. of water in the ninth week to 260 mOsm./kg. of water at term. Their data suggest a fairly abrupt fall in osmolarity at the 32nd week. The more extensive studies by Makepeace et al. (1931) show a more steady decrease in osmolarity with advancing human gestation. In an extensive review of the subject by Seeds (1965) it is evident that the tonicity of amniotic liquid can vary greatly even at the same gestational age, as a function in part of the state of hydration of the mother. For example, Lind et al. (1969) report osmolalities of 255 to 280 at 32 to 34 weeks gestation, and 230 to 280 at term (Fig. 2–2).

Amniotic fluid has slightly less Na^+, K^+, and Cl^- than maternal or fetal serum. The sugar is usually much lower than in serum, averaging 32 mg./100 ml. compared to 79 mg./100 ml. in maternal serum (Makepeace, 1931). The most striking difference is in the much lower total protein in amniotic fluid, 0.23 mg./100 ml. compared to 6.1 gm./100 ml. in serum. The electrophoretic distribution of proteins in the amniotic fluid shows greater similarity to that of the fetal serum rather than maternal serum (Brzezinski et al., 1961; Abbas and Tovey, 1960; Mentesti, 1959). In its low concentration of large molecules such as lipoproteins, fibrinogen, and some gamma globulins, the amniotic fluid is similar to interstitial fluid. Albumin comprises more than 60 per cent of the amniotic fluid protein (Brzezinski et al., 1961).

The turnover of amniotic fluid, studied with isotopes, is very rapid, about 26 moles of water per hour (Hutchinson et al., 1955; Plentl, 1959). This large volume of water would carry 68 mEq. Na^+

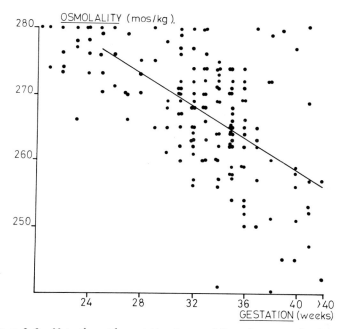

Figure 2–2. Note the wide variation in osmolality of amniotic fluid at any given gestational age. The trend is indicated by the solid line. (Courtesy of T. Lind et al., 1969.)

and 1.19 mEq. K$^+$. Since only 15 mEq. Na$^+$ and 0.5 mEq. K$^+$ are exchanged per hour, they must be "turned over" by specific independent mechanisms. One route of turnover is by way of fetal swallowing, a phenomenon that occurs as early as 12 weeks in the human and may reach 500 ml. in a 24-hour period (Pritchard, 1965). The role of the fetus in exchange rates of amniotic liquid in the rabbit, at least, is about one-half of the total transfer in that species. This estimate is based on studies in which the fetus was crushed, and the exchange rate of liquid reduced (Paul et al., 1956).

The source and fate of the fluid have puzzled investigators for years, and even now only fragments of the story are known. Makepeace et al. (1931) reasoned that the fluid at term must be diluted with a hypotonic substance, probably fetal urine which is present in small amounts from the third to fourth months of gestation. At six months' gestation, the urine is hypertonic with respect to its tonicity at term and is present in only small amounts, but later the volume increases and the tonicity decreases.

The possibility that the lung could contribute to the amniotic fluid was proposed by Jost and Policard (1948) after they observed an increase in lung volume of the rabbit fetus after tying the trachea. More recently Lanman et al. (1971) ligated the tracheas of fetal lambs near mid-gestation. The pregnancies continued, and on delivery at term the lungs of lambs with tracheal ligation weighed nearly ten times that of sham-operated controls or nonoperated twins. Maturation of the lung with distention of the alveoli with fluid was also noted in an infant with an anomalous lung not connected with the trachea (Potter and Bohlender, 1941). Secretions from the nasopharyngeal and buccal cavities as well as the lung itself contribute to the amniotic fluid. Reynolds (1953) found 30 to 40 ml. of fluid accumulated per hour in a bag applied over the nose of a fetal lamb. Setnikar et al. (1959) cannulated the tracheas of fetal goats and guinea pigs and collected fluid from the airways. They compared the osmotic pressure and protein content of tracheal effluent and amniotic fluid and found them to be very similar; however, in lambs the osmolarity of the tracheal effluent is closer to that of plasma than amniotic fluid (Ross, 1963).

The actual volume of liquid from lung that enters the amniotic pool is probably relatively small compared to the contribution of the kidney. Goodlin and Rudolph (1970) found very low flows in stable fetal goat and sheep preparations, whereas Pitkin et al. (1968) documented the major contribution of the kidney by labeled Diodrast injected into the fetal circulation. In the living animal, the dye appeared promptly in the amniotic fluid; none appeared after fetal death. Measurements of alveolar liquid formation in the exteriorized fetal lamb were made by Normand et al. (1971). They estimated the alveolar liquid volume as well as rate of formation from dilution of inulin put in the liquid. Their results were 30 ml. alveolar volume per kg. body weight, produced at a rate of 0.036 ml./min./kg. The amount entering the amniotic pool per day from a 3-kg. lamb would be 144 ml.

The more detailed studies of Adams et al. (1963) on the nature and origin of fluid in the fetal lung have shown that the tracheal fluid of lambs differs from amniotic fluid in having a lower pH (6.43 compared to 7.07 of amniotic fluid) and a lower CO_2 level (4.4 mEq./liter compared to 18.4 mEq./liter for amniotic fluid). Moreover, tracheal effluent contains the surface-active material normally found in the airspaces of the lung. I^{131} and $Na^{22}Cl$ injected into the fetal blood were excreted by both the lung and the kidney. These studies suggest that fetal tracheal fluid may be an ultrafiltrate of blood, with selective reabsorption or secretion by the lung. Evidence for active secretion of lung liquid was provided by Strang (1967), who measured the ratios of cations and anions between lung liquid and plasma. He further noted that the protein content of 300 mg. per cent would require uptake by the lymphatic vessels on the initiation of breathing.

Alterations in the viscosity of amniotic fluid in the ewe have been noted, and there was a high correlation with the ability of the lamb to survive. The outcome was poor for those with viscous amniotic fluid and viscous secretions from the mouth which presumably contributed to it. The responsible substance was a mucoprotein, which apparently impeded lung expansion at birth (Moss et al., 1966).

(For discussion of phospholipids in amniotic fluid, see p. 200.)

INTRAUTERINE RESPIRATION

A question that has aroused considerable investigation and some controversy is whether respiratory movements are initiated at birth, or are a continuation of intrauterine respiration. Although the lung is not the organ of gas exchange for the fetus, rhythmic movements of the thorax have been observed in sheep, dog, cat, guinea pig, rabbit, and human fetuses (Snyder and Rosenfeld, 1937; Barcroft and Karvonen, 1948; Ahlfeld, 1888; Bonar et al., 1938; Dawes, 1973).

The evidence that the neural regulatory apparatus is capable of initiating and sustaining respiratory activity at an early stage of human development is unequivocal in that infants weighing 600 gm. at birth have survived, and fetuses weighing 400 gm. may have sequential gasps, which, while ineffective in gas exchange, testify to the organization of respiratory activity.

The experimental studies that have resulted in controversy about intrauterine respiration have been well reviewed by Schaffer (1956) and Smith (1959). The investigations fall into two main categories; first, direct observations through the abdominal or uterine walls, and second, the injection of radiopaque material or dyes into the amniotic sac, with subsequent study of the lung for evidence of aspiration of the injected material.

Observations of fetal respiratory activity through the abdominal wall of the pregnant woman date at least from 1888 when Ahlfeld published his observations, and have been extended by Bonar (1938) and Dietel and Dietel (1957). Many observations on rabbits, cats, and guinea pigs by Snyder and Rosenfeld (1937) testify to the occurrence of respiratory activity in fetal animals. However, not all fetuses show rhythmic respirations at all times. Barcroft and Karvonen (1948) in their studies on sheep of different gestational ages noted rhythmical movements after the 40th day of gestation; however, by the 90th day of gestation there were no spontaneous respiratory movements. In fact, fetal respiratory activity could not be induced by anoxia or hypercapnea in fetuses near term (147 days in the sheep). Harned et al. (1962) studied the chemical control of respiration in the sheep fetus, exteriorized near term, and found no respiratory activity despite wide changes in pH, Pco_2, and Po_2. The combined stimulus of a low Po_2 and low pH, achieved by perfusion of the exteriorized fetal lamb carotid artery, did evoke sustained respirations (Harned et al., 1966; Pagtakhan et al., 1969). Cord occlusion per se, in the absence of blood gas alterations, did not stimulate breathing. Thus, fetal respiratory activity may be seen in some fetuses, but it is not always present.

Although the anesthetized, exteriorized fetus need not breathe and remains viable, apparently in the more physiologic intrauterine environment, rhythmic respiratory movements are present at least 40 per cent of the time. Dawes et al. (1972) described high frequency respiratory movements in unanesthetized fetal lambs associated with rapid eye movements. Little fluid shift occurred in the airway, even with an occasional gasp. The fetal respiratory movements were unaffected by section of the cervical vagi.

Respiratory movements can occur in the human early in gestation with sufficient force to introduce radiopaque material from the amniotic cavity into the lungs. Reifferscheid and Schmiemann (1939) demonstrated the presence of radiopaque material in the lungs of human infants after injection of the material into the amniotic sac 24 hours before section. Davis and Potter (1946) also found evidence of fetal aspiration in all infants exposed to the foreign material more than 17 hours, although very few were studied with shorter exposures. The fetuses, including one of only 115 gm., were studied at intervals before the therapeutic abortion. The evidence of human fetal respiration near term is convincing in the observation by Potter of radiopaque material in the lung of a 3.25-kg. infant delivered by cesarean section. However, many other studies have failed to show radiopaque material in the lungs after injection into the amniotic cavity (Windle et al., 1939; McLain, 1964). It can no longer be argued that under many circumstances the fetus does make respiratory movements, although they are not sustained as rhythmic respirations throughout the last part of gestation.

Chapter Three

THE AERATION OF THE
LUNG AT BIRTH

THE INTRODUCTION OF AIR

The forces required for the first breath must overcome the viscosity of fluid in the airway, surface tension, and tissue resistive forces (Fig. 3–1). Agostoni et al. (1958) found the viscous resistance to the movement of amniotic fluid in the airway of a guinea pig to be 58 cm. H_2O at a flow of 0.7 ml./sec. He reasoned that viscous forces would be maximal at the beginning of the first breath, since the greatest displacement of fluid would occur in the trachea. On the other hand, surface forces would be maximal where the radii of curvature of the airways are the smallest, presumably at the terminal bronchioles, at which point viscous forces are minimal. Probably the greatest resistance to the initial inflation of the lungs is from surface forces. Opening pressures of infants' lungs which are inflated step-wise post-mortem are about 20 to 25 cm. H_2O in birth weights of 1 kg. to 3 kg., and are about 30 cm. H_2O in lungs of infants weighing under 1 kg. (Gruenwald, 1963). While pressures measured post-mortem may not be the same as would prevail during life, these data suggest that the pressures required to overcome surface tension are high. The magnitude of tissue resistance forces is not known at the time of the first breath. In view of the small pressures required to change the size of the lung after respiration is established, tissue forces are probably not great at birth (Enhorning and Adams, 1965).

The concern about the presence of fluid in the fetal lung, its origin and composition, discussed in the previous section, arose in part from observations that such fluid enhances the introduction of air into the

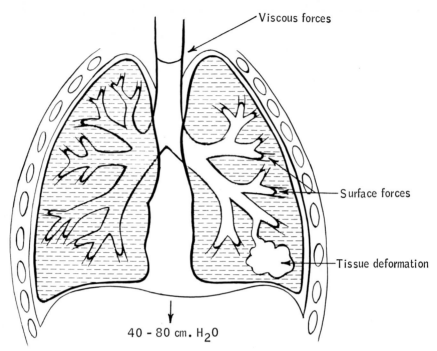

Viscous forces

Surface forces

Tissue deformation

40 - 80 cm. H₂0

Figure 3–1. Schematic representation of forces that oppose the introduction of air into the airless lung. The lung on the left is filled with fluid, the one on the right side of the picture shows air at different levels. Each terminal airspace will inflate fully before the next "opens."

airless lung (Avery et al., 1959). If fluid is present in an amount equal to one-half of the functional residual capacity, inflation will occur at about 5 cm. H_2O pressure lower than it will in the fluid-free airless lung (Fig. 3–2). This effect may be from changes in the configuration of the smaller units of the lung. Fluid, by enlarging the radii of curvature of the alveolar ducts, for example, could facilitate expansion in accord with the LaPlace relationship, which states that the pressure in a tube is directly proportional to tension and inversely proportional to radius ($P = t/r$). In the case of air entering a liquid-filled tube, the pressure required would be determined by the surface tension at the liquid-air interface, and the formula would then be $P = 2t/r$ (Avery et al., 1959; Avery, 1962). An alternative explanation for the observation of a lower opening pressure in lungs with fluid in them is that in-spissated material is less likely to obstruct the airway if fluid is present.

It is not at all clear where the fluid goes. Only three routes seem possible: out of the airway, into the circulation directly from alveolus to capillary, or into the circulation by way of lymphatics. Some infants appear to spit or drool a considerable volume of fluid at birth, perhaps from the oropharynx, esophagus, or lung. The thorax is subjected to pressures up to 95 cm. H_2O during vaginal delivery, and

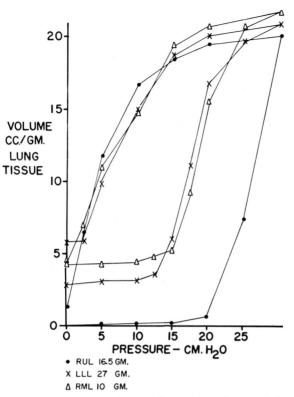

VOLUME
CC./GM.
LUNG
TISSUE

PRESSURE – CM. H$_2$O

• RUL 16.5 GM.
X LLL 27 GM.
Δ RML 10 GM.

Figure 3–2.   Static-pressure-volume relationships of excised dog lungs. Note that when some fluid is present in the lungs (curves X and Δ), the opening pressure is lower than it is when the airways do not contain added fluid. (From Avery et al.: J. Clin. Invest. 38:456, 1959.)

when the head is delivered before the thorax, some fluid is probably thus expressed from the lungs. As much as 20 ml. has been measured coming from the infant's mouth during vertex delivery (Karlberg et al., 1962). To some extent the elastic recoil of the thorax may suck in air, at least into the upper airways, and displace fluid more distally into the lung.

Karlberg (1960) made the interesting observation that the high intrathoracic pressure during the expiratory phase of the first breath occurs initially with the glottis closed. He thought this might facilitate absorption of the fluid by the capillaries. There should, however, be no pressure difference between alveolus and capillary when both would be exposed to the same positive intrathoracic pressures.

It is probable that the low protein content of amniotic fluid in comparison to that of fetal blood favors the movement of fluid into the blood by osmotic pressure as capillary perfusion increases at birth. The argument becomes difficult, however, if we assume that it is the incoming air which oxygenates the blood and reflexly dilates the pulmonary vascular bed (pp. 42–43). How can the fluid be removed by the capillaries before they are perfused, and how can they be perfused before the alveoli are ventilated? There is no answer to this question at this time, unless it is that sufficient gas exchange can occur across the upper airways to oxygenate the blood enough to cause a fall in pulmonary vascular resistance.

The lymphatics may carry into the circulation as much as one-third of the lung liquid and probably all of the protein. Histological study of lungs of rabbits sacrificed at intervals after birth showed engorgement of the lymphatics for several hours (Aherne and Dawkins, 1964). Direct measure of lymph flow from the thoracic duct of the lamb showed an increase with the initiation of breathing, which was more marked in mature than in immature animals (Boston et al., 1965). The relative importance of lymph drainage and clearance by the blood stream and the consequences of difficulty with either route, remain to be established.

The pathways of egress of lung liquid have been explored with the use of horseradish peroxidase (molecular weight, 40,000) administered via the airway before the onset of ventilation at birth in fetal rabbits. Gonzalez-Crussi and Boston (1972) found that transfer of the marker from the alveolar space took place in part by slow pinocytotic uptake across type I pneumonocytes and diffusion between stromal cells in the interstitium. There was also some diffusion across epithelial or endothelial basement membranes. They did not find any transcellular channels, although they did note occasional deep invaginations into the type I pneumonocyte. They felt they could not rule out the possibility of channels, although they must be infrequent, if present at all. It was of interest that the transfer of the marker was through the type I pneumonocyte rather than the type II cell (Fig. 3–3).

In an elegant series of studies on exteriorized fetal lambs, the group at University College Hospital, London, have contributed significantly to understanding of aspects of lung liquid movement. They studied the permeability of lung capillaries to macromolecules in immature and mature fetuses by measuring their relative concentration in alveolar liquid, plasma, and lung lymph. The resorption of large molecules was examined by instilling them into the alveolar liquid and then recording their uptake in lymph and plasma.

In brief, their data show that capillaries are more permeable than alveolar walls; significant changes in alveolar wall permeability occur with the introduction of air; the permeability becomes relatively greater in premature than term lambs. The investigators think of the alveolar barrier as "rupturing" with the introduction of air, and the rupture is more profound in the case of the premature infant. No anatomical evidence exists to support the concept of pores or rupture of alveolar walls; however, alterations in permeability are documented and may represent changes in pinocytic activity or other properties that affect diffusion (Boyd et al., 1969; Normand et al., 1970, 1971).

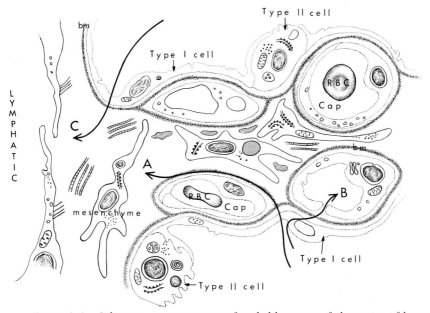

Figure 3–3. Schematic representation of probable routes of absorption of lung liquid. Arrow A shows a pathway along the basement membrane; arrow B points to an entrance into a capillary, across interendothelial cell junctions as well as a type I cell; arrow C enters a lymphatic. Studies based on electron microscopic observations with horseradish peroxidase. (From Gonzalez-Crussi and Boston: Lab. Invest. 26:114, 1972.)

THE COURSE OF LUNG EXPANSION

The inflation of the lung of a normal infant at birth is probably nearly accomplished with the first good cry, although some further changes occur over the next hours or days. The opening of alveoli necessarily occurs serially, each unit going to full inflation before the next opens. This "pop, pop, pop" phenomenon is understandable in the light of the LaPlace expression, and is illustrated in Figure 3–4.

The evidence for the rapidity of lung inflation is in part roentgenographic (Fawcitt et al., 1960). The lungs look well inflated one-third of a second after the onset of breathing. Further indications of the rate of aeration of the lung after birth come from several different kinds of measurements. The volumes of the first breaths in term infants vary from about 10 to 70 ml. The residual volume may be 20 to 30 ml. after the first expiration (Karlberg, 1957; Karlberg et al., 1962). Serial measurements of the functional residual capacity show this volume at 10 minutes of age to be about 17 ml./kg. body weight, and by 30 minutes, 25 to 35 ml./kg., or about the same as at 96 hours of age (Klaus et al., 1962; Geubelle et al., 1959). The volume of a cry—"crying vital capacity"—at 30 minutes of age was about 77 per cent of that

The relation of pressure (P) to radius (r) and surface tension (T) is $P = \dfrac{2T}{r}$

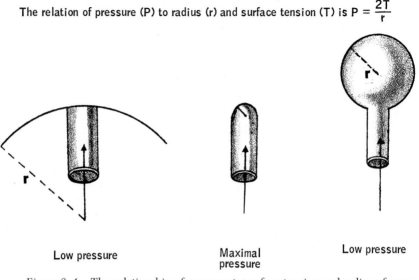

Low pressure   Maximal   Low pressure
                            pressure

Figure 3–4. The relationship of pressure to surface tension and radius of curvature of a bubble on a tube. Once the radius of the bubble exceeds the radius of the tube, it will proceed to enlarge until it encounteres another force from surrounding tissue or an increase in tension in its wall.

obtained in the same infants at 72 hours (Sutherland and Ratcliff, 1961). Serial measurements of lung compliance show a gradual increase over the first week of life, from 2 to 4 ml./cm. H_2O (Drorbaugh et al., 1963). The distribution of ventilation, estimated from nitrogen wash-out curves, is as even in the first hour of life as on the third or fourth day (Klaus et al., 1962).

PRESSURES REQUIRED FOR FIRST BREATH

Pleural pressures, as recorded from a sensing device in the esophagus, are from 10 to 70 cm. H_2O subatmospheric during the first breath. The large pressure is applied transiently for only 0.5 to 1 second according to the tracings published by Karlberg (1962) (Fig. 3–5). During the first expiration there is a high positive pleural pressure of 20 to 30 cm. of water. With increasing age, the same volumes may be achieved with less applied pressure, although the second and third breaths often resemble the first breath. By one to two days of age, the compliance of the lung is four to five times greater than it was at the time of the first few breaths, and flow resistance is decreased by one-half to one-fourth of the earlier values. Calculations show the total work of the first breath to be about the same as that of a cry in an infant several days of age.

The large changes in pleural pressure are the result of changes

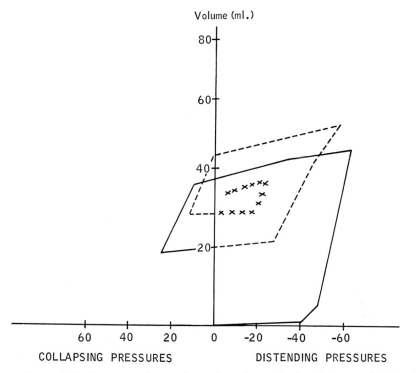

Figure 3–5. Pressure-volume relationships during the first (−), second (---), and third (xxxx) breaths as recorded from an esophageal catheter and a reverse plethysmograph. (Adapted from tracings of Karlberg et al.: Acta Paediat. *51*:121, 1962.)

in the volume of the surrounding thoracic cage. The chief muscle responsible for the large change in thoracic volume must be the diaphragm, although the intercostal muscles and accessory muscles of respiration doubtless participate. Jäykkä (1957) proposed that pulmonary vascular engorgement precedes the first breath and that the associated erectile force on the capillaries acts to distend the lung and "suck in" air. However, the pressure change that can be achieved in the airway in association with acute distention of pulmonary vessels in the airless dog lung is less than 5 cm. H_2O subatmospheric, or far lower than that required to "open" an airless lung (Avery et al., 1959). Vascular engorgement tends to increase the size of the airspaces slightly if the lung is at minimal volume. Since the lung contains a finite volume of fluid at the initiation of breathing, the effect of vascular engorgement in facilitating the first breath is probably negligible.

STIMULI FOR THE INITIATION OF RESPIRATION

Although it is not possible to assign priorities to the multiple chemical and physical stimuli that accompany birth and could initiate respiration recent systematic studies have contributed greatly to our understanding of the process. (See Chapter 5.)

The first breath may be thought of as a gasp, triggered by tactile and thermal changes. Release of the lamb from immersion in liquid and a change in temperature are significant stimuli to respiratory activity (Harned et al., 1970). In a series of studies on the chemical control of respiration, Harned and colleagues (1971) demonstrated that rhythmic breathing could occur in the fetal lamb in whom carotid and aortic bodies had been denervated. Vagotomy, on the other hand, seriously compromised respiratory activity. Central chemosensing mechanisms are probably operative in fetal and neonatal life as shown by Biscoe and Purves and also by Harned et al. When the fetus was denervated and the vagi divided, an increase in ventilation occurred with CO_2 administration. The sudden changes in fetal blood gases associated with the introduction of air into the lungs and the subsequent oscillations in gas tensions in carotid arterial blood are probably more potent stimuli to the peripheral chemoreceptors than are the relatively slow changes in blood gases which occur in utero (Avery et al., 1965; Purves, 1966). When steep changes in blood gases (mean decrease in $P_aO_2 = 10$ mm. Hg; increase in $P_aCO_2 = 26$ mm. Hg) were produced at the level of the carotid body in mature fetal lambs, a ventilatory response was noted, although after a longer time lag than that found after birth. Woodrum et al. (1972) interpreted their findings as suggestive that rapid asphyxial changes in either arterial oxygen or carbon dioxide tensions may be key factors in the initiation of gasping. Purves has suggested that the lack of sympathetic activity in the fetus may permit a relatively large blood flow to the carotid body. The increase in sympathetic discharges which he measured in the lamb at birth could reduce the blood flow and hence increase the sensitivity of the carotid body to small changes in gas tensions (Purves and Biscoe, 1966).

The intrinsic rhythmic activity of central respiratory neurons is enhanced by nonchemical stimuli. It seems probable that they play a central role in the first breath, since their activity would be augmented by physical stimuli at birth. It is also evident that the interaction of peripheral chemoreceptor activity is essential. The relative importance of central chemosensitive areas in the initiation and maintenance of respiration requires further study. (See page 53.)

CONTRIBUTIONS OF PHARYNGEAL MOTION

Serial roentgenograms of the oropharynx at birth reveal a swallowing motion associated with the first breath in some infants. Initially, the hyoid is displaced caudally, and the dorsal wall of the pharynx moves in the dorsal direction as the pharynx fills with air. The head is usually slightly extended, as is the spine. After the diaphragm descends with the first inspiratory effect, the pharynx is occluded, and the hyoid and larynx move ventrally. These sequential acts are similar to those seen in some paralyzed individuals who learn to propel air into the lung with their glossopharyngeal musculature. This participation of the upper airway in the first breath, sometimes referred to as "frog-breathing," may augment the inspiratory force of diaphragmatic descent. Occasionally, air is swallowed into the esophagus before it is visible in the lower airways (Bosma and Lind, 1960).

Chapter Four

PERINATAL CIRCULATION

by ROBERT L. WILLIAMS

Consideration of the fetal circulation and the changes that occur at birth and during the first days of life are fascinating not only to the student of cardiovascular physiology but to the clinician as well. It is obvious at once that successful growth of the fetus depends on tissue oxygenation and that the placenta is the organ of gas exchange. The dramatic circulatory adjustments that accompany birth are not matched at any other time of life. Small wonder that occasionally they do not occur smoothly and that clinical signs and symptoms may accompany delayed or inadequate circulatory adjustments.

The fetal circulation has been the subject of several recent reviews (Lind et al., 1964; Dawes, 1968; Rudolph, 1970; Heymann and Rudolph, 1972). It has traditionally been studied during acute experiments in exteriorized fetal lambs or goats which have been removed from the uterine cavity and placed in water baths with the placental circulation intact (Huggett, 1927). These fetuses survive the procedures necessary to allow measurements of pressures and blood flow in the systemic and pulmonary vessels, and the circulatory changes associated with the initial artificial inflation of their lungs may be observed. Blood pressure, heart rate, and the distribution of the cardiac output have also been studied in acute experiments on previable human fetuses delivered by hysterotomy while the placenta was still attached (Rudolph et al., 1971).

The chronic fetal lamb preparation was developed (Meschia et al., 1965) to obviate the effects of exteriorization of the fetus on its cardio-

38

vascular function (Heymann, 1967) and to allow repeated physiologic measurements in the same fetus during the last half of gestation. This technique has opened new vistas in the study of the fetal circulation, for it is now possible, for example, to examine the development of the changes in the cardiac output and its distribution, the maturation of reflex control of the circulation, and the changes resulting from surgically created cardiovascular lesions.

FETAL CIRCULATION

The fetal circulation is characterized by a low systemic and a high pulmonary vascular resistance and the presence of large "right-to-left" shunts through the foramen ovale and the ductus arteriosus. These are probably the major determinants of the difference in oxygen content of the blood perfusing the various fetal organs (Fig. 4–1).

Highly oxygenated blood ($PO_2 = 28$ to 30 mm. Hg) returns from the placenta in the umbilical vein and reaches the heart either by passing through the ductus venosus or the parenchyma of the liver. The factors determining the relative proportions of ductal flow remain to be elucidated; however, it appears that in the fetal lamb from 20 to 80 per cent of umbilical venous flow can bypass the liver.

The anatomical configuration of the right atrium and atrial septum is such that a large proportion of the inferior vena caval blood (containing all the highly oxygenated umbilical venous blood plus the less oxygenated blood from the lower body) passes directly into the left atrium where it is joined by the pulmonary venous return, and together they flow into the left ventricle. A smaller proportion of inferior vena caval flow plus most of the less oxygenated superior vena caval blood passes primarily across the tricuspid valve into the right ventricle. Thus, it is seen that the oxygenation of the blood is different in the two cardiac ventricles. The various factors controlling atrial shunting are poorly understood, and it must be remembered that the human infant has a proportionately larger head and upper body than the fetal lamb, and this almost certainly alters the pattern of right atrial flow distribution. Lind and Wegelius (1954) have shown with cineangiographic techniques that qualitatively similar streaming occurs in the human infant.

The more highly oxygenated ($PO_2 = 23$ to 26 mm. Hg) left ventricular blood perfuses the coronary vessels [which contribute to the blood supply of the ductus arteriosus (Dawes, 1968)] and the upper body, including the brain.

In the fetal lamb the main pulmonary artery is in direct continuity with the widely patent ductus arteriosus and almost all of the right ventricular output ($PO_2 = 17$ to 20 mm. Hg) streams preferentially

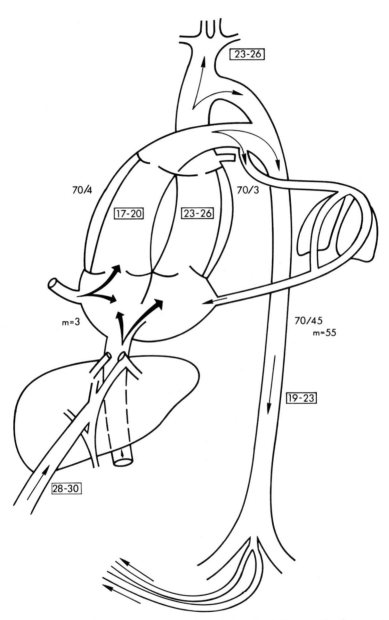

Figure 4–1. Schematic representation of the circulation in the late gestation fetal lamb. Arrows denote the direction of blood flow: oxygen tension (mm. Hg) enclosed in boxes and fetal pressure (mm. Hg) labeled outside the cardiac chambers and blood vessels. (Modified from Heymann and Rudolph, 1972.)

into the descending aorta. This large communication equalizes perfusion pressures in the fetal arteries and dictates that the blood flow to each organ be a function of its vascular resistance. Thus, blood flow is much greater through the noninnervated placental vessels than in the pulmonary circulation.

Experiments utilizing the distribution of radioactive microspheres injected into the neck and hindlimb veins of chronic fetal lambs have shown that cardiac output and its distribution change throughout gestation. These experiments have also confirmed earlier studies showing that the large placental blood flow (40 to 50 per cent of combined ventricular output) is in striking contrast to the low pulmonary blood flow (3 to 7 per cent of combined ventricular output) during fetal life (Rudolph and Heymann, 1970).

The range of cardiac output in near-term monkeys (*Macaca mulatta*) was 370 to 630 ml./kg./min. as determined by Behrman et al. with microspheres (1970). During fetal distress in both lambs and monkeys, there is a significant redistribution of cardiac output with the maintenance of blood flow to the heart, brain, and adrenal glands at the expense of pulmonary and placental flow. Normally in the fetal primate about 47 per cent of the total cardiac output perfuses the placenta.

FETAL BLOOD GASES

The degree of oxygenation of the human fetus in utero is not known, since it has not been possible to sample major arteries in utero without risk to the pregnancy. Most investigators have attempted to infer the degree of fetal oxygenation from samples of blood taken from the umbilical cord (MacKay, 1957; Pennoyer et al., 1956), or from the intervillous space at the time of cesarean section (Prystowsky, 1957). In full-term infants of normal pregnancies, umbilical artery saturation averaged 31 per cent and umbilical vein saturations 65 per cent (MacKay, 1957). Blood from the intervillous space in normal pregnancies varied from 45 to 97 per cent saturated, with an average of 66 per cent. Measurements of human fetal scalp blood at the beginning of labor give values for pH of approximately 7.30, with a standard bicarbonate of 19 mEq./L. and a PCO_2 of 44 mm. Hg (Beard and Morris, 1965). Oxygen saturation is about 26 per cent (Saling, 1964). Newman et al. (1967) report a mean fetal scalp pH of 7.28, a PCO_2 of 46.5 mm. Hg, and a PO_2 of 23 mm. Hg. When mothers are given added oxygen to breathe, the fetal scalp PO_2 can rise to 35 mm. Hg.

It is possible to know the state of fetal oxygenation in monkeys before labor begins, since catheters can be inserted, for long intervals, into fetal vessels without interruption of the pregnancy. Arterial oxygen saturation is between 80 and 95 per cent, pH 7.37 to 7.40, and a P_{CO_2} in the range of 35 mm. Hg (James, 1966). In lambs, umbilical venous oxygen saturations are 75 to 85 per cent, with a P_{O_2} of 20 to 35 mm. Hg (Stahlman, 1966).

REGULATION OF THE FETAL CIRCULATION

Recent experiments have shown that the fetal circulation, especially in late gestation, is capable of complex patterns of responses to various physiologic and pharmacologic stimuli and that many of these responses are mediated by the autonomic nervous system.

Sympathetic efferent nerve endings have been demonstrated histochemically in the fetal myocardium, although there is considerable variation in the time course of development (Friedman, 1968; Lipp, 1972). Epinephrine has an effect on the cardiovascular system of the two-day chick embryo (Hoffman, 1971), and the intravenous infusion of isoproterenol into the 60-day gestation fetal lamb is associated with cardioacceleration (Barrett, 1972). The lamb fetal myocardium is under vagal influence by at least 85 days' gestation (Vapaavuori et al., 1972). In these chronic preparations atropine administration produced an increase in fetal heart rate, and the response was much greater in fetuses near term.

The baroreceptor reflex is present in the fetal lamb by at least 85 days of gestation, and the amount of vagal bradycardia in response to the acute elevation of fetal blood pressure increases toward term (Shinebourne et al., 1972). Fetal hypoxemia without acidemia is associated with profound alterations in the circulation, for when a ewe breathes low-oxygen mixtures there is an increase in fetal arterial pressure and a decrease in heart rate. Cardiac output and umbilical blood flow are maintained; however, the blood flow to brain, heart, and adrenal glands increases at the expense of flow to the rest of the body (Cohn, 1972).

Dawes (1972) has recently described cardiovascular changes associated with fetal eye movements, rapid irregular breathing, and alterations in fetal cerebral cortical activity. Electrical stimulation of the hypothalamus of the chronic fetal lamb can produce marked changes in blood pressure, heart rate, and respiratory movements (Williams et al., 1972). It would appear that the pathways for central autonomic regulation of the circulation are developed in the fetal lamb as early as 90 days of gestation.

Severe asphyxia is associated with the release of adrenaline and noradrenaline from the fetal adrenal medulla (Comline and Silver, 1961, 1965); however, the contribution of these endogenous catecholamines to the cardiovascular changes during hypoxemia and acidemia is not known.

The pulmonary blood flow, as previously mentioned, is only 3 to 7 per cent of the combined ventricular output in the fetus. It should be stated, however, that the fetal lungs (3.2 per cent of the total fetal weight near term) are metabolically active, for their oxygen consumption is 5.4 per cent of the total fetal oxygen consumption (Dawes, 1954). This may provide an important clue to the mechanism of the high pulmonary vascular resistance in fetal life.

An anatomical explanation for this high fetal pulmonary vascular resistance was offered by Reynolds (1956) who suggested that the small pulmonary blood vessels were kinked and tortuous and subsequently unfolded at birth when the lungs were expanded. Lung expansion, irrespective of the nature of the gas used, does indeed result in a decrease in pulmonary vascular resistance (Campbell, 1968); however, the changes are most pronounced with an oxygen-containing mixture (Cook, 1963).

It is now thought that the low PO_2 in the blood perfusing the lungs is the major determinant for maintaining the fetal pulmonary arterioles in a state of tonic vasoconstriction (Cassin, 1964). Recent observations by Rudolph and Heymann (1972) suggest that the fetal pulmonary blood vessels are exquisitely sensitive to PO_2 changes of a few mm. Hg in the normal fetal range.

Whereas the pulmonary arterial injection of catecholamines, acetylcholine, bradykinin, and histamine as well as alterations in fetal pH and PCO_2 are associated with changes in pulmonary vascular resistance, the precise role of these substances in the normal control of the pulmonary circulation is not known. Under certain circumstances a sympathetic nervous influence on the pulmonary blood vessels can be demonstrated. Campbell (1967) observed pulmonary vasodilatation when the sympathetic nerves to the lungs were sectioned in acute experiments on fetal lambs. They also suggested that the pulmonary arterioles participated in an aortic body chemoreceptor reflex, for fetal asphyxia was associated with pulmonary vasoconstriction which could be abolished by either bilateral thoracic sympathectomy or the administration of hexamethonium.

THE TRANSITIONAL CIRCULATION

Profound alterations in the cardiovascular system occur as the newborn adapts to an extrauterine life. Some of these changes occur immediately at the time of birth, and others occur more gradually during the early neonatal period. After delivery, the cardiovascular system must quickly adjust to: (1) a sudden increase in systemic vas-

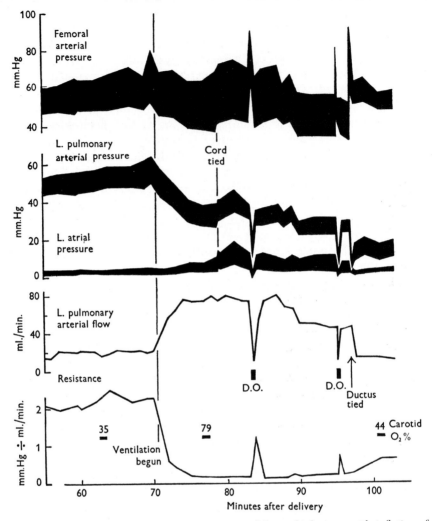

Figure 4–2. Changes in blood pressures and flow which occur with inflation of the lungs of the newborn lamb. (From Dawes, G. S.: J. Physiol. *121*:141, 1953.)

cular resistance as the cord is clamped and the large, low-resistance placental circulation is removed; (2) a rapid decrease in pulmonary vascular resistance and increase in pulmonary blood flow associated with the onset of ventilation; and, (3) a variable blood volume which depends, in part, on the size of the placental transfusion (Buckels and Usher, 1965) (Fig. 4–2).

As in fetal life, the anatomy of the atrial septum allows blood flow patterns to determine the nature of the atrial shunt during the immediate neonatal period. When placental blood flow to the right atrium ceases and pulmonary venous flow to the left atrium increases, the mean pressure in the left atrium becomes greater than that in the right, and the valve of the foramen ovale is pushed against the septum secundum functionally closing the interatrial communication. It should be realized that the normal anatomical sealing of the foramen is delayed, and the potential for interatrial shunting in either direction exists for some time after birth. This depends on the mean and phasic atrial pressure differences and the size of the valve in relation to the diameter of the foramen. A small right-to-left atrial shunt was demonstrated by cineangiograms in "normal" newborns under 12 hours of age (Lind and Wegelius, 1953). This shunt has been found most frequently in asphyxiated babies or during crying (Prec and Cassels, 1952). Left-to-right shunting after birth is probably related to an incompetent foramen ovale (Hoffman et al., 1972) and has been noted in asphyxiated babies in the first few hours of life (James et al., 1961).

Systemic cardiac output in the neonatal period has been difficult to measure. Krauss and Auld (1972) adapted a rebreathing method to measure mixed venous oxygen tensions. In newly born low birth weight infants, values of 50 to 100 ml./kg./min. were obtained, and in term infants the values were 300 to 500 ml./kg./min. Venous admixture was under 30 per cent in most instances. A right-to-left ductus shunt was excluded, since the arterial sampling site was the right radial or temporal artery.

There is now general agreement that the increase in pulmonary blood flow occurring at birth is primarily related to the pulmonary arteriolar dilatation brought about by the expansion of the lungs with air. Although it has been shown by Staub (1963) that blood in the arteriole can be oxygenated by diffusion from surrounding alveoli, the exact mechanism by which an increased PO_2 is associated with pulmonary vasodilatation remains unexplained. Locally produced chemical mediators may be of importance, since a cuff of pulmonary parenchyma surrounding the arteriole is necessary for the demonstration of the oxygen effect in vitro (Lloyd, 1968). The potent pulmonary arteriolar dilator, bradykinin, may play a role, for it has been found in high quantities in the left atrial blood of lambs when the lungs were inflated with oxygen but not nitrogen (Heymann et al., 1969).

The pulmonary arterioles in the newborn are extremely reactive. In newborn calves hypoxia and acidemia produced marked increases in pulmonary vascular resistance and the hydrogen ion effect was greatest in the low oxygen range (Rudolph, 1966). In the asphyxiated lamb, little change in pulmonary vascular resistance follows acute correction of the acidosis. Greater improvement is seen with infusion of liquids that increased blood volume (Johnson et al., 1972).

Pulmonary vascular resistance decreases progressively in the normal infant born at sea level (Rudolph, 1961). The first phase occurs rapidly with the onset of respiration and is followed by a second slower decrease lasting about five days as the medial muscle mass in the pulmonary arterioles regresses (Naeye, 1961). There is a final further decrease which progresses until three to five weeks of age, by which time the arterioles have an adult configuration. These changes roughly parallel the time course of the decrease in pulmonary artery pressure. The alveolar PO_2 is undoubtedly a determinant, for this regression is attenuated in infants with chronic alveolar hypoxia from pulmonary or central nervous system diseases (Naeye and Letts, 1962), and children born and living at altitude have a persistently high pulmonary vascular resistance (Sime et al., 1963). In the first hours of life the pulmonary artery/aorta pressure ratio is higher in infants who have had a larger placental transfusion at birth (Arcilla et al., 1966).

The pulmonary blood flow in the first hours of postnatal life is difficult to measure, since the persistence of shunts through the foramen ovale or the ductus arteriosus complicates the measurement. In the absence of shunts, the uptake of an indicator gas will measure pulmonary blood flow. Cotton et al. (1971) used this method in 32 normal infants (weight 2.03 kg. to 4.35 kg.) in whom they doubted the presence of significant shunts. Before age 24 hours, the mean "effective" pulmonary blood flow was 138 ml./kg./min. and rose to 166 ml./kg./min. ±25.6 S.E. at a mean age of 81 hours. Brady and Rigatto (1969) used the N_2O uptake technique in normal infants and demonstrated an increase in "effective" pulmonary blood flow between ages 10 hours and eight days.

Whereas in fetal life almost all the right ventricular output crosses a ductus arteriosus which is large enough to allow equal pressures in the pulmonary artery and descending aorta, this structure is normally functionally closed by about 15 hours of age (Rudolph et al., 1961; Moss et al., 1963) and is anatomically closed by about three weeks (Mitchell, 1957). The ductal shunt is probably bidirectional in the first few hours of life (Moss et al., 1963) and then, as pulmonary artery pressure decreases further, becomes a left-to-right shunt until closure occurs (Prec and Cassels, 1955). Several studies with various techniques (Prec and Cassels, 1955; Condorelli and Ungari, 1960; Rudolph et al., 1961; Jeiger et al., 1964) have shown left-to-right ductal shunting several days after birth, and it is probable that transient changes in ductal diameter and aortic and pulmonary artery pressures can be associated with ductal shunting until anatomical closure occurs.

Although catecholamines can produce ductal constriction in the fetal lamb, it is generally conceded that the major factor associated with closure of the ductus arteriosus is the postnatal increase in the arterial PO_2 (Born et al., 1956). This may explain, in part, the delayed ductal closure reported in prematures (Danilowicz et al., 1966) and the increased incidence of patent ductus arteriosus in children born at altitude (Alzamora-Castro et al., 1960).

The mechanism of the ductal oxygen response is under intense study at the present time. In the fetal lamb it is not dependent on the extrinsic nerves (Born et al., 1956). In vitro experiments with fetal lamb ductus show that the oxygen response is greater in late gestation and is not affected by alpha- or beta-adrenergic blockade. There is in vitro evidence that the oxygen response may be mediated by acetylcholine and blocked by atropine (Oberhänsli-Weiss et al., 1972), whereas Fay (1971) suggests that in the guinea pig oxygen triggers the constriction of ductal smooth muscle by increasing the rate of oxidative phosphorylation as a result of a direct effect on a terminal cytochrome component.

It would appear that the increase in arterial PO_2 that normally occurs postnatally is associated with widely divergent effects on various segments of vascular smooth muscle: constriction of umbilical arteries and the ductus arteriosus; pulmonary arteriolar dilatation; and little, if any, effect on systemic arterioles.

Cardiac murmurs are sometimes noted in normal full-term babies. On prolonged auscultation, crescendo systolic murmurs can be heard in the first few hours of life in about one-third of normal infants and even more frequently in babies who are asphyxiated or premature (Burnard, 1958, 1959). The precise origin of these murmurs is poorly defined; however, many are probably related to changing hemodynamics during ductal closure. Ejection systolic murmurs that radiate well to the axillae may be due to transient physiologic branch pulmonary artery stenosis. The right and left branch pulmonary arteries retain their fetal configuration with small relative diameter and an acute angle of origin from the main pulmonary artery until about four months of age (Danilowicz et al., 1972). The continuous murmur at the left base, a classic sign of a patent ductus arteriosus in older infants, is rarely present in the neonatal period, for pulmonary artery pressure can be very similar to aortic pressure; and turbulent flow, sufficient to produce a murmur, may occur only during systole. Kitterman et al. (1972) diagnosed patent ductus arteriosus in 17 of 111 premature infants (1750 gm. or less) and noted a harsh systolic murmur best heard at the middle to lower left sternal border. In most, there was some extension of the murmur into early diastole.

Chapter Five

REGULATION
OF RESPIRATION

FETUS

The lack of responsiveness of the sheep fetus, exteriorized near term, to a change in pH, P_{CO_2}, and P_{O_2} might lead to the conclusion that the chemical regulation of respiration is not operative before birth. Fetal lambs also fail to show respiratory excitation after injections of cyanide, whereas lambs one to two days of age will show increased respiratory activity after small doses of cyanide (Reynolds and Mackie, 1961). Rosenfeld and Snyder (1938) did find newborn rabbits delivered at 28 days to be unresponsive to carbon dioxide, but at 29 days' gestation they responded. Clearly, responsiveness to chemical stimuli is not impressive in the fetal animal. Similar studies on human fetuses are, of course, not available.

Chemoreceptors are present in the human fetus from early in gestation (Boyd, 1937). In fact, richly vascularized glomus tissue is present between the aorta and pulmonary artery at 50 to 60 days of gestation. This chromaffin tissue with the histologic attributes of chemosensitive tissue, known as the inferior aorticopulmonary body, is perfused by blood from the pulmonary artery and from branches of the coronary arteries. After birth, the blood supply from the pulmonary artery retrogresses (Boyd, 1961). No function has been ascribed to this glomus tissue in the human fetus. Whatever its role, it would appear to play this in utero, since it disappears after birth.

The evidence that some chemosensitive tissue is responsive in the sheep fetus was provided by the measurements of electrical activity from the cut end of the nerve from the carotid sinus. Electrical discharges ceased when the ewes were given 100 per cent oxygen (Cross

48

and Malcolm, 1952). It appears that the peripheral chemoreceptors are present and capable of discharge. Whether the medullary centers fail to respond to the signals, or the respiratory effector apparatus (lungs and muscles of respiration) fails to respond or is under active inhibition from other sources, is not known. (See Chapter 3.)

NEWBORN

The qualitative responses of ventilation in the newborn infant to changes in the concentration of inspired gases, tactile and thermal stimuli, and drugs can be readily evaluated. The quantitative aspects of the responses, particularly with reference to comparisons with adult responses, are difficult because of the problem of sizing. A per cent increase in ventilation may be used, but it is difficult to interpret since resting ventilations differ so greatly. A change per unit surface area or per unit body weight may give different answers without any assurance as to which is the most physiologically meaningful comparison. An evaluation of the ventilatory responses of infants is further complicated by the probability that they are not exactly the same on the first day of life as they might be at the end of the first week, nor are the responses of a 1.0-kg. infant necessarily the same as those of a 3.0-kg. infant.

Table 5–1 lists the known factors which in some way alter or regulate the respiration of adults. Not all of these have been carefully evaluated in infants. Perhaps the most extensively studied factors are the chemical ones.

Chemical Stimuli to Respiration

Interest in the role of carbon dioxide in the control of respiration dates from the classic studies of Haldane and Priestley (1905). Since then innumerable carefully reviewed investigations confirm the central importance of blood gas tensions in the regulatory mechanism (Schmidt and Comroe, 1940; Heymans, 1950; Gray, 1950; Dejours, 1959). The increase in ventilation in infants with acidosis was appreciated years ago, and in fact the measurement of a low P_{CO_2} in the expired air of these infants by Howland and Marriott in 1916 preceded the first measurements of a decreased CO_2 content in the blood.

Studies of the ventilatory response of newborn infants to increased amounts of carbon dioxide in the inspired air, done chiefly during the past 15 years, show that the infants do increase their ventilation (Wilson et al., 1942; Howard and Bauer, 1950; Cross et al., 1953; Miller, 1954; Stahlman and Sexton, 1961; Tooley et al., 1962; Avery et al., 1963).

Table 5–1.   Factors Known to Influence Respiration

Stimuli	*Depressants*
Chemical	
Arterial P_{CO_2} up to about 80 mm.Hg	Arterial P_{CO_2} over 80 mm.Hg
Arterial pH 7.0–7.4	Arterial pH less than 6.9 or over 7.5
Arterial P_{O_2} less than about 80 mm.Hg	Profound hypoxia
(in adults)	
(Newborn infants with only mild hypoxemia are stimulated by inspired oxygen.)	
Pharmacological	
Epinephrine	Morphine
Lobeline	Barbiturates
Nicotine	Chloramphenicol
Salicylates	Neomycin, etc.
Picrotoxin	
Nikethamide	
Progesterone	
Pulmonary Reflexes	
Deflation receptors (Hering-Breuer)	Stretch receptors
Stretch receptors (Head's reflex)	Aortic arch and carotid sinus stretch receptors
Pressoreceptors	
Decrease in blood pressure	Increase in blood pressure
Bones and Joints	
Stretch receptors in muscles	
Tactile responses	
Thermal	
Fever	Hibernation
Sudden chilling	
Cortical	
(Voluntary control of breathing is possible within limits.)	

There is no unanimity on the quantitative aspects of the ventilatory response of the newborn infant to carbon dioxide. Cross concluded that the ventilatory response to a given P_{CO_2} was greater in the infant than in the adult, at least at low inspired mixtures; Stahlman found the response to be less in the early days of life than later; Tooley felt that the response was similar in infants and adults. The problem is again chiefly in terms of how infants are compared with adults. Avery et al. found that the ventilation of infants at a given P_{CO_2} was greater than that of adults, but that the change in ventilation expressed as liters/kg. body weight for a change in alveolar CO_2 tension was the same (Fig. 5–1). The greater ventilation at a given P_{CO_2} was thought to be a function of the higher CO_2 output per kg. and the slightly lower bicarbonate levels, hence poorer buffering of infants. The observation of the similarity of the change in ventilation/kg./unit change in CO_2 tension in infants and adults suggests that their neural

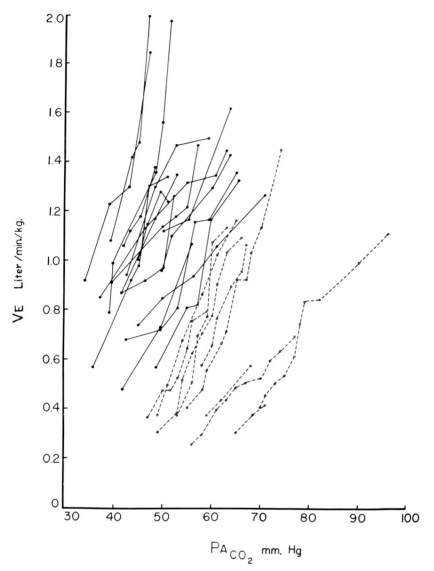

Figure 5–1. The relation of ventilation per kg. body weight to alveolar carbon dioxide tensions in infants (solid lines) and adults (dotted lines). The mean slope of the infant curves is the same as that of the adults. The shift to the left in infants is thought to be the combined effect of lower buffering, greater metabolism per kg. body weight, and the tactile stimuli from application of a mask. (From Avery et al.: J. Appl. Physiol. 18:895, 1963.)

regulatory apparatus has the same sensitivity, but that the output of the effector apparatus — the lungs — is a function of body mass. The effects of a depletion in buffering and an increase in metabolism appeared to be additive to the stimulus of increased inspired carbon dioxide to respiration.

The role of P_{O_2} in the regulation of respiration can be studied by measuring the effects of 100 per cent oxygen breathing. As Dripps and Comroe noted (1947), it is probable that the normal adult has some "tonic" chemoreceptor activity from air breathing. One hundred per cent oxygen will in a sense denervate the oxygen receptors, and a temporary decrease in ventilation is observed. Studies in infants show that there is a decrease in ventilation if 100 per cent oxygen is given after air breathing, and an even greater decrease if 100 per cent oxygen is given after a period of 15 per cent oxygen (Cross and Warner, 1951; Cross and Oppe, 1952; Miller and Behrle, 1954; Brady et al., 1964). Reinstorff and Fenner (1972) found an average reduction in ventilation of 15 per cent in a study of 15 infants from 28 weeks to term. They exposed the infants to 8 to 15 seconds of 100 per cent oxygen, and measured ventilation for a 10-second interval after $P_{A}O_2$ increased. All of their infants were under three days of age. These studies would support the concept that even in the first day of life ventilatory responses to changes in P_{O_2} occur.

The effects of hypoxia as a ventilatory stimulus may differ on the first day of life from those at a later age. Miller and Behrle's studies (1954) show a tendency for infants under 24 hours of age to hypoventilate in a 12 per cent oxygen environment, whereas those six to 11 days of age hyperventilate for the first few minutes of exposure to low oxygen, then hypoventilate to some extent over the next few minutes. These findings have been difficult to interpret since it is now clear that the responses are critically dependent on environmental temperature and may be effected by persistent fetal circulatory pathways (Purves, 1966). During the first week of life, transient hyperventilation can be induced in a 12 per cent oxygen environment only if the infants are kept warm. After the first week, sustained hyperventilation occurred regardless of environmental temperature (Ceruti, 1966).

In the newborn rabbit, Dawes and Mott (1959) found an increase in minute volume after injections of sodium cyanide and abolished the effect after denervation of the carotid sinus. They concluded that oxygen-sensitive chemoreceptors were functional soon after birth in this animal.

The effects of changes in CO_2 and O_2 on respiration are not additive (Lloyd et al., 1958). The ventilatory response to a given alveolar P_{CO_2} is greater at a lower P_{O_2}; moreover, the slope of the relationship between ventilation and $P_{A}CO_2$, usually referred to as the CO_2 response curve, is an inverse function of the alveolar oxygen tension. In a series of studies on newborn lambs from four hours to 10 days of age, Purves found the enhancement of the response to carbon dioxide in the presence of low oxygen tension the same as in adults. He further showed that the response was less after bilateral section of the carotid sinus nerves. Denervation of the chemoreceptors abolished the ventilatory response to hypoxia (Purves, 1966).

The relative importance of peripheral and central chemosensitive areas in the regulation of respiration has been under intense investigation in recent years. Changes in cerebrospinal fluid hydrogen ion concentrations are of central significance in steady state conditions. The pH of spinal fluid is acid 7.32 with respect to blood, 7.40 in the resting state, with a bicarbonate gradient maintained by an active transport system. The fetal and neonatal lambs show acid-base relationships between spinal fluid and blood similar to those found in ewes, adult dogs, and man (Hodson et al., 1968). The fetal lamb under spinal anesthesia seems relatively unresponsive to an increase in hydrogen ion concentration in the spinal fluid, as judged from studies of Herrington et al. (1971).

Nonchemical Stimuli to Respiration

Clinical experience testifies to the powerful effects of nonchemical stimuli to respiration in the newborn. The traditional spanking after birth, the ease with which a cry is elicited, the increase in oxygen consumption with a fall in body temperature (Brück et al., 1962; Karlberg et al., 1962), and the increase in ventilation with handling and mask application (Avery et al., 1963) illustrate nonchemical respiratory stimulants.

The recent work of Burns (1963) has elucidated in the experimental animal some of the respiratory responses from nonchemical stimuli, or "neuronal traffic" through the medulla. He has recorded discharges from the respiratory neurons with microelectrodes in the medulla. Those discharges, which are synchronous with respiration, are thought to arise in the inspiratory and expiratory centers (Fig. 5–2). After section of the medulla, the output of these neurons de-

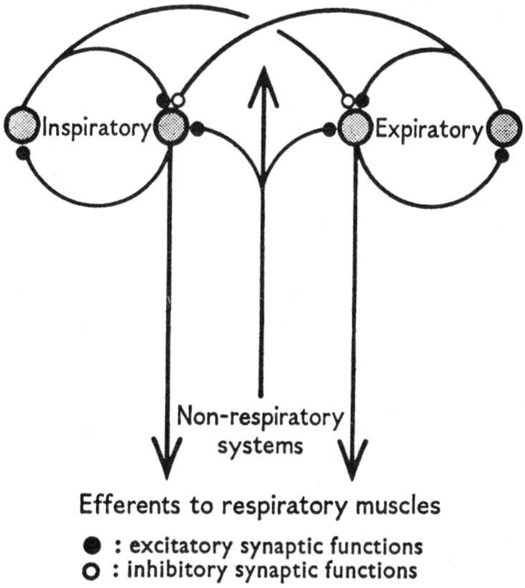

Figure 5–2. Schema of respiratory center. The nonchemical stimuli increase the output of the inspiratory and expiratory centers. (From Burns, B. D.: Brit. Med. Bull. *19*:7, 1963.)

creases. They increase, with stimulation of the distal cut end of the medulla, as if their output depended on a background of nonchemical neuronal traffic.

Pulmonary Reflexes

The Hering-Breuer and Head reflexes, thought to arise from receptors in the lungs and to be mediated through the vagus nerve, are probably active in the newborn. Few studies have been done on human infants; however, Cross et al. (1960) provided evidence that Head's reflex, or the induction of a gasp on lung inflation, is present in the first days of life. They found it less frequently in infants from two to six days of age. Whether this is a reflex unique to the newborn period, or is associated with stretch of deflation receptors in atelectatic lung at any age, deserves further investigation. In the newborn rabbit, Dawes and Mott (1959) have found well-marked inflation and deflation reflexes which are not present after vagotomy. The role of these reflexes in the rhythmicity of respiration in the newborn period, as at any age, remains a matter of conjecture.

Respiratory Patterns

Periodic Breathing.   One of the most common respiratory patterns in premature infants is known as periodic breathing, which denotes brief recurring periods of apnea in a sequence of breaths. In fact, it is so common as to be considered normal in premature infants; this implies that the majority do it, as they surely do, or that it is harmless, which is not established.

In one series of premature infants the incidence of irregular breathing was 75 per cent, and of definitive periodicity, 29 per cent (Bouterline-Young and Smith, 1950). Others have found periodic breathing in 44 per cent of infants (Graham et al., 1950), but rarely in the first 24 hours of age (Deming and Washburn, 1935).

Some clinical observations may be summarized as follows:

1. Periods of apnea last five to 10 seconds.
   Periods of ventilation last 10 to 15 seconds.
   Average rate is 30 to 40/min.
   Rate during ventilatory interval is 50 to 60/min.
2. An infant may have regular respirations, then periodic, then regular again within a given hour. In general, periodic breathing appears during a more wakeful state, regular breathing during deep sleep.
3. Periodic breathing is rarely seen in the first 24 hours of life, and is uncommon before five days of age.
4. It may persist for six weeks in small infants, but it is unusual after 2 kg. weight or 36 weeks' gestational age.
5. It is more common and lasts longer in smaller infants.

Measurements of the pH of arterialized capillary blood during periodic breathing reveal that infants who show periodic breathing most of the time tend to be slightly alkalotic (mean pH, 7.44) compared with the more regular breathers (mean pH, 7.39). This observation was confirmed by the finding that the P_{CO_2} of end-tidal air was slightly lower during phases of periodic breathing than during regular breathing. However, Rigatto and Brady (1972) found no difference in end-tidal CO_2 during periodic or regular intervals among infants who showed both patterns. The group which was usually periodic had a mean P_ACO_2 of 40 mm. Hg, compared to 34 mm. Hg in the regular group. More striking was the lower arterial oxygen tensions in the periodic (P_aO_2 = 57 mm. Hg) group compared to 66 mm. Hg in the regular group.

No significant changes in heart rate or body temperature occur during periodic breathing, in contrast to infants with more prolonged apneic spells in whom bradycardia and hypothermia frequently occur (Fig. 5–3).

It has been known for some years that an increase in the inspired oxygen concentration or carbon dioxide will convert periodic breathing to regular breathing. No threshold value has been established, as infants seem to differ in the amounts required. On the other hand, the arterial oxygen saturation of infants who show periodic breathing is not lower than that of other infants (Graham et al., 1950). The first suggestion that low oxygen may contribute to the incidence of periodicity is a comparison of the report of Deming and Washburn (1935) in Denver with that of Murphy and Thorpe (1931) in Philadelphia. In Denver, where the barometric pressure averages 625 mm. Hg, Deming and Washburn found that half of their term infants showed periodic breathing. In Philadelphia, at a barometric pressure of 760 mm. Hg, periodicity is rare in term infants, as it is in Baltimore, also at sea level. More recently, Rigatto and Brady (1972) added significant confirmatory evidence that low arterial oxygen tensions may be a significant factor in periodic breathing and apneic spells.

It is tempting to try to interpret periodic breathing in premature infants in the light of studies on adults with Cheyne-Stokes or Biot type breathing. It is at once apparent that the intervals of apnea and ventilation are briefer in infants, and a crescendo-decrescendo pattern is not the rule in them. The hypotheses put forth to explain periodicity in adults include those of a prolonged lung to brain circulation time (Guyton et al., 1956; Lange and Hecht, 1962) and lesions in the medulla or pons which interfere with the central integration of respiratory stimuli (Brown and Plum, 1961). The subsequent normal development of many infants who show periodic breathing makes either explanation unlikely. Moreover, Rigatto and Brady (1972) found normal lung to ear circulation times during periodic breathing. One possible basis for the phenomenon in infants derives from its associa-

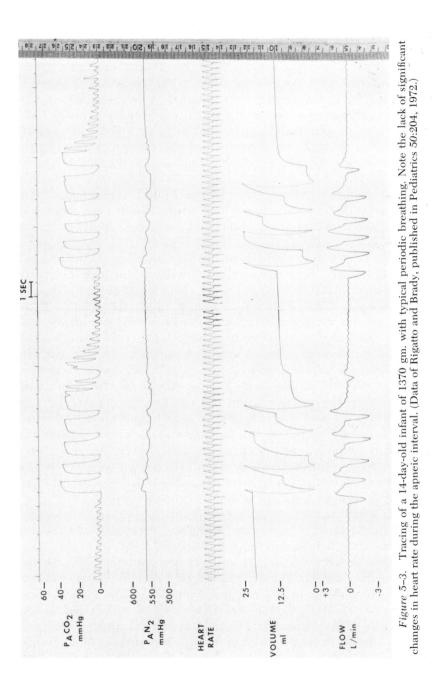

Figure 5–3. Tracing of a 14-day-old infant of 1370 gm. with typical periodic breathing. Note the lack of significant changes in heart rate during the apneic interval. (Data of Rigatto and Brady, published in Pediatrics 50:204, 1972.)

tion with immaturity. It seems probable that the central nervous system integrating pathways are not well established in those babies. Further studies are needed to clarify this point.

Apneic Spells. One of the more frequent and alarming experiences in a premature nursery is the occurrence of apneic spells of more than 20 seconds' duration. The etiology in some infants is obvious when the larynx is inspected with a laryngoscope and milk or mucus can be seen occluding it. At times, prolonged apnea is associated with other forms of respiratory distress, such as hyaline membrane disease, pneumonia, or pulmonary hemorrhage. There is a measurable decrease in oxygen saturation during prolonged apnea from 95 per cent to 81 per cent saturation after 25 seconds of apnea in one of the patients of Miller et al. (1959). Blystad (1956) noted a respiratory acidosis in infants with apneic spells. Bradycardia is usually present in prolonged apnea, in contrast to its absence in periodic breathing.

Prolonged apneic spells may occur at any day of life, may be repetitive, and tend to be more common in smaller infants. They occurred three times as often in infants of less than 1.25 kg. with respiratory distress compared with infants of more than 1.5 kg. birth weight in Miller's series (1959). Steinschneider (1972) reported five infants seen between five and 40 days of age because of recurrent cyanotic and apneic episodes. He carried out systematic studies on these infants recording rapid eye movements and respiration during sleep and wakefulness. Although the majority of the episodes of apnea were brief, occasionally they were prolonged, and the infants became cyanotic. Two of the five infants ultimately died during similar episodes. The apneic episodes were noted when the infants were free of any other evident disease. However, it was also observed that during upper respiratory infections the frequency of the spells increased. The apneic intervals were most frequently noted during REM sleep. Steinschneider speculates that this may have something to do with the sudden unexpected death which is known to occur most frequently between four and 16 weeks of age.

We have observed infants similar to those described by Steinschneider and remain puzzled. The usual reason for coming to the hospital is that the infant was observed to be cyanotic and was aroused by a parent who hastens to the hospital. By the time the child is examined, everything seems perfectly normal, but because of the disturbing nature of the experience, hospitalization has been advised. During several weeks of hospitalization of such infants, we have seen these cyanotic attacks occur during sleep, but always without any clear-cut triggering episodes. They are unrelated to meals and thus are readily distinguished from the cyanosis and choking that accompany aspiration.

The seriousness of apneic spells is apparent from the high mortality of infants who have them. Illingworth (1957) reviewed his ex-

Table 5–2. Deaths in the First Month of Life among Severely
Apneic and Nonapneic Infants*

Infants	Birth Weight (kg.)		
	1.0–1.25	1.25–1.50	1.50–1.75
Apneic			
Number born	16	5	9
Number died	9	2	7
Nonapneic			
Number born	7	22	41
Number died	3	4	3

* From Miller et al.: Pediatrics, 23:676, 1959.

perience with 170 infants with apneic spells, 60 per cent of whom
were premature. Seventy per cent of the premature infants with spells
died, and 15 per cent of term infants with spells died. Miller (1959)
tabulated the mortality in infants with apneic spells (Table 5–2).

Increased concentrations of inspired oxygen do not always prevent apneic attacks, although infants remain better oxygenated during
such attacks when they breathe enriched oxygen mixtures. The duration of apneic spells may actually be prolonged with added oxygen.
Tactile stimuli such as turning the infant or slapping the feet often
result in the resumption of regular respiration.

Experimental production of apneic spells in infant monkeys was
reported by French et al. (1972). During the first week of life, some of
the infant monkeys made no respiratory efforts during nasal occlusion
and would remain apneic thereafter. When retested at 10 to 12 weeks
of age, the monkeys readily established mouth breathing. A "diving
reflex" was elicited in some of the monkeys. Immersion of the face in
water led to apnea and bradycardia with an increase in blood pressure.
In the young monkeys, the response persisted after immersion ended.
The authors suggest that obligate nose breathing and a diving reflex
may be responsible for sudden infant deaths, regardless of the initiating factors.

It is tempting to speculate that the apneic spells denote intracranial pathology. Their occurrence during respiratory distress, and
the association of intracranial hemorrhage and hyaline membrane disease, suggest that the spells may be a clinical expression of central
nervous system depression. While no careful correlations of apneic
spells and intracranial hemorrhage have been reported, our few observations make it clear that they need not go together. Only 33 per
cent of Illingworth's patients had cerebral hemorrhages (1957). The
higher incidence of apneic spells in the very small infants suggests
immaturity with respect to the integration of multiple stimuli to
respiration. Delineation of the mechanisms awaits further study.

Chapter Six

METHODS OF STUDY OF PULMONARY FUNCTION IN INFANTS

At first thought, it may be surprising that nearly every aspect of pulmonary function which has been measured in adults has also been measured in newborn infants. Of course, those procedures which require active patient cooperation cannot be applied to infants; however, those determinations which depend on a resting patient can be measured, and when a cry will suffice for a deep breath, this too can be elicited. It is much easier to evaluate pulmonary function in a newborn infant than in a two-month- or two-year-old child, since children tend to object actively to test situations beyond the newborn period.

BLOOD GASES

Perhaps the most useful single measure of ventilatory adequacy at any age is the partial pressure of carbon dioxide in the arterial blood (PCO_2). This measurement has become much more feasible since it has been ascertained that free-flowing capillary blood from a warmed extremity or ear lobe has the same gas tensions as arterial blood. If the hand or foot of a normal infant is warmed to 40°C for three minutes, and a single clean puncture made so that blood flows freely, the gas tensions in the capillary blood will be the same as those in blood sampled directly from arteries. After the first hours of life, or when acrocyanosis is no longer present, no warming is necessary if the infant is in an incubator. In the event of shock or heart failure, tensions in capillary blood will differ from those of central arterial blood because of stasis in the periphery. The validity of a capillary sample in sick infants has been confirmed by a study reported in 1972 by Glasgow et al. Their technique consisted of using a vasodilating cream (constituents—histamine dihydrochloride 0.01 per cent, methyl nicotimate 1.0 per cent, glycol monosalicylate 10 per cent, and capsicum oleoresin 0.1 per cent—Whitehall Laboratories Ltd., Cooksville, Ontario, Canada), applied to the infant's heel for 15 to 20 minutes. The heel was then cleansed with alcohol and a 3-mm. skin puncture made with a number 15 surgical blade. Blood was collected directly into preheparinized glass capillary tubes, sealed, and mixed. The values for pH and P_{CO_2} were nearly identical. The values for P_{O_2} corresponded to those in the descending aorta as long as the oxygen tension was 60 mm. Hg or below. There was no prediction possible at higher oxygen tensions. The value of using a digital arteriole as the site of sampling was made apparent by the studies by Corbet and Burnard (1970). Temporal and radial artery punctures are feasible (Bucci et al., 1966; Wunderlich and Reynolds, 1972). Digital blood can be used with confidence for determinations of pH and carbon dioxide tensions since arterial-venous differences are so small, and sequential changes are often of more clinical importance than single values.

Micro methods are available for the determination of pH, P_{CO_2}, and P_{O_2}. With suitable nomograms, the bicarbonate concentration can be calculated. While these determinations are not universally used because adequate instruments have only recently become available and remain expensive, the simplicity of the methods and the great value to be gained from such information warrants their use. It is essential to make the measurements within 15 minutes of drawing the sample and to keep the sample anaerobic in order to measure accurate gas tensions.

The feasibility of continuous monitoring of ear-lobe tissue oxygen tension was shown by Strauss et al. (1972). The correspondence with arterial P_{O_2} was excellent in the range of 34 to 162 mm. Hg. The method is not widely used in part because of the complexity of the equipment, the need for calibration every six hours, and the potential

Table 6–1. Normal Values for Umbilical Arterial Blood

	20 minutes	*1 hour*	*4 hours*
pH	7.33–7.36	7.40–7.42	7.39–7.42
P_{CO_2}	33–37	32–33	34–35
P_{O_2}	52–68	49–66	64–68

(From Stephenson et al. J. Pediat., 76:848, 1970. The lower values of P_{O_2} and pH are in chilled infants.)

Table 6–2.

Infants	Bag Volume (ml.)	Rebreathing Time (secs.)	Final Equilibration Time (secs.)
1.5–2.5 kg.	100	30	10
Over 2.5 kg.	200	60	10
1–24 mos.	200–300	60	10–15

local complications from the inserted wire. It has great potential in investigative studies in animals.

The arterial P_{CO_2} can be estimated in infants without drawing blood or using expensive apparatus. A rebreathing technique, originally used by Howland and Marriott in 1916 and modified by many investigators for adults, has recently been adapted for use in infants and young children (Lertzman and Ciner, 1965; Hodson et al., 1966). It uses the lung as a tonometer to bring mixed venous blood gases into equilibrium between the air in the lung and the air in a bag from which the patient rebreathes. The carbon dioxide tension in the air in the bag can be analyzed. Since arterial carbon dioxide tensions are about 6 mm. Hg lower than mixed venous tensions, the subtraction of 6 mm. Hg from the measured value gives arterial tensions. The bag volumes and appropriate time intervals for rebreathing in infants are noted in Table 6–2.

The reason for special interest in the P_{CO_2} in the newborn infant is the relative frequency of pulmonary insufficiency in the first minutes and days of life. A measure of the carbon dioxide combining power is an adequate index of the degree of acidosis in most clinical pediatric problems after the newborn period, since metabolic disorders are much more frequent than pulmonary disorders. However, the carbon dioxide combining power or bicarbonate concentration may be quite normal in the newborn infant, and a severe respiratory acidosis still be present. If the pH as well as the bicarbonate concentration is measured, the P_{CO_2} can be calculated from the Henderson-Hasselbalch equation:

$$pH = pk + \log \frac{(HCO_3^-)}{0.03\ P_{CO_2}}.$$

The degree of acidosis and the relative contributions of the metabolic and respiratory components can be assessed when all three of the variables in this equation are known. It is useful to consider the HCO_3^- as being under renal regulation, and the P_{CO_2} as being controlled by the lung; thus the pH $\sim \dfrac{\text{kidneys}}{\text{lungs}}$. Rapid changes in pH are possible by changes in the degree of ventilation. Since the lung is a kind of tonometer that mixes atmospheric air with blood, the gases in the blood come into equilibrium with the gases in the alveoli. Thus when normal individuals are horizontal, the end-tidal sample of expired air contains carbon dioxide at the same tension as arterial blood. Moderate hyperventilation will result in a decrease in arterial carbon dioxide tension (P_aCO_2), hence an increase in pH. Hypoventilation from breath holding, apneic spells, central nervous system depression, or pulmonary insufficiency will raise the P_aCO_2 and hence lower the pH so that respiratory acidosis ensues. Renal compensation by adjustments of bicarbonate which tend to keep the pH normal is achieved less quickly than are the changes in PCO_2 induced by respiratory maneuvers, but may take place within an hour or so if the ventilation is persistently altered in one direction or another. Thus a measure of the bicarbonate concentration suggests the duration of the ventilatory abnormality. For example, no significant changes in bicarbonate levels occur during an episode of crying in which the pH may rise to 7.50 and the PCO_2 fall to 20 mm. Hg. The course of acid-base adjustments in the first hours of life in normal infants has been documented by the studies of Oliver et al. (1961), Weisbort et al. (1958), and Reardon et al. (1960) (Fig. 6–1).

Umbilical Artery Catheterization

In a newborn infant sufficiently distressed to require significant increase in inspired oxygen concentrations, serial measurements of arterial oxygen tensions are necessary to guide therapy. The problem arises as to the site of sampling for the determination. Temporal or right radial artery samples are in many respects ideal, since they represent blood going to the brain and retinal vessels. Bucci et al. (1966) have described a technique for radial artery sampling that is widely employed. In very small infants who require repeated measurements, the umbilical artery has been advocated as a reasonable site. Although it is below the level of the ductus arteriosus, and hence may have some venous admixture, aortic blood from the umbilical artery usually approximates that of blood proximal to the ductus and is useful in monitoring the sick infant (Murdock et al.). The catheter tip may be relatively safely located between T6 and T10, which is 0.33 times the heel-crown length of the infant. Weaver and Ahlgren (1971) report that by using that formula they locate the catheter tip within the thoracic aorta and avoid dangers of location near the celiac, renal, or mesenteric arteries. This position carries the risk of air embolism if the infant cries at a time when the catheter is exposed to atmospheric pressure; it avoids the dangers of occluding an artery to a vital organ, and thus appears justified. Complications of umbilical artery catheterization have been of the order of 10 per cent, according to Cochran et al. (1968) and Gupta et al. (1968). Major thromboses were noted in

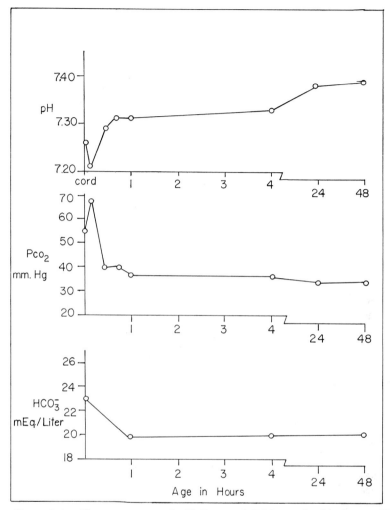

Figure 6–1. Changes in arterial pH, Pco₂ and HCO₃⁻ in the first hours of life. (Based on data of Oliver et al.: Acta Paediat. 50:346, 1961; and Reardon et al.: J. Pediat. 57:151, 1960.)

some infants by Wigger et al. (1970). The duration of catheterization and the use of the catheter for infusion of hypertonic solutions increase the dangers. The most common complication is a temporary blanching of the leg, which is usually reversed by removal of the catheter or warming of the contralateral leg. Serious complications such as major thromboses occur in about 2 per cent of infants. Clinically silent thromboses, demonstrated by aortography, were found in 18 of 19 infants who had had umbilical artery catheterization. Neal et al. (1972), who conducted that study, emphasize the need for careful selection of patients for umbilical artery catheterization. (For discussion of radiographic evaluation of catheter placement, see page 104.)

EVALUATION OF SHUNTS

The degree of visible cyanosis is a function of the arterial oxygen saturation, the hematocrit value, and the peripheral circulation. The experienced observer who considers all of these as he approaches an infant can estimate the severity of cyanosis fairly well. On the other hand, he is helped by a direct measure of arterial oxygen saturation or the partial pressure of oxygen in the blood. The latter is essential to quantify mild degrees of hypoxia, since the shape of the oxyhemoglobin dissociation curves requires a large decrease in oxygen tension before significant unsaturation is present.

The arterial oxygen tension depends on the ventilation, diffusing capacity of the lung, distribution of ventilation and perfusion within the lung, and right-to-left shunts in the cardiovascular system. To distinguish which of these is responsible for the cyanosis in a given infant requires a variety of tests. It is usually simplest and most informative to distinguish the effect of right-to-left shunt from all of the others. This can be done by having the infant inhale 100 per cent O_2. After 15 to 20 minutes, the alveolar oxygen tension will be the same as barometric pressure minus the partial pressure of water vapor at body temperature and the partial pressure of carbon dioxide. The high alveolar oxygen tensions are sufficient to overcome any barrier to diffusion, so that persistent arterial tensions below alveolar tension mean that some portions of the circulating blood are bypassing ventilated spaces in the lung.

Since the calculation of right-to-left shunts has come into general use in the evaluation of infants with respiratory distress, a few words about the derivation of the equations follow.

The amount of oxygen in the arterial blood must equal the amount that comes from the pulmonary capillaries which perfused ventilated alveoli, plus the amount that comes through nonventilated alveoli or anatomic shunts such as the ductus arteriosus or foramen ovale. This can be written $Q_T C_a O_2 = Q_{c'} C_{c'} O_2 + Q_S C_{\bar{v}} O_2$ here

$$Q_T = \text{total blood flow}$$
$$C_a O_2 = \text{oxygen content of arterial blood}$$
$$Q_{c'} = \text{pulmonary capillary blood flow}$$
$$C_{c'} O_2 = \text{oxygen content of the pulmonary capillaries}$$
$$Q_S = \text{shunted blood flow}$$
$$C_{\bar{v}} O_2 = \text{mixed venous oxygen content.}$$

Since $Q_{c'} = Q_T - Q_S$ the expression can be written
$$Q_T C_a O_2 = (Q_T - Q_S) C_{c'} O_2 + Q_S C_{\bar{v}} O_2 \text{ or}$$

$$\frac{Q_S}{Q_T} = \frac{C_a O_2 - C_{c'} O_2}{C_{\bar{v}} O_2 - C_{c'} O_2}$$

The only value which is usually measured is $C_a O_2$ or the oxygen content of arterial blood. If the partial pressure of oxygen is measured, the content can be determined from the oxyhemoglobin dissociation curve at known pH (Fig. 6–2).

The values of $C_{C'O_2}$ or oxygen concentration in pulmonary capillary blood from ventilated alveoli is the oxygen capacity plus 1.8 volumes of oxygen, the amount dissolved in blood at 600 mm. Hg oxygen tension. (Each 100 ml. of blood contains 20 ml. of oxygen combined with hemoglobin plus the 1.8 ml. dissolved in the blood or 21.8 ml. of oxygen.) The concentration of oxygen in mixed venous blood is usually assumed on the basis of an arterial-venous oxygen difference of 4 ml. oxygen per 100 ml. of blood. Measured differences have varied from 15 per cent in well babies to 10 per cent in sick infants (Rudolph et al., 1961), or 2 to 6 ml. oxygen per 100 ml. in other studies (Strang and McLeish, 1961).

Since the calculation of the shunt requires several assumptions, and the use of a nomogram, it seems practical to omit the calculation and report the oxygen tensions achieved under specified conditions. In small infants who are not seriously distressed, it seems unwise to give 100 per cent oxygen to make this calculation. Serial measurements of oxygen tensions at known inspired concentrations, such as 40, 50, or 60 per cent, are just as useful in following a given infant (Fig. 6–3).

Measurements of the right-to-left shunt in normal newborn babies show that about 15 to 20 per cent of the cardiac output is shunted; in infants with hyaline membrane disease up to 80 per cent may be shunted right-to-left, compared to less than 7 per cent in healthy adults (Prod'hom et al., 1962; Strang and MacLeish, 1961; Nelson et al., 1963).

OXYGEN TRANSPORT

The delivery of oxygen to the tissues depends on the amount of oxygen in the blood, the cardiac output, and the distribution of the circulation. The high affinity of human fetal blood for oxygen was first noted by Anselmino and Hoffman in 1930. This interesting property was thought to be an adaptation to intrauterine life appropriate to the fetus acquiring oxygen across the placenta. Subsequently it has become apparent that fetal hemoglobin is not essential to normal intrauterine life, since infants given intrauterine transfusions are capable of normal growth. More recently some have questioned whether the high affinity of fetal hemoglobin for oxygen might impair oxygen delivery to the tissues in postnatal life.

New insight into the reasons for differences in the amount of oxygen held by a given amount of hemoglobin at any given PO_2 came in 1967 when Benesch and Benesch demonstrated that the affinity of a solution of adult hemoglobin for oxygen was dependent on the concentration of organic phosphates, 2,3-diphosphoglycerate (DPG) and

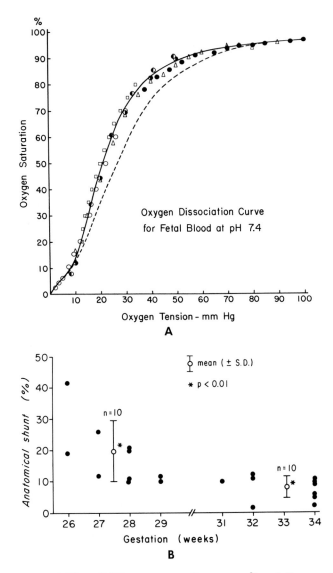

Figure 6–2. A, The solid line represents the oxygen dissociation curve predicted from the formula by Gomez (Gomez, D. M.: Amer. J. Physiol. *200*:135, 1961). The broken line is the curve observed in adult blood by Dill (Dill, D. B.: *Handbook of Respiration.* W. B. Saunders Co., Phila., 1958, p. 73). The points along the solid line are in vitro data from many authors, tabulated by Nelson and co-workers. (From Nelson et al.: J. Clin. Invest. *43*:606, 1964.)

B, Individual and group means (± S.D.) of anatomical shunt in relation to gestational age. The infants were free of cardiorespiratory distress and were studied between 12 and 84 hours of age. (Data of Parks et al.)

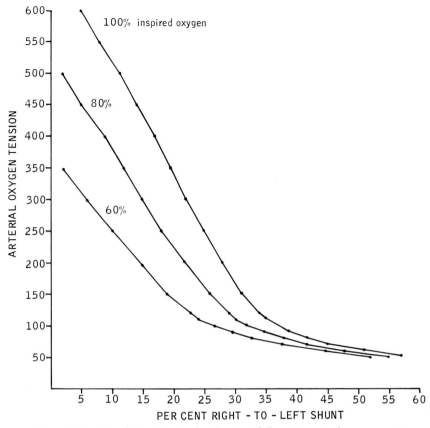

Figure 6–3. Graph to estimate the shunt at different inspired oxygen mixtures. The calculations were based on an assumed hemoglobin of 16 gm./100 ml., an arteriovenous difference of 4 volumes per cent, a respiratory quotient of 0.8, and an arterial P_{CO_2} of 40 mm. Hg. Constructed with the aid of a Severinghaus nomogram. (Courtesy of Dr. Scott Faulkner.)

adenosine triphosphate (ATP). However, fetal hemoglobin does not show as great an interaction with 2,3-DPG and ATP. In infants, the oxygen affinity of hemoglobin is dependent on the interaction of the amount of adult hemoglobin present in the cell and 2,3-DPG. The oxygen affinity of fetal blood decreases during gestation and depends on the relative proportions of adult and fetal hemoglobin as well as on the level of DPG (Orzalesi and Hay, 1971).

The significance of the differences in oxygen affinity of infants' and adults' blood for hemoglobin was shown by Delivoria-Papadopoulos et al. (1971) (Figs. 6–4 and 6–5). They noted in normal infants a shift to the right in the oxyhemoglobin dissociation curve from the first day of life through the first months, as fetal hemoglobin became proportionately less. They also demonstrated the effect on oxygen delivery of exchange transfusion with adult blood. For a given arterial-

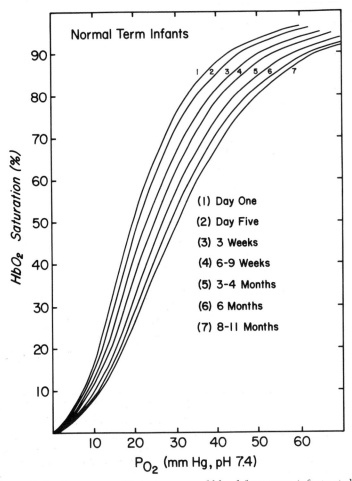

Figure 6–4. Oxygen equilibrium curves of blood from term infants at different postnatal ages; each curve represents the mean value of the infants studied in each age group. (Courtesy of Delivoria et al:: Pediat. Res. 5:235, 1971.)

venous difference (in the range of 40 to 80 mm. Hg) two to three times as much oxygen was given up by adult hemoglobin as by fetal hemoglobin. They suggest that in some distressed infants, blood replacement could improve oxygen delivery to the tissues.

DEAD SPACE AND ALVEOLAR VENTILATION

Each breath is distributed to a portion of the lung in which little or no gas exchange occurs—the airways—and to a portion in which oxygen is absorbed and carbon dioxide is released by the blood which perfuses it—the alveoli. The air that does not undergo gas exchange

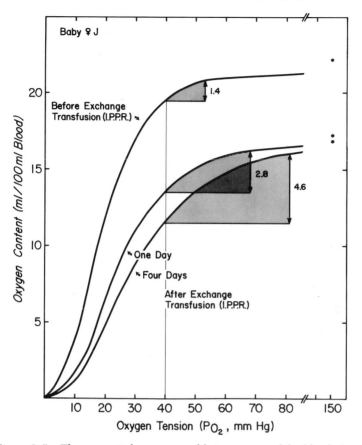

Figure 6–5. The sequential oxygen equilibrium curves of the blood of an infant with severe respiratory distress syndrome treated with exchange transfusion and intermittent positive-pressure respiration. The double arrows represent the oxygen unloading capacity between a given "arterial" and "venous" P_{O_2}. The points corresponding to 150 mm. Hg on the abscissa are the O_2 capacities. In this infant the oxygen delivery increased from 1.4 to 4.6 ml. during the course of one week. (Courtesy of Delivoria et al.: Pediat. Res. 5:235, 1971.)

with the blood is considered as dead space ventilation, and that which participates in gas exchange is alveolar ventilation. The magnitude of the respective portions of each breath depends on the method by which it is measured. For example, the dead space can be calculated from measurements of the fraction of carbon dioxide in the expired air, the fraction in the alveolar air or end-tidal sample, and the amount of air expired per minute. The Bohr equation which relates these values is

$$\dot{V}_D = \frac{(F_A CO_2 - F_E CO_2)}{F_A CO_2} \dot{V}_E$$ where V_D = dead space ventilation per min-

ute, $F_A CO_2$ = the alveolar carbon dioxide concentration, $F_E CO_2$ = the concentration of carbon dioxide in the expired sample, and $\dot{V}_E$ = the total ventilation per minute. The alveolar ventilation V_A is related to V_E and V_D as follows: $V_E = V_A + V_D$ which says simply that the whole is equal to the sum of the parts. The size of the dead space calculated from an end-tidal sample may differ from that calculated from the carbon dioxide tension in the arterial blood. If the discrepancy is large, it suggests that portions of the lung are like dead space in that they may be ventilated but poorly perfused. A third method of measurement is to monitor the nitrogen concentration in the air which is expired after a single breath of oxygen. The expired nitrogen will be zero, until a volume equal to the dead space has been exhaled. A variation of this method is to follow the concentrations of nitrogen in expired air after air-wash-in following oxygen breathing.

All three of these methods have been used to measure the dead space and alveolar ventilation in newborn infants. The first method, which involves measuring the end-tidal carbon dioxide and expired volume and its carbon dioxide concentration, was used by Nelson et al. (1962), who also measured the arterial carbon dioxide tension and thus compared the findings by the two methods. In normal infants there were no significant differences in the arterial PCO_2 and the end-tidal PCO_2, so the dead space calculated by the two methods was similar. They found the average dead space to be 4.4 ml. for infants of average weight of 2.58 kg., which was 30 per cent of a single breath. These measurements agreed with those of Cook et al. (1955), who used arterialized capillary blood to measure the carbon dioxide tension and found the dead space to be 5.0 ml. in term infants. Strang (1961) measured the end-tidal carbon dioxide with a mass spectrometer and calculated the dead space to be 9.2 ml., or about one-half of a tidal volume. In a subsequent study, Strang and McGrath (1962) studied the nitrogen concentration of expired air after a period of oxygen breathing. They found the dead space to average 8.5 ml. in infants whose weights averaged 3.22 kg.

The alveolar ventilation per unit of lung volume of infants is about twice that of adults, or 378 ml./min. when the tidal volume is 18 ml. (Strang, 1961). This is not surprising, since the oxygen consumption of the infants is nearly twice that of the adult, when expressed per kilogram body weight (Cross et al., 1966) (Table 6–3).

One of the problems in collecting expired air from infants is to construct a suitable low-resistance valve. Figure 6–6 shows such a valve with negligible resistance and with a dead space of less than 0.8 ml.

LUNG VOLUMES

The total volume of air in the lungs can be measured, and subdivisions of it are designated as lung volumes. The maximum amount of

Table 6–3. Representative Values in Normal Infants at Term[*]

	Umbilical vein	30 min.	1–4 hrs.	12–24 hrs.	24–48 hrs.	96 hrs.	Reference
				Arterial Blood			
pH	7.33		7.30	7.30	7.39	7.39	Reardon et al. (1960)
P_{CO_2} mm. Hg	43		39	33	34	36	Oliver et al. (1961)
HCO_3 mEq./liter	21.6		18.8	19.5	20	21.4	Nelson et al. (1962,
P_{O_2} mm. Hg	28 ± 8		62 ± 13.8	68	63–87		1963)
O_2 saturation			95%	94%	94%	96%	
Crying vital capacity ml. (for 3 kg. infant)		77 range (56–110)			92 (69–128)	100	Sutherland and Ratcliff (1961)
Functional residual capacity, ml./kg.		22 ± 8	25 ± 8	21 ± 1	28 ± 7	39 ± 9	Klaus et al. (1962)
Lung compliance ml./cm. H_2O/kg.		1.5 ± 0.05		2.0 ± 0.4		1.7	Cook et al. (1957)
Lung compliance/FRC ml./cm. H_2O/ml.			0.04 ± 0.10	.053 ± 0.009		0.065	Chu et al. (1964) Cook et al. (1957)
Right to left shunt as percentage cardiac output			22% (range 11–29%)	24% (17–32%)			Prod'hom et al. (1964)

		Comment	Reference
Respiratory frequency	34/min. range 20–60	1–2 days 1–11 days	Cook et al. (1955) Cross (1949)
Resistances cm. H_2O/liter/second	29, 26 18 ± 6/3	Total lung resistance Airway resistance	Cook et al. (1949), Swyer et al. (1960), Polgar (1962)
Flow rates ml./second	48–37 161–106	Max. insp., max. exp. rest crying	Swyer et al. (1957), Long and Hull (1961)
Ventilation ml./kg./min.	200		Cook et al. (1955), Nelson et al. (1962)
Dead space ml.	4.4–9.2	Term infants	Nelson et al. (1962), Cook et al. (1955), Strang (1961)
Alveolar ventilation ml./kg./min.	120–145	First 3 days of life	Nelson et al. (1962)
O_2 consumption ml./kg./min.	6.2	At neutral temperature	Oliver and Karlberg (1963)
CO_2 production ml./kg./min.	5.1	At neutral temperature	Oliver and Karlberg (1963)
Alveolar-arterial O_2 differences mm. Hg	28 ± 10, room air 311 ± 70, 100% O_2	Age 7 hrs. to 42 days Age 6 to 58 hrs. 3 infants	Nelson et al. (1963)
Arterial-alveolar CO_2 differences mm. Hg	1.8 ± 3.8	Age 3 to 74 hours	Nelson et al. (1962)

[*] From Avery, M. E., and Normand, C.: Anesthesiology *26*:510, 1965.

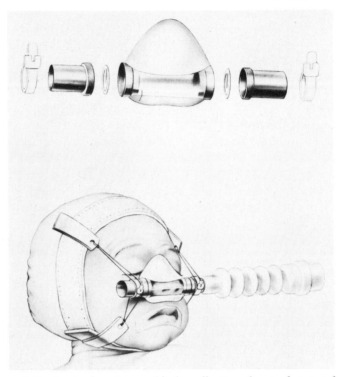

Figure 6–6. A valved mask assembly for collection of expired air in infants. The upper portion shows the acrylic shell and silastic flap valves, threaded couplings, and nylon straps. The assembly is shown in position below. It can be purchased from J. Ben Buck, 616 Fifth Street, Ames, Iowa. (From Silverman et al.: J. Pediat. 68:468, 1966.)

air that can be contained in a lung without rupture is the total lung capacity. The amount that remains after a forced expiration is the residual volume, and the difference between the two is the vital capacity. Normal breathing takes place with the lung at about 40 per cent of peak volume. Each breath is a tidal volume, and the amount of air present at the end of a quiet expiration is the functional residual capacity. Figure 6–7 shows the volume subdivisions of the lung of a normal 3.0-kg. infant on the left, with those found in infants with respiratory distress on the right. The spirogram beside each bar diagram indicates the types of tracing from which some of the lung volumes are measured.

Body Plethysmograph

An infant can be placed in a box with his head or face outside. Since it is difficult to make an airtight seal around the neck, it has been found preferable to expose the face (Fig. 6–8). A lightweight and well-balanced spirometer may be attached to the box to record volume changes; alternately, pressure changes in the box may be measured with suitable sensitive pressure transducers. If the box is calibrated

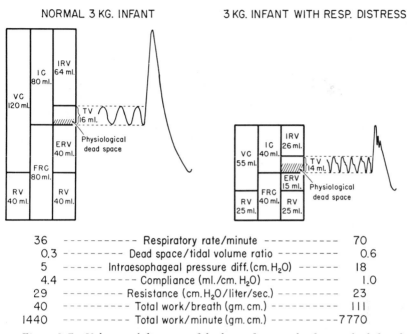

Figure 6–7. Volume subdivisions of the lung of a normal infant on the left and of one with hyaline membrane disease on the right. (Cook, C. D.: Respiration and Metabolism of Newborn Infants. Exhibited at VIII International Congress of Pediatrics, Copenhagen, 1956.)

with a syringe delivering known volumes, the respiratory volumes may be calculated from the pressure changes. The accuracy of the techniques that record volume spirographically is ±5 per cent (Drorbaugh and Fenn, 1955). The method of pressure measurements is probably more accurate since there is minimal inertia in the recording apparatus, although this has not been precisely determined. It is important to calibrate at respiratory frequencies to correct for the adiabatic effect, since there will be a temperature change with expansion and compression of the gas.

A whole body plethysmograph suitable for infants between 680 and 3400 gm. was described by Polgar and Lacourt (1972). Lung volumes and airway resistance can be measured with such instrumentation. Modifications of total body plethysmography for measurement of lung volume and airway resistance in infants of one month to five years of age were reported by Doershuk et al. (1970). Their subjects were supine and lightly sedated.

Reverse Plethysmography

After a few breaths the volume of a cry can be measured very simply by reverse plethysmography. In this procedure, a mask is

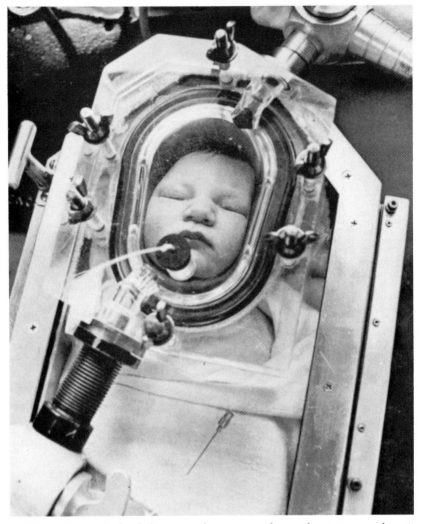

Figure 6–8. A body plethysmograph to measure lung volumes in a newborn infant. (Courtesy of W. Tooley; from Comroe, J. H.: Am. Rev. Resp. Dis. 85:179, 1962.)

applied over the nose and mouth of the infant, and attached by wide-bore tubing to a large box or bottle of 50 to 60 liters capacity. The pressure changes in the container can be measured with a pressure transducer, which can convert the small changes in pressure to an electrical signal, suitably amplified and recorded. The changes in pressure with introduction of known volumes into the container are measured to calibrate the plethysmograph (Karlberg et al., 1960). Since the volume of the container exceeds that of the cry of an infant about 500 to 600 times, the increase in pressure in the container is only one part in 500, or only 1.5 mm. Hg. The accuracy of this method is within ±5 per cent. If a few tidal volumes are all that are needed, a

20-liter container suffices. A noticeable effect from the buildup of carbon dioxide during rebreathing limits this method to recording for less than one to two minutes (Avery and O'Doherty, 1962).

Volumes by Barometric Methods

Drorbaugh and Fenn (1955) described a method for measurement of lung volumes in small animals and infants which has the advantage of having the subject completely enclosed in a box. Pressure changes in the box will result from the exchange of heat from air warmed in the lungs of the infant as the expired air enters the box. The authors noted that the limitations to this method were (1) the inability to get an accurate reading when the infant moved, (2) the time required for vapor pressure and temperature equilibrium, and (3) the necessity to open the chamber at intervals to prevent fall in oxygen. The method has not been widely used, since other methods are equally satisfactory. The one potential advantage of having the infant unrestrained is offset by the inability to get reliable measurements when he moves.

Volumes from Air Flow

Since flow is volume per unit time, volume itself is the integral of flow. It is possible to measure volume by measuring the area under a flow curve or by electrical integration of flow.

Air flow can be measured with a pneumotachygraph. This instrument consists of a fine-mesh screen that provides a known resistance to the flow of air through it. A screen of 400 mesh/sq. in. is suitable for infants; flows of 10 ml./sec. will create a pressure difference across it of about 0.1 mm. H_2O. Since the pressure difference is directly proportional to flow at a constant resistance, flows can be readily calculated (Swyer et al., 1960). A modified pneumotachygraph, suitable for measurements of spontaneous breathing as well as assisted ventilation, was described by Gregory and Kitterman (1971). They adapted plastic endotracheal tube connectors (internal diameter, 11 mm.) with a 400 mesh stainless steel wire screen as the resistor. The instrument is lightweight, has a volume of only 2 to 3.4 ml., and a low resistance.

"Crying Vital Capacity"

One of the most useful measurements of pulmonary function in adults is the vital capacity, which assesses the degree to which the lung can be stretched by a voluntary effort. The "crying vital capacity" may be thought of as a measure of the degree to which the lung of an infant can be stretched by an involuntary effort or an induced cry. In serial studies on normal newborn infants, Sutherland and Ratcliff

(1961) found the volume of a cry at about seven minutes of age to be from 56 to 110 per cent of that measured on the third day of age. The absolute volume was a function of body weight; about 50 ml. in a 1.5-kg. infant, nearly 100 ml. at 2.5 kg., and approximately 150 ml. at 4.5 kg.

Functional Residual Capacity

The volume of gas in the lungs at end expiration serves as a buffer of inspired gases so that large changes in gas tensions in alveoli are reduced. It further serves to keep the airways open, so that air may flow freely and not have to duplicate with each inspiration the forces that are required to open an airless lung.

Three methods have been used to measure the functional residual capacity (FRC) in newborn infants. One is the closed-circuit helium method (Berglund and Karlberg, 1956). A closed system is filled with 21 per cent oxygen, 19 to 20 per cent helium, and the remainder nitrogen. The baby breathes into this system until the concentrations of helium in the spirometer and his lungs are the same; this usually requires five to seven minutes. At the end of this period, the volume and concentration of helium in the spirometer can be measured, and the volume of the lung calculated. Suitable corrections for the dead space of the apparatus and gas volumes at body temperature and pressure saturated (BTPS) are required.

The second method uses a plethysmographic technique to measure the total thoracic gas volume. This method, first described by DuBois et al. (1956), depends on the change in volume that takes place when an infant makes a forced expiration against an obstruction. A single determination requires only a few seconds and thus can be used to follow changes in FRC over a period of time. Klaus et al. (1962) found the FRC to be nearly the same in the first minute after birth as it was by three days of age, with an average of 25 ml./kg. body weight. In infants under 1750 gm., Krauss and Auld (1971) found the volumes by plethysmography in excess of those by nitrogen washout in the first week of life. The third method involves estimation of the FRC from the slope of the nitrogen wash-in curve after oxygen breathing. Strang and McGrath (1962) described the details of this procedure and analyzed the errors inherent in it. Their value for FRC in infants whose weight averaged 3.22 kg. was 49.5 ml., which is lower than the values obtained by other methods. Similar values, with the same method were reported by Hanson and Shinozaki (1970). Strang and McGrath found, in accord with other studies, that the FRC was about the same at six or seven hours of age as it was over the ensuing five days in normal infants. Hanson and Shinozaki noted some normal infants in whom a progressive increase in FRC occurred after the initial 12 hours of life.

FLOW RATES

Just as some investigators have sought to measure volumes by integration of flow, others have studied air flow by electrical differentiation of volume (Long and Hull, 1961). The advantages of electrical differentiation of the signals recorded by reverse plethysmography are the lack of inertia in the system and the lack of resistance at high flows. The average maximum inspiratory flow in a crying term infant during the first three days of life is 161 ml./sec., and the maximum expiratory flow is 106 ml./sec.

The pneumotachygraph described on page 75 can be used to study air flow during quiet breathing. Swyer's findings (1960) on term infants show an average inspiratory flow of 48 ml./sec. and an expiratory flow of 37 ml./sec. These measurements of flow during quiet breathing are important if one wishes to sample expired air for measurements of end-tidal gases. The sampling device should not be set at flow rates higher than 35 ml./sec., or some room air will mix with expired air.

COMPLIANCE

The compliance of the lung, or change in volume per unit change in pressure at points of no air flow, is a measure of the distensibility of the lung. Since the volume measured is the air moved out of the mouth, any reduction in lung volume — such as after aspiration of particulate matter — will reduce the measured lung compliance without any necessary change in the properties of the lung that is ventilated. Thus large reductions in lung compliance are found in hyaline membrane disease, for example, since so much of the lung is atelectatic and so little of it is ventilated. This determination has been used by many investigators to study the changes in the lung after birth and to follow the course of hyaline membrane disease. Lung compliance is not an easy determination to make and it is even more difficult to interpret, so there is some doubt that it will ever achieve wide usage.

The calculation of lung compliance requires a measure of tidal volume and of the changes in pleural pressure associated with it. Since it is not practical nor safe to put a needle in the pleural space, pressure changes are measured in the esophagus, which is so compliant that changes in pressure in it are adequate indices of pleural pressure (Fig. 6–9) (Dinwiddie and Russell, 1972). Either a saline-filled catheter (Cook et al., 1957) or a thin-walled balloon (Swyer et al., 1960) in the esophagus can be attached to a pressure transducer to record changes in pressure. The saline-filled catheter has the two

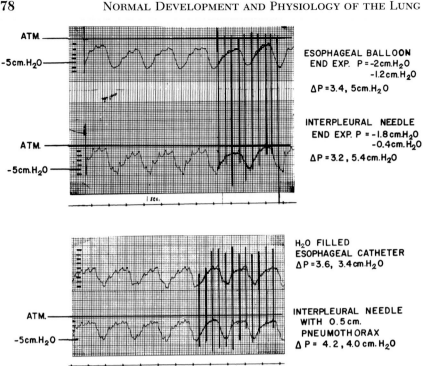

Figure 6–9. Comparison of pressure changes measured simultaneously with a needle in the pleural space and a catheter or balloon in the esophagus in an anencephalic newborn infant. (Data of R. F. Hustead and M. E. Avery.)

limitations that the orifice may become plugged with mucus and that only changes in pressure can be accurately determined. Absolute pressures could be measured if it were possible to determine a zero reference pressure. The balloon must be very thin and have suitable pressure-volume characteristics of its own, so that pressures in the regions measured will not reflect tension in the wall of the balloon. For example, if a portion of the balloon is in the stomach, gas may be under tension in the portion still in the esophagus and false readings obtained. Despite these limitations, useful measurements have been made with esophageal catheters and balloons. The average compliance of the lung of the normal newborn infant in whom breathing is established is 4 to 6 ml./cm. H_2O. Since the average tidal volume is 16 to 20 ml., it is obvious that the infant applies about the same pressures to achieve a tidal volume as an adult. In the range of quiet breathing, the distensibility of the lung of the infant is also about the same as that of the adult, when sized per unit body weight. Thus a 70-kg. adult has a tidal volume of 500 ml. and a compliance of 125 ml./cm. H_2O. A 3-kg. infant is $1/23$ the weight of the adult, and the compliance of his lung is reduced by the same amount.

The compliance of lungs and thorax together in apneic, paralyzed infants five to 76 days of age was 4.9 ml./cm. H_2O on the average during quiet breathing, and 5.2 ml./cm. H_2O after forced inflations.

The similarity of these values to those measured on lungs alone suggests that the compliance of the thorax of infants is very large (Richards and Bachman, 1961). Somewhat lower values for the dynamic compliance of lungs and thorax were found in anesthetized infants, with a mean of 2.8 ml./cm. H_2O (range 1.5 to 4.9). Static compliances were similar to dynamic compliances in this study, which differed from the previous one cited by the omission of prolonged inflations just before the measurements were made (Reynolds and Etsten, 1966).

If the lung compliance is studied over the full range of lung volumes, and the volumes are compared on the basis of lung weight, the lungs of infants do not compare favorably with those of adults. It is evident at least in goats that peak distensibility of the lung, at 30 cm. H_2O, is less in the young goat compared to the older ones, if the comparison is made on the basis of lung weights (Avery and Cook, 1961). In humans too, Stigol et al. (1972) found an increase in distensibility with age up to approximately eight years. In their study of 27 excised lungs, they noted little change in the overall shape of the static pressure-volume curve when lung volumes were expressed as a percentage of that obtained at 20 cm. H_2O distending pressure. These findings suggest that there is more parenchyma per unit of potential airspace in the young lung than in the old lung. Such a finding would be expected, since bronchi and vessels are not as small, relatively, as airspaces in the infant.

The compliance of the trachea and bronchi in infants of differing maturity was studied by Burnard et al. (1965). Infants of approximately 1 kg. weight had more compliant airways than those of 2 and 3 kg., in that they were relatively more distensible and less able to resist collapse (Fig. 6–10).

AIRWAY RESISTANCE

The resistance of the airways to the flow of air through them depends on their radii, length, and numbers. It can easily be deduced that airway resistance would be larger in smaller individuals. It can also be assumed that airways in infants could not be reduced in size proportionally to body mass, since bronchioles $1/20$ the diameter of those of adults would impose too great a resistance to airflow. While accurate measurements of airway dimensions at known distending pressures are not available for all ages, the studies of Engel (1947) suggest that bronchiolar diameter doubles from infancy to adulthood, while tracheal diameter increases about threefold (Fig. 6–11). Even the modest proportional reductions in size are significant in increasing airway resistance, since resistance is an inverse function of the fourth or fifth power of the diameter of the airway, depending on whether flow is laminar or turbulent.

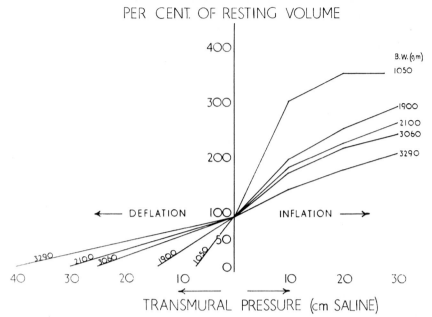

Figure 6–10. Pressure volume relations of tracheobronchial segments from infants of differing birth weights. Note the much greater distensibility and lower resistance to collapse of airways in the smaller infants. (From Burnard et al.: Austr. Paed. J. *1*:12, 1965.)

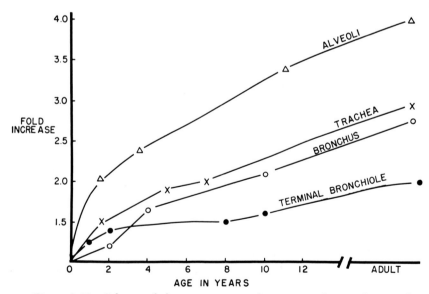

Figure 6–11. Schema of changes in airway diameters with age. These studies were not done at constant distending pressures and hence can be only estimates of changes in size. The data of Dunnill (1962) show only a doubling of alveolar diameter from infancy to adulthood. (From *Handbook of Respiration*, W. B. Saunders Co., Phila., 1958. Data of Scammon and Engel.)

Measurements of airway resistance in newborn infants have been done by several means. In one method, resistance is measured as the ratio of the total pressure change to the corresponding total flow change between points of each volume. This method measures total resistance, which includes airway and tissue resistance. Pleural pressures and volume changes in the lung are recorded during quiet breathing. It is possible to measure flow from the slope of the volume tracing, since flow is volume per unit time (Fig. 6–12). The average flow resistance calculated by this method in normal newborn infants in the first days of life is 29 cm. $H_2O/L./sec.$ (Cook et al., 1957). Measurements from infants up to two years of age show considerable variation, but their average was also 20 cm. $H_2O/L./sec.$ with a standard deviation of ±20 (Krieger, 1963). The contribution of the upper airway to total resistance is substantial, of the order of 12 cm. $H_2O/L./sec.$, or nearly one-half (Polgar and Kong, 1965).

Another method of measurement of airway resistance is a plethysmographic method in which changes in airflow are plotted electronically against the simultaneous changes in pressure in the body plethysmograph. With this method airway resistance can be measured as a function of lung volume. In infants, as in adults, airway resistance is reduced at large lung volumes. The average value for airway resistance in normal newborn infants with this method is 18 cm. $H_2O/L./sec.$ (Polgar, 1961). In a series of infants in which both total pulmonary resistance and total airway resistance were measured, it was possible

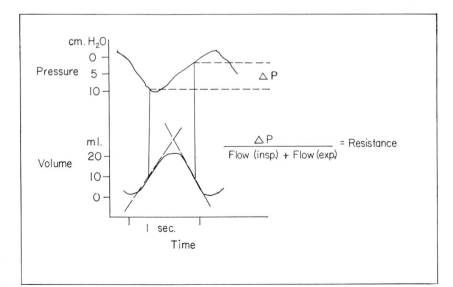

Figure 6–12. Airflow can be calculated from the slope of the volume tracing versus time. Airway resistance can be calculated if the change in pressure and flow is known as illustrated on the right. (Modified from Cook et al.: J. Clin. Invest. 36:440, 1957.)

to calculate the difference, or viscous resistance, of the lung tissues. Viscous resistance averaged 8.7 cm. $H_2O/L./sec.$, or about twice that found in adults (Polgar and String, 1966). In a group of infants between one month and 24 months of age, Doershuk et al. (1970) found a mean airway resistance of 17.7 cm. $H_2O/liter/sec.$ (range = 8.7 to 30). Their infants were supine, sedated, and nose breathing.

DIFFUSION

The exchange of gases between pulmonary capillary blood and alveoli is by diffusion. The physical principle that governs diffusion of gases across a membrane, stated by Fick, is that the quantity of a substance which crosses a membrane will depend on the properties of the membrane and the substance which crosses it, the surface area of the membrane, its thickness, and the partial pressures of gases on either side of it. Since neither the surface area nor thickness of the alveolar membrane is known precisely, the diffusion capacity of the lung cannot be expressed per unit surface area, but rather is expressed in the units of ml. of gas/mm. Hg pressure/min. The measurement of diffusion capacity is further complicated by the difficulty of assigning a mean pressure to alveolar gases or pulmonary capillary gases, since they change as blood flows past the alveolus.

Only two gases have been used to measure diffusion capacity, and they are the two that have an affinity for hemoglobin so that pressure gradients will be measurable, namely, oxygen and carbon monoxide. Stahlman (1957) chose a steady-state method with 0.1 to 0.2 per cent carbon monoxide in her studies on newborn infants. She measured carbon monoxide uptake and alveolar carbon monoxide tensions. Since hemoglobin combines so quickly with carbon monoxide, she assumed the partial pressure of the gas in the blood to be negligible. In a series of 31 normal newborn infants from nine to 96 hours of age, she found the diffusion capacity to be between 0.87 to 3.10 ml./mm. Hg/min. Stahlman's studies (1960) on infants with respiratory distress thought to have hyaline membrane disease showed a reduction in diffusing capacity in four, and normal results in two who were less severely affected.

UNIFORMITY OF VENTILATION

The uniformity of ventilation can be assessed by pulmonary nitrogen washout after the inhalation of oxygen. During these measurements, FRC can also be calculated, since the rate of decline in expired nitrogen concentration depends on the volume of the space being washed out.

Hanson and Shinozaki (1970) found that the majority of normal infants will wash out the nitrogen from their lungs after 20 to 35 breaths, or in one to one and one-half minutes. Improvement in the uniformity of ventilation occurred through the first six days. The authors conclude that the normal infant may have some poorly ventilated or perhaps atelectatic areas for variable periods after birth, a conclusion consistent with measurements of "trapped gas" for some days (Nelson et al., 1963).

VENTILATION-PERFUSION RELATIONSHIPS

The efficiency of gas exchange depends on the nearly perfect matching of blood flow and alveolar ventilation within the millions of terminal airspaces. Intrinsic regulatory mechanisms are directed toward preservation of the ideal ventilation-perfusion ($\dot{V}_A/\dot{Q}$) ratio of 0.8. In regions of high ventilation, the low carbon dioxide tensions lead to local airway constriction and tend to reduce ventilation to that area. In regions of low ventilation, the lowered alveolar oxygen tensions cause local vasoconstriction which shunts blood to the better ventilated areas. In pulmonary disease, it is not surprising that the compensatory regulation mechanisms may be overcome; and derangements in ventilation-perfusion relationships are common.

The method of choice in quantifying $\dot{V}_A/\dot{Q}$ disturbances is to measure the alveolar-arterial nitrogen tension gradient. Regions of the lung that are relatively poorly ventilated, but still perfused, will have an elevated alveolar nitrogen tension, since more oxygen will be absorbed than carbon dioxide excreted. On expiration the small amount of ventilation from those regions will mix with larger amounts from normally ventilated regions and will not raise the end-tidal nitrogen tension significantly. However, the nitrogen tension in the blood will increase. Since nitrogen is inert, and neither consumed nor produced by the tissues, the nitrogen tension in all body liquids will be the same. Thus it can be measured by gas chromatography in a specimen of urine collected under anaerobic conditions. Measurements in newborn infants on the first day of life showed a mean gradient of 25 mm. Hg, which fell over the course of the next few days to values of less than 10 mm. Hg, which is in the normal range for older children. The conclusion from those studies was that it may take the newborn infant several days to match ventilation and perfusion appropriately (Ledbetter et al., 1967). Subsequently, Nourse and Nelson (1969) measured the arterial-alveolar nitrogen difference, and found in a group of normal infants of diabetic mothers that the difference was about 40 mm. Hg within the first hour of life but usually was less than 10 mm. Hg by four hours of age. Krauss et al. (1971) studied the urinary-alveolar nitrogen gradient in 20 normal term infants and reported it to be less than 10 mm. Hg within the first day of life. In infants with meconium aspiration, it was significantly elevated (as high as 40 mm. Hg for the first few days of life).

Chapter Seven

ROENTGEN
EVALUATION OF
THE CHEST

Radiologic examination is an integral part of the diagnosis and management of newborn infants with respiratory distress. In most instances, only plain films are required, and complex special procedures are unnecessary. However, all too frequently improper exposure of the radiographs renders the resultant information useless or misleading. The key to proper radiography of the neonate lies in careful attention to technical details, proper equipment, and most importantly the interest and competence of the radiologic technologist and cooperation of the nursery personnel.

TECHNICAL FACTORS

X-rays are generated in an evacuated tube which contains a filament (cathode) and a metal (usually tungsten) target, or anode. Electrons are produced by applying a current of electricity to the filament. By applying a potential difference (kilovoltage) between the cathode and anode, electrons are accelerated across the tube to the anode. The x-rays are then emitted when the electrons rapidly decelerate in the anode. The resultant exposure is dependent on the kilovoltage, the milliamperage applied to the cathode, and the duration of exposure.

Equipment

The best equipment for making roentgenograms of infants permits rapid exposures at high milliamperage (ma.) and moderate kilovoltage (kv.). Roentgenographic machines with 1000 ma. three-phase generators are ideal. Single-phase x-ray generators are adequate if exposures can be made consistently at 1/60 of a second or less.

Few mobile x-ray machines permit exposures at high milliamperages. Those which will make exposures at 200 to 250 ma. and at 1/120 of a second are readily available and permit excellent films to be made in the nursery where a distance of 6 feet is rarely possible and a distance of 40 inches is used. These machines require 220 volt mains, and when new hospitals are constructed and old ones renovated, it is important to install appropriate outlets. Condenser-discharge and battery-operated mobile x-ray units which are now coming into use do not require outlets.

Different radiographic machines vary considerably in power, and it is not possible to list exposure factors that are correct for all installations. Of greater importance is the avoidance of excessive exposure times in order to minimize the effects of motion. Ideally, exposure time should be no more than 1/120 of a second.

Radiography

In order to minimize geometric magnification and distortion of the image, the patient is placed as close as possible to the film, and the x-ray tube is removed as far as possible from the film. Since the intensity of the radiation varies inversely with the square of the distance between the tube and the film, there are practical limits to how far the x-ray tube can be placed from the film. The conventional distance when making chest roentgenograms of older patients is 6 feet. However, because of the infants' small size, image distortion is minimized and a shorter distance is acceptable. Actually it is difficult to see any difference between chest roentgenograms of the same infant made at 6 feet and at 3 feet (Davis, 1967). By halving the distance, the exposure time may be cut to one-fourth. Therefore, while it may be administratively simpler to make all chest roentgenograms in a radiology department at the same 6-foot distance, when equipment with adequate power is not available in the nursery, the distance must be decreased.

In order to keep the radiation dose as small as possible, the kilovoltage should be relatively high (Fendel, 1967). If it is too high, however, roentgenograms with insufficient contrast result. The range of kilovoltage that is practical will depend upon the film employed and other factors; in most departments exposures in the 60- to 85-kv. range are satisfactory.

Although the use of rapid exposures allows motion of the chest to be stopped during respiration, it is difficult to obtain films at known phases of the respiratory cycle, particularly when respiratory rates are abnormally rapid. The use of nasal thermistors, which utilize the warm exhaled air to initiate x-ray exposure at the beginning of expiration, has been advocated by some (O'Hara et al., 1965) but are cumbersome and have not been widely adopted. Evaluation of lung volume and heart size may be enhanced by the use of simultaneous anteroposterior vertical and lateral horizontal beam radiographs (Grossman et al., 1970). Scattered radiation from the two x-ray tubes is reduced by special lead filters or grids.

Positioning

Correct positioning and immobilization are even more important than adequate equipment. There are many commercial devices for holding infants for chest roentgenograms. While most of them permit good films to be obtained by a skilled technologist, their very multiplicity attests that none of them is completely satisfactory, and they have little use in radiography of newborn infants. Because of the severity of illness of many of the infants requiring chest radiographs, many films are exposed in the nursery. This is most efficiently carried out using portable x-ray equipment which allows radiographs to be taken without removing the infant from the incubator. After the film cassette is placed in the incubator and the patient positioned, the incubator is closed and exposure is made through the plastic top and sides.

Both frontal and lateral views should be obtained. These are made with the infant in the supine position, the frontal (AP) projection being made with a vertical beam (Fig. 7–1) and the lateral with a horizontal beam (Fig. 7–2A). Decubitus views, also made using a horizontal beam, are extremely helpful, particularly when pneumothorax (see also page 248) is suspected (Fig. 7–2B).

The infant must be straight, not bent to one side or slightly rotated. For the films obtained in the supine position, extending the infant's arms above the head facilitates correct positioning and exposure on inspiration. Methods of examination in the radiology department and immobilization devices are illustrated by Davis (1967).

Protecting the Infant

Good protection from excess radiation is mandatory. All examinations should be done with an x-ray tube having a well-constructed collimator that incorporates a variable rectangular diaphragm to limit the radiation beam and a light localizer to show exactly where the radiation will strike the patient. Since a small amount of radiation gets through even the best collimator, a thick piece of lead-rubber should be placed over the gonads during each exposure. In a carefully collimated examination of the chest, the amount of radiation to the

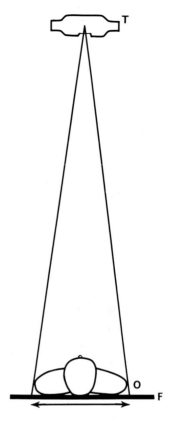

Figure 7-1. Geometric arrangement of x-ray tube, patient, and film for standard radiography using a vertical beam. This is the position for an AP supine projection. T = x-ray tube, O = object, F = film.

lungs is small, to the thyroid even less, and to the gonads almost negligible (Fendel, 1967).

It is important that the radiologic technologists adhere to all hospital rules for handling infants so that the infant is not exposed to infection or to unnecessary trauma. If the infant is brought to the radiology department, the antiseptic conditions of the nursery must be duplicated as closely as possible. While the infant is out of the nursery, every effort should be made to minimize his contacts with those who may carry infection. The infant should not be left unattended in the radiographic room. Hospitals with large nurseries find it advantageous to install a radiographic room in the nursery.

Fluoroscopy

Fluoroscopy is not used frequently in examination of newborn infants but can be useful in specific circumstances for the study of the nasal passages, trachea, esophagus, etc. The fact that the infant must be removed from his environment for fluoroscopic examination is of importance. Newman and Poznanski (1970) have solved the problem

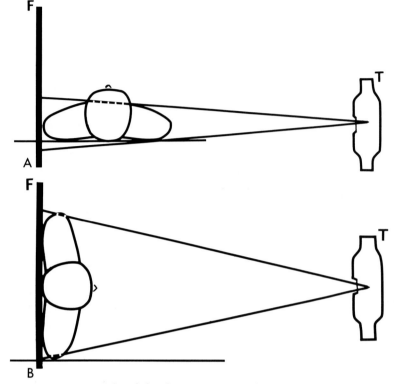

Figure 7–2.   Lateral and decubitus projections for use in the nursery. *A*, Horizontal beam. T = x-ray tube, F = film. *B*, Right lateral decubitus.

of hypothermia with a simple, home-made radiant heating device. Oxygen, when necessary can be supplied by mask.

Fluoroscopy should be done only with an image intensifier which provides a better image with less radiation to the patient than the now obsolete fluoroscopic screen. The image from the intensifier may be relayed to a television monitor for viewing by a group and simultaneously recorded on videotape without additional radiation to the patient. Cine film provides better detail than video tape recording, but since the photographic film must be exposed from the output phosphor of the image intensifier at high levels of light intensity, there is a considerable increase in the amount of radiation which the patient receives. Kinescopic motion pictures recorded directly from the television image provide somewhat less detail than cine film, but at lower radiation levels. Most fluoroscopic equipment also has the capability for individual "spot" films or 70 or 90 mm. rapid filming.

Details of special fluoroscopic procedures will be discussed with the appropriate subject.

Magnification Radiography

Direct radiographic magnification is accomplished by increasing the distance between the patient and the film (object-film distance) (Greenspan et al., 1967). The object becomes magnified because of divergence of the x-ray beam (Fig. 7–3). In Ablow's (1969) series of patients, magnification of approximately 2.5 resulted in the best resolution of pulmonary densities in newborn infants. Magnification with maximum resolution and minimum distortion due to penumbra is accomplished by reducing the site of emission of x-rays on the anode to approach a point source as closely as possible by the use of x-ray tubes with small focal spots in the order of 0.2 to 0.3 mm. diameter as compared with standard focal spot sizes of 1 to 2 mm.

Magnification radiography cannot be carried out unless the patient can be removed from the incubator and may therefore be impractical in more severely ill infants. This problem is partially solved by installation of the radiographic equipment in the intensive care nursery (Ablow and Markarian, 1972) or modification of portable x-ray machines. Since this technique results in increased levels of absorbed radiation, it is not recommended for routine use. The advantages and disadvantages of magnification radiography have been reviewed by Bookstein (1971).

Figure 7–3. Magnification radiography. Placing the patient closer to the x-ray source and remote from the film results in magnification because of divergence of the x-ray beam.

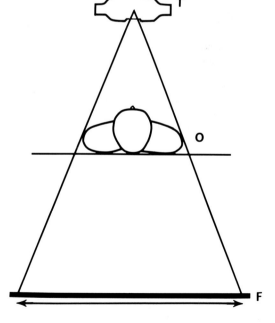

Contrast Media

Opacification of the esophagus is of value in the elucidation of mediastinal masses, vascular anomalies, and causes of aspiration pneumonia such as swallowing disorders and tracheoesophageal fistulas. Under any of these circumstances, the contrast medium used may enter the lung. Dunbar et al. (1959) examined the effects of barium sulfate, aqueous dionosil (propyliodone), and lipiodol on the lungs of rats. All produced an early cellular reaction. The most marked late changes were caused by lipiodol and the least reaction was caused by dionosil. Lipiodol is quite easily aspirated (Neuhauser and Wittenborg, 1953), and particularly when the infant is in the supine position, it tends to enter the right upper lobe (Castilla et al., 1971). Thirteen of 100 infants examined by DeCarlo et al. (1952) aspirated iodized oil, but none of these same infants aspirated barium. The chief disadvantage of barium is that it may cause airway obstruction and that it tends to be retained in the lung longer than other contrast media (Reich, 1969).

The frequently requested "gastrografin swallow" should be avoided under all circumstances, since it and similar diatrizoate water-soluble contrast media may lead to severe pulmonary edema if aspirated (Reich, 1969). Also, because of its high osmolarity (1900 mOsm./liter), gastrografin will cause a marked decrease in plasma volume when swallowed because of movement of fluid into the lumen of the bowel (Harris et al., 1964; Rowe et al., 1971). The perfect contrast medium for gastrointestinal studies in infants has not yet been discovered, but barium sulfate, when used under careful fluoroscopic control, is perhaps the least damaging to the lung and has some advantages over other media even when used for bronchography (Clement, 1969).

Bronchography is an infrequent examination in the neonatal period but may be useful in the investigation of tracheal and bronchial anomalies. Dionosil in either an aqueous or oily base is the most frequently used contrast medium for this purpose but probably is more damaging to the surfactant than barium. Powdered tantalum is a new agent which adheres firmly to the airway mucosa, and since it does not fill the lumen, will not interfere with pulmonary function (Nadel et al., 1970). It has been used successfully in infants under one year of age but is still in the experimental stage (Gamsu et al., 1973).

PITFALLS

Motion

In interpreting roentenograms of infants, there are many factors that may be confusing. The most common is slight respiratory motion.

In normal portions of the lungs, the vessels should register as exquisitely sharp markings on the roentgenograms. If the images of the vessels are not sharp, there was undue respiratory motion during the exposure. Slight motion may blur the images of the vessels sufficiently to suggest abnormal pulmonary densities when none are present. With more motion, the converse may occur: small densities will not be registered clearly on the film and may be overlooked. Thus, respiratory motion can lead to errors of both underdiagnosis and overdiagnosis. When there is sufficient respiratory motion during the exposure to blur the images of the diaphragm or the ribs, or when the infant physically moves during the exposure, the examination is clearly unacceptable.

Lordosis

If the infant is radiographed in a lordotic position—for example, with his back arched—the ribs appear to be unduly horizontal and the images of the anterior ends of the upper ribs may be superior to the images of their posterior ends. The cardiac apex appears to be elevated and unduly round, suggesting ventricular enlargement. The degree of lordosis is likely to vary on serial roentgenograms of the same infant, and the observer must be aware of these variations if he is not to misinterpret them as pathologic changes.

Rotation

Slight degrees of rotation of the infant are common. To judge rotation by the relationship of the medial ends of the clavicles to the spine is of little worth in evaluating infants, who may twist the lower part of the body in one direction and the upper part in the other. It is more satisfactory to judge rotation by comparing the distances from the costochondral junctions to the midline of the spine on each side at various levels of the chest. Rotation will cause a spurious shift of the mediastinal structures in the direction of rotation of the patient and will magnify the normal bronchovascular markings on the side of the chest closest to the x-ray beam (Fig. 7–4).

Degrees of Inspiration

Roentgenograms made during expiration suggest cardiomegaly and pneumonia (Fig. 7–5). It is traditional to evaluate the degree of inspiration at the moment of exposing the roentgenogram by relating the level of the diaphragmatic domes to the posterior portions of the ribs. Actually the domes are considerably nearer to the anterior than the posterior chest wall, and it is more reliable to relate the position of the diaphragm to the anterior ends of the ribs. Roentgenograms taken during good inspiration will show the diaphragmatic domes at

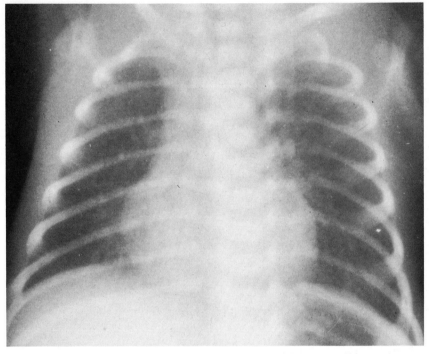

Figure 7-4. Effects of rotation. Rotation to the right posterior oblique position causes the apparent shift of the mediastinum to the right and partially obscures the right lung. Note the differences in position of the anterior rib ends on either side.

about the level of the anterior ends of the sixth ribs. The left dome is usually slightly lower than the right.

Costal and diaphragmatic respiration is frequently somewhat asynchronous in the infant, and two roentgenograms may show considerable variation in pulmonary ventilation and in apparent heart size with the diaphragmatic domes at the same height. A full evaluation of the degree of inspiration at the time of filming includes evaluation of the height and contour of the diaphragm, the slope of the ribs, whether the lungs appear to bulge into the intercostal spaces, the thickness of the thoracic soft tissues, and the separation of the pulmonary blood vessels.

Skin Folds

The skin of an infant is relatively loose and is likely to be pushed into folds as the infant is placed against the film cassette. Such skin folds are usually longitudinally oriented and may mimic pneumothorax. Careful observation will usually disclose that the folds can be followed beyond the rib cage, clearly differentiating them from pneumothorax (Fig. 7-6).

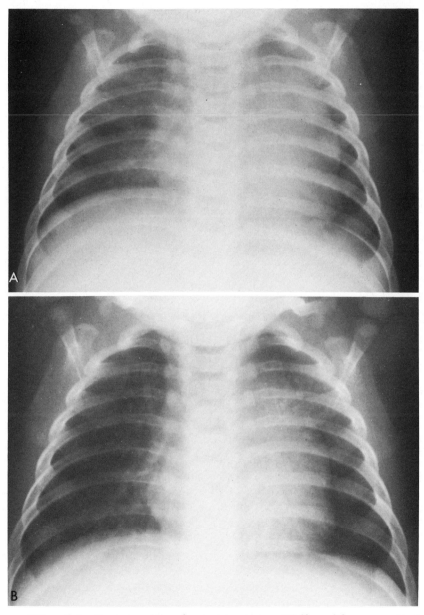

Figure 7–5. Expiratory (A) and repeat inspiratory (B) films of the same patient. It was impossible to exclude pathologic changes in the lungs in A. On inspiration, the lungs are shown to be clear and the heart is normal.

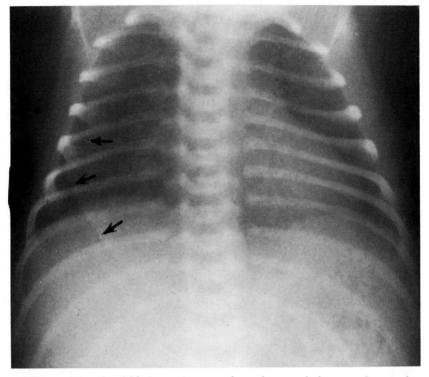

Figure 7-6. Skin folds (arrows) projected over lower right lung may be mistaken for a pneumothorax. Note lung markings lateral to folds. The folds extend below the limits of the lung bases.

THE NORMAL CHEST

Lungs

Interpretation of chest radiographs in the early postnatal period is dependent on knowledge of the changes which occur during transformation of the fetal to the newborn lung. The fetal lung contains liquid which occupies the potential airspaces and which is largely a secretory product of the lung (Strang, 1967). It has been suggested that part of the liquid is expelled by compression of the thoracic cage during its passage through the birth canal and that the subsequent passive expansion of the chest wall after delivery contributes to the early aeration of the lungs (Karlberg et al., 1962). The remainder of the liquid is displaced by active respiration and is resorbed by the pulmonary vascular and lymphatic systems (Humphreys et al., 1967). Radiologic evidence for liquid displacement rather than expansion of atelectatic lungs at birth was produced by Lind et al. (1966) who demonstrated that the thoracic cage and lungs maintained the same size and configuration after pulmonary aeration as in the fetal state and that there is no sudden increase in lung volume with aeration.

Radiologic studies have also demonstrated that pulmonary aeration is rapid and complete during the first few breaths of life (Fawcitt et al., 1960).

It is not surprising, however, that the fetal-neonatal transition is not always complete during the first few days of life and that retention of lung liquid may explain the transient pulmonary densities in clinically normal newborn infants described by Harris (1967) and the appearance of pulmonary vascular congestion on radiographs made in the delivery room (Berdon and Baker, 1966). Nadelhaft and Ellis (1957) have reported a 5 per cent incidence of pathologic appearing pulmonary densities in 1000 full-term newborn infants. In the series of Peterson and Pendleton (1955), 37 of 41 infants without respiratory distress showed clear lungs within five hours of life. Thirteen of the 41 infants were premature. The only pattern evident in the normal lungs was the bronchovascular tree. Interlobar fissures were frequently visible.

The normal markings in the lungs are composed almost entirely of the images of the pulmonary arteries and veins. Interlobar fissures may cast images, as may the walls of the central bronchi.

Premature infants are subject to a much higher incidence of pulmonary abnormalities, notably hyaline membrane disease. However, even very small premature infants may survive with completely normal appearing lungs (Fig. 7–7). The physiologic data of Burnard et al. (1965) suggest that hyperinflation of the lungs of some low birth weight infants may be noticeable. This may be explained by normal lung compliance associated with increased collapsibility of small airways in premature babies (see also page 80).

Diaphragm

The image of the diaphragm of the normal newborn infant is usually rounded smoothly on both frontal and lateral roentgenograms

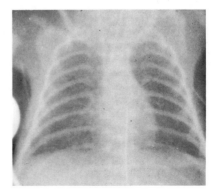

Figure 7–7. A 21-week gestation, 350-gm. infant who was the product of abortion. In spite of severe prematurity, the infant lived for five hours during which time chest radiographs showed no abnormalities. Chest radiograph printed exact size.

of the chest. The anterior costophrenic angle is quite shallow, and the apex of each hemidiaphragm is located moderately anterior and slightly medial to its mid-portion. During quiet breathing the domes are usually at the level of the anterior portions of the fourth ribs or intercostal spaces, and the excursion is less than one interspace. When the infant cries the excursion is much greater (Burnard and James, 1961).

Trachea

In a normal infant, the trachea is displaced slightly to the right of the midline by the left aortic arch (Fig. 7–8). The distance from the thoracic inlet to the carina varies considerably between deep inspira-

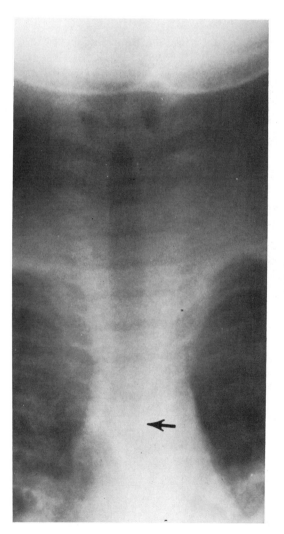

Figure 7–8. Normal tracheal air column. Note slight deviation to the right at the level of the aortic arch (arrow).

tion and deep expiration. In deep inspiration the trachea lies close to the midline, whereas on expiration it buckles to the right in the chest and anteriorly in the neck.

The caliber of the trachea varies with respiration. Variations are greatest in the anteroposterior diameter and thus are best recognized by roentgenographic or fluoroscopic examination with the patient in the lateral position. Wittenborg et al. (1967) found that changes in the caliber of the trachea of the normal infant are barely measureable during quiet breathing, whereas with breath holding, crying, or struggling the anteroposterior diameter of the lumen varied by 20 to 50 per cent.

Thymus

Perhaps the greatest source of confusion even for the observer experienced in interpreting roentgenograms of the infant chest is the thymus. It may be sufficiently large to extend to the diaphragm, obliterating both borders of the heart on the frontal projection. At times, the presence of a large thymus may be deduced from extension of the thymus into the minor fissure, producing the well-known "sail sign," with a notch between the lower margin of the thymus and the heart, or by its characteristic wave-like contour (Mulvey, 1963).

The thymic shadow is usually more prominent on the right than on the left. The thymic "sail sign" was found in less than 5 per cent of patients with prominent thymuses by Tausend and Stern (1965). The thymic border is differentiated from an upper lobe pneumonia by absence of air-containing bronchi within it and typical undulations of its lateral border (Fig. 7–9A). Frequently, however, the presence of a large thymus rather than a large heart cannot be established with certainty from the frontal chest roentgenogram. Consequently, the best evaluation of heart size in an infant is made on a correctly positioned lateral chest roentgenogram obtained during good inspiration. If the heart is more than minimally enlarged, it will almost always extend abnormally close to the spine (Fig. 7–9B).

The large thymus of infancy frequently fills the relatively clear space that is present above the heart in older children and adults. When this space is small or lacking but the heart does not appear to be enlarged posteriorly on the lateral film, significant cardiomegaly is probably not present, no matter how large the central mediastinal shadow may be on the frontal roentgenogram. For this reason, the concept of the thymicocardiac image, rather than that of the cardiac silhouette, is probably preferable in the evaluation of chest roentgenograms of infants and children (Caffey, 1967).

The thymus may appear to be small or absent when the lungs are hyperinflated, and it involutes rapidly under conditions of stress. Congenital absence may, however, be suspected when no thymic shadow is seen on serial radiographs during the first three to four days

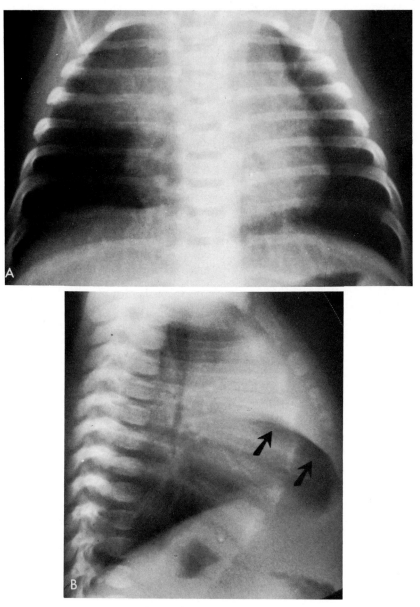

Figure 7–9. A, Typical thymic sail sign due to large lobe of thymus obscuring the right upper lobe. Note the undulations of the lateral border of the thymus. *B*, The inferior border of the thymus (arrows) is clearly delineated in the anterior mediastinum on the lateral projection. The heart is not enlarged posteriorly.

of life (Kirkpatrick and Capitanio, 1972). This finding is of particular importance in the presence of neonatal tetany due to associated absence of parathyroids which also develop embryologically from the third and fourth pharyngeal pouches (DiGeorge, 1965). Anomalies of related anlage, such as right aortic arch, are also recognizable in this syndrome (Kirkpatrick and DiGeorge, 1968).

Other immune deficiency diseases may lead to the appearance of an "empty" mediastinum due to hypoplasia of thymic tissue (Presberg and Singleton, 1968) (Fig. 7–10). Thymic dysplasia (Swiss type agammaglobulinemia) is occasionally associated with bone abnormalities resembling mild achondroplasia (Alexander and Dunbar, 1968).

Heart Size

Variations in size of the thymic shadow and differences in timing of x-ray exposures during phases of the respiratory and cardiac cycles may interfere with accurate interpretation of heart size in newborn infants. However, cineradiographic studies of normal infants during quiet breathing have shown surprisingly little variation in transverse diameter of the heart during the respiratory and cardiac cycles (Burnard and James, 1961). A greater variation occurred in crying babies in which the greatest transverse diameter of the heart was found on inspiration before a cry, but which was not usually greater than that of the resting baby. In normal full-term newborn infants, the transverse diameter of the heart as measured on frontal roentgenograms is usually slightly greater than 50 per cent of the transverse diameter of the thorax measured at the level of the right diaphragmatic dome, and it decreases slightly during the first three days of life (Martin and Friedell, 1952) (Table 7–1). Similarly, Kjellberg et al. (1954) found a significant decrease in heart size during the first two days of life in both mature and premature infants which was thought to reflect changes in blood volume associated with the cessation of placental circulation.

Another possible explanation for the change in the cardiothymic image during the first days of life is a reduction in the size of the thymus. It has been demonstrated that the normal thymus usually shrinks in response to the administration of adrenal corticosteroids or to stress (Caffey and di Liberti, 1959; Caffey and Silbey, 1960). Thymic shrinkage caused by the stress of birth and mediated by endogenous corticosteroid production may account for the change in the thymic/cardiothoracic ratio in the first two days of life.

Vessels

The undivided pulmonary artery and the first portion of the thoracic aorta are usually covered by the thymus in the newborn infant and therefore are difficult to discern. The side of the aortic arch

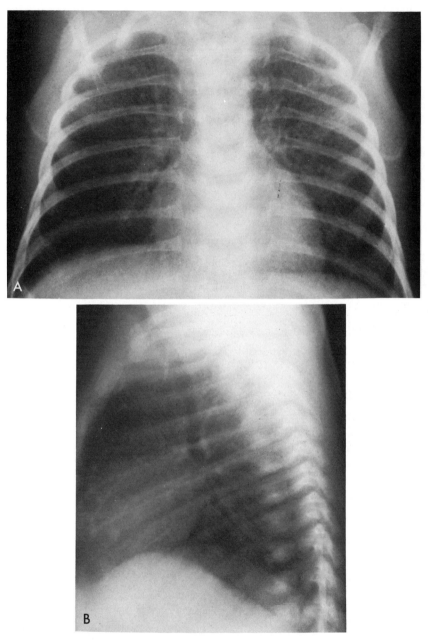

Figure 7–10. Thymic alymphoplasia in two-month-old infant. Note narrow upper mediastinum on frontal projection (*A*). There is mild bilateral pneumonia. Serial films showed a consistently "empty" anterior mediastinum on lateral views (*B*).

Table 7–1. Cardiothoracic Ratios (Per Cent). Mean ± One
Standard Deviation*

Day	1	3	5
	.556 ± .037	.525 ± .033	.526 ± .031

* Antero-posterior projection, 40-inch distance, recumbent position, inspiration.
(From Martin and Friedel: Amer. J. Roentgen. 67:905, 1952.)

can usually be determined by its displacement of the trachea (see Fig. 7–8), and the descending aorta can sometimes be identified through the thymicocardiac image.

Occasionally, a small mass, which was termed "the ductus bump" by Berdon et al. (1965), is seen in the left upper mediastinum.

Interpretation of Pulmonary Abnormalities

It is beyond the scope of this presentation to elaborate the numerous radiologic signs by which pulmonary disease can be recognized and differentiated. Basic pulmonary roentgenology is discussed by Felson (1960), and a detailed description of the anatomical bases of fundamental roentgen signs has been recently offered by Fraser and Paré (1970). It is useful to differentiate airspace disease due to consolidation or collapse from interstitial infiltration. These roentgen patterns will be elaborated in the descriptions of the specific diseases of the newborn lung to which they apply.

RADIOGRAPHY OF MONITORING
AND TREATMENT DEVICES

Endotracheal Tubes

Resuscitation of infants with respiratory failure and ventilatory assistance with intermittent positive-pressure respirator therapy requires the use of endotracheal tubes. Particularly in small premature infants, the position of the tube can alter easily when the patient is moved. Most endotracheal tubes are, however, radiopaque, and their position can therefore be easily checked from radiographs.

The tip of the tube should be well below the vocal cords but approximately 2 cm. above the carina. A tube which is too low in position will usually fall into the right main bronchus (Kuhns and Poznanski, 1971). Its wall will thus occlude the left main bronchus, and if the catheter extends to the right lower lobe bronchus, occlusion of the right upper lobe and middle lobe bronchi will occur, leading to rapid atelectasis (Fig. 7–11). Because of its more horizontal course, the left main bronchus is less frequently entered.

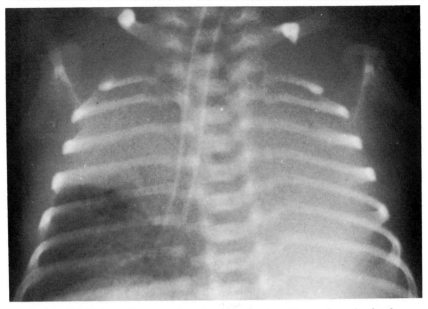

Figure 7–11. Complication of tracheal intubation. The endotracheal tube extends into the right lower lobe bronchus, occluding the left main bronchus and right upper and middle lobe bronchi, resulting in atelectasis.

Accidental esophageal intubation (Stool et al., 1971) is identifiable on radiographs by the posterior position of the tube, poor pulmonary aeration, and intestinal distention (Fig. 7–12).

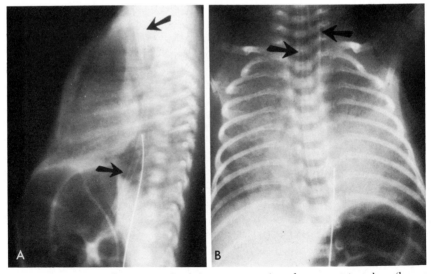

Figure 7–12. The nasotracheal (upper arrows) and nasogastric tubes (lower arrows) are both in the esophagus on lateral projection (*A*). Note their side-by-side position in the esophagus on the AP view (*B*). The lungs are poorly aerated and there is gastrointestinal distention with air.

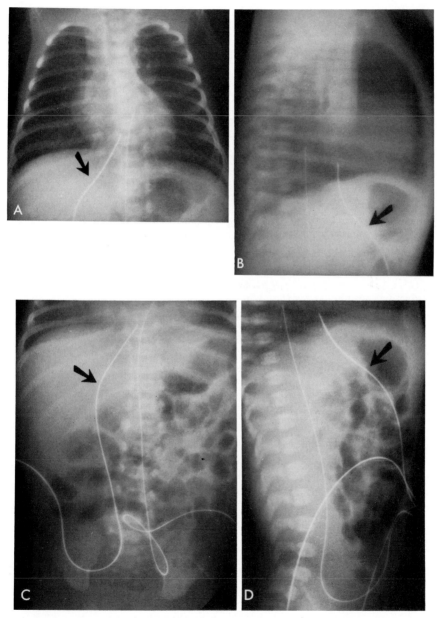

Figure 7–13. Course of umbilical venous (arrows) and arterial catheters in chest (*A* and *B*) and abdomen (*C* and *D*) of newborn. The venous catheter passes through the ductus venosus into the intrathoracic portion of the inferior vena cava. The tip of the arterial catheter is in the thoracic aorta adjacent to the sixth thoracic vertebra.

Umbilical Catheters

Umbilical catheters are now widely used in order to monitor acid-base balance and blood gas tensions in newborn infants with respiratory distress. On occasion, the umbilical arterial catheters are also utilized for aortic and cerebral angiography (Emmanoulides and Hoy, 1967). The small, flexible polyethylene catheters should contain a radiopaque stripe so that their position can be monitored either during placement under fluoroscopic control or, more practically, by means of abdominal and chest radiographs taken immediately following positioning of the catheter (Fig. 7–13). Baker et al. (1969) have stressed the necessity of lateral films in addition to anteroposterior projections in order to avoid catheter misplacement.

The umbilical arterial catheter passes through one of the paired umbilical arteries to the internal iliac artery and into the abdominal aorta. The catheter tip should be remote from the celiac, renal, and mesenteric arteries because of the danger of thrombosis. According to Phelps et al. (1972), the celiac axis is usually adjacent to the top of the 12th thoracic vertebra. The optimal position of the tip of an end-hole catheter is probably in the lower thoracic aorta, opposite T6 to T10.

Umbilical venous catheters are utilized mainly for administration of blood. The umbilical vein ascends in the inferior border of the falciform ligament toward the porta hepatis and left portal vein from which the ductus venosus originates. The catheter can then pass through the ductus venosus and hepatic veins to enter the inferior vena cava and right atrium. The optimal position of the catheter tip is in the intrathoracic portion of the inferior vena cava. Rosen and Reich (1970) and Campbell (1971) have discussed the anatomical details of catheter placement and malposition.

The radiologic findings of hepatic calcifications (Ablow and Effman, 1972) and gas in the portal veins (Schmidt, 1967) have been attributed to umbilical vein catheterization. Complications may be reduced by avoidance of fluid infusions through large-vessel catheters. (For discussion of other complications caused by catheters, see also pages 62 and 63.)

Other Hardware

Superimposed hemostats, temperature sensors, and electrocardiographic leads can cause unnecessary confusion, and because of their relatively large size, electrocardiographic leads may obscure vital areas of the chest and should always be removed prior to radiography.

PART

II

Disorders of Respiration in the Newborn Period

Chapter Eight

NORMAL AND
ABNORMAL AIRWAYS

The upper and lower airways of the infant may be the sites of a variety of disorders, congenital or acquired. Obstruction of the upper airway is classically associated with forced inspiratory efforts of little effect. When the nares are obstructed at birth, as in bilateral choanal atresia, the infant shows profound retractions and ultimately apnea and cyanosis occur unless an oral airway is insured. Laryngeal narrowing may give inspiratory stridor as well as expiratory prolongation if it is severe. Airway narrowing within the thorax is associated with expiratory prolongation, and a compensatory increase in lung volume. When the lesion is localized, the effect of mediastinal shift may be more significant than the wheeze or prolongation of expiration. A complete obstruction, of course, leads to airlessness of the portion of the lung distal to it.

The following sections describe some of the conditions associated with airway obstruction in infants.

RADIOLOGIC EVALUATION OF NORMAL AIRWAYS

In the normal neonate, the observation of preferential nose breathing (Cook et al., 1956) has been demonstrated radiologically by Ardran and Kemp (1970), who have shown that the oral airway remains closed during sleep due to apposition of the tongue and soft palate. The oral air passage may open during crying. Recognition of air in the nasal cavities may be difficult, but air content of the naso-

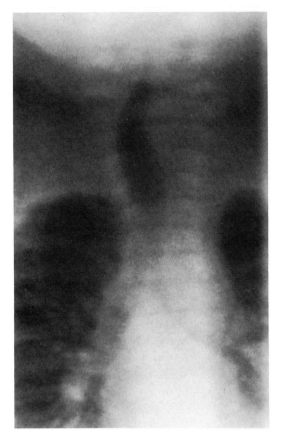

Figure 8–1. A high kilovoltage radiograph of the neck shows normal redundancy of the trachea, resulting in slight deviation of the cervical trachea to the right. The aortic arch is responsible for the deviation of the intrathoracic portion of the trachea.

pharynx is well demonstrated on a lateral radiograph. The nasopharynx is well suited for the passage of air in the newborn, since adenoidal tissue is lacking during the first month of life, and the total thickness of nasopharyngeal tissues is rarely more than 0.5 cm. during the first three months (Capitanio and Kirkpatrick, 1970).

In the infant the cervical portion of the trachea is redundant (Ardran and Kemp, 1968) and may be normally deviated to the right (Fig. 8–1). Anterior tracheal buckling can occur on expiration and on flexion of the neck (Fig. 8–2). This should not be misinterpreted as the result of a retropharyngeal mass. A lateral view or fluoroscopy of the neck in a position of extension and during inspiration will help to exclude pathologic thickening of the retropharyngeal tissues.

Excellent evaluation of the tracheal and central bronchial air column is obtained by making roentgenograms with high kilovoltage (130 to 150 kv.) and heavy filtration (1 mm. copper or brass) (Maguire et al., 1966). This technique is especially useful for demonstrating endotracheal lesions such as polyps and subglottic hemangiomas (Tefft, 1966) (Fig. 8–1).

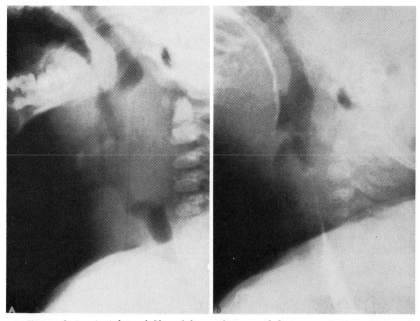

Figure 8–2. *A*, A lateral film of the neck exposed during expiration suggested a retropharyngeal mass. *B*, A repeat film, made in deep inspiration, shows the retropharyngeal region to be normal.

CHOANAL ATRESIA

Obstruction of the nasal airway may be unilateral or bilateral, membranous or bony. If the obstruction is complete and bilateral, the infants are often in great distress at birth, although breathing is usually initiated through the mouth with the first good cry. Thereafter, their distress is episodic, most marked when they are fed or disturbed, at which time there are deep retractions and even cyanosis. The diagnosis, which may be suspected from the symptomatology, becomes highly probable when the mouth is held closed and respiratory effort moves no air and is confirmed by inability to pass a probe through the nares. Some infants survive as mouth breathers; Medovy and Beckman (1951) commented on a number of adults in whom the diagnosis was first made after the age of 20 years. Other infants may die from inability to tolerate feedings and aspiration.

There is a familial tendency to this disorder, evident in most large series reported from the occurrence in several generations and in siblings. Associated congenital malformations include Treacher-Collins syndrome, palatal abnormalities, colobomas, tracheoesophageal fistula, and congenital heart disease (Flake and Ferguson, 1964). The abnormality is twice as frequent on the right side as on the left, and twice as frequent in girls as in boys (Hobolth et al., 1967).

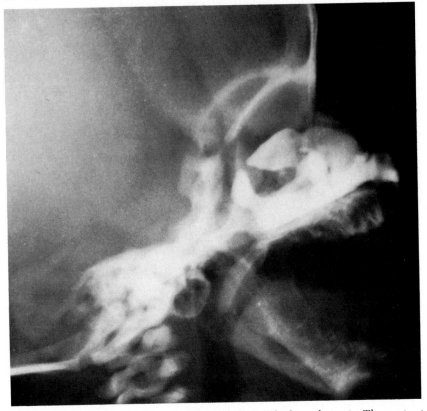

Figure 8–3.   Lateral view of face of an infant with choanal atresia. The contrast medium in the nares does not enter the nasopharynx.

The diagnosis may be confirmed by the instillation of a few drops of methylene blue into the nostril; if the choanae are patent, the dye can be seen in the pharynx. It is also possible to visualize the obstruction by the use of radiopaque material such as dionosil in the nasal cavity and by lateral or occipitomental views of the nose and nasopharynx with the patient in the supine position (Fig. 8–3). The use of a few drops of a nasal decongestant such as ephedrine prior to the examination is an aid to accurate radiologic interpretation.

The treatment of bilateral choanal atresia consists of establishing a communication between the anterior and posterior nares (Beinfield, 1959). Pending definitive operation, an oral airway should be inserted and taped in position to permit the infant to breathe at all times. A rubber nipple with a large hole in it, strapped by tapes over the ears, is a useful aid. The infant usually requires two to three weeks before he can mouth breathe successfully. Feedings may be by intermittent gavage or indwelling polyethylene catheter. These measures permit the selection of an optimal time for the creation of a nasal passage.

Two operative approaches are widely used. In the event of membranous obstructions, intranasal perforation of the membrane can be accomplished. The intranasal route can also be used to drill through bony obstructions, and catheters can be placed in the nostrils until healing occurs. Many surgeons now prefer the transpalatal approach in which the mucosa is reflected and the hard palate perforated (Walker, 1954; Flake and Ferguson, 1964). The intranasal procedure has been carried out successfully on the first day of life; the transpalatal procedure as early as two weeks of age. The general condition of the infant and the presence of other problems may require deferment of the definitive procedure. Operative correction of unilateral choanal atresia may be postponed until the child is several years old.

Laryngeal Webs

A membranous obstruction may be present at the level of the true vocal cords or just above or below them. Although this lesion was seen by Holinger et al. (1954) in 19 infants, its rarity is suggested by the diagnosis of only nine cases over a 17-year period in a hospital with 4000 admissions a year (Hudson, 1951). If the web is complete, the infant will gasp for air, but none enters the lungs, and death ensues. More commonly, the web only partially obstructs the airway, in which case the infant shows stridor and a hoarse or very weak cry. Given these symptoms, direct laryngoscopy is indicated. Occasionally, the web can be perforated if it is totally obstructive; if it is only partly obstructive, laryngeal dilatations may suffice. A tracheotomy would be lifesaving if the web were obstructive. Voice disturbances may persist even after the web is perforated or excised (Baker, 1954).

Laryngeal atresia is far less common but has been seen in one of twins (Rankin and Mendelson, 1956).

The association of congenital laryngeal webs with interventricular septal defects was reported by Shearer et al. (1972) in three children. The webs were anterior in location and at the level of the glottis. The mild nature of the problem in one of their patients resulted in detection at age five years, although the mother had noticed a high-pitched weak voice from birth. In another infant, aphonia and respiratory distress were significant in the first weeks of life, necessitating tracheostomy at 13 weeks of age.

Other anomalies may be associated with congenital webs of the larynx: 11 per cent of McHugh and Loch's series of 133 cases had associated malformations (1942).

STRIDOR

The symptom of stridor in the newborn period has been mentioned in association with vocal cord paralysis (page 113), vascular rings (page 115), and tumors that compress or narrow the upper airway. In addition, there are infants who have stridulous respirations in the absence of any of these conditions (Wilson, 1952).

One group appears to have an elongated or floppy epiglottis. On laryngoscopy, an exaggerated folding backward of the epiglottis can be seen (Baker, 1954). Whether or not symptoms can be attributed to the abnormal epiglottis is not established; however, infants in whom we have entertained that diagnosis characteristically recover by several months of age, and almost always by one year. This condition, often referred to as congenital laryngeal stridor, is the most common cause of noisy breathing in infancy. In a review of the clinical features in 39 infants (25 male, 14 female) Arthurton (1970) noted the onset at birth in two-thirds of them, but onset was delayed up to four months in others. Usually the stridor persisted for less than a year, but in eight infants it lasted more than two years. The effect of sleep was variable.

This type of stridor can be convincingly demonstrated radiologically (Dunbar, 1970). With the patient in the supine position, horizontal beam lateral views of the neck are made with spot films or high speed cinerecording. During the time when stridor is present, anteroinferior displacement and vibration of the aryepiglottic folds and posterior indrawing of the epiglottis can be seen on inspiration.

Laryngeal spasm with stridor may accompany tetany of the newborn or may be the first symptom of hypoparathyroidism. Wilson (1952) says that of 48 cases of neonatal tetany at the Rotunda Hospital in Dublin only one developed stridor. Our impression concurs with his that neonatal tetany is rarely associated with laryngeal spasm. On the other hand, a serum calcium determination is in order in stridor that is unexplained on an anatomical basis.

Stridor in association with apneic spells and cyanosis has been called "neurogenic stridor in infancy" by Allen et al. (1954). Their two infants responded to treatment with phenobarbital and Dilantin. They attributed the condition to overactive autonomic reflexes triggered in the upper respiratory and gastrointestinal tracts. We have not recognized this entity and suspect the diagnosis should be entertained only after all other causes of stridor have been ruled out.

An interesting, but rare association of inspiratory stridor beginning at birth with calcification of laryngeal and tracheal cartilages has been reported (Nabarro, 1952; Russo and Coin, 1958). In the patient described by Goldbloom and Dunbar (1960), diminution in severity of the stridor corresponded to a decrease in density of the calcifications. None of the infants appeared to have chondrodystrophia calcificans congenita (Fig. 8–4).

Causes of expiratory stridor are less clearly defined. In some patients, narrowing of the upper thoracic trachea can be detected radiologically during expiration. When this coincides with audible stridor, a diagnosis of "tracheomalacia" may be made. In some infants the narrowing is most likely due to the so-called "anomalous" innominate

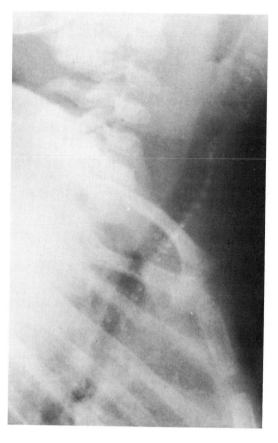

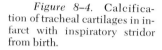
Figure 8–4. Calcification of tracheal cartilages in infarct with inspiratory stridor from birth.

or common carotid artery (see also page 117), but in others, the etiology and significance of this finding are unknown. Wittenborg et al. (1967) observed only minimal changes in tracheal caliber during the respiratory cycle in normal resting infants and a decrease in caliber of up to 50 per cent during exertion. Exaggerated degrees of expiratory collapse of the intrathoracic trachea occurred in conditions such as bronchiolitis, in which peripheral airway obstruction was present. It is unlikely that expiratory stridor is often due to an intrinsic abnormality of the tracheal cartilage.

VOCAL CORD PARALYSIS

Paralysis of the vocal cords in the newborn infant may be unilateral or bilateral, and in either event it may be symptomatic. Bilateral paralyses are thought to be central in origin, perhaps related to nuclear aplasia or injury. The occurrence of persistent stridor in four siblings, one of whom died, suggests a hereditary basis in some instances of laryngeal abductor paralysis (Plott, 1964). Unilateral paralyses are seen more frequently on the left side and are thought to be associated with pressure on the recurrent laryngeal nerve at the time of birth. A rare cause of paralysis of the left vocal cord in association with paralysis of the left hemidiaphragm is an aneurysm of the ductus arteriosus (Berger et al., 1960). Occasionally, right vocal cord paralysis may be found, but the etiology is not always clear. The condition occurred only once or twice in 3000 deliveries in our nursery.

The symptoms are an inspiratory stridor and a hoarse cry. Retractions are present occasionally. A tracheotomy may be required if the infant has difficulty moving air.

Laryngoscopy should be done to rule out other causes of stridor. Occasionally, it is possible to identify a paralyzed cord; more commonly, it is difficult to be sure if an apparent fixation of a cord is from spasm or the effect of the laryngoscope itself, which can hold a cord in a fixed position.

Sometimes the symptoms are transient; occasionally they persist. As the child grows, the airway narrowing is less apparent, but noisy, stridulous respirations may persist for several years; they are particularly prominent with exercise or in the presence of mild infections.

MALFORMATIONS OF THE GREAT VESSELS

The changes in the configuration of the great vessels which occur during embryonic life, discussed by Congdon (1922), are so complex that it is surprising that vascular malformations occur in the mediastinum as infrequently as they do. Many are of no clinical significance; others interfere with swallowing or respiration or both, and may be amenable to operative correction. Gross (1953) discussed in detail the clinical features and operative techniques based on his experience with 57 infants and children referred for operation. He thought that the clinically significant anomalies fell into five categories: double aortic arch, right aortic arch with a left ligamentum arteriosum, anomalous innominate artery, anomalous left common carotid artery, and aberrant subclavian artery. Occasionally the left pulmonary artery arises as a branch of the right pulmonary artery and compresses the trachea and esophagus as it crosses between them. Associated cardiac and pulmonary lesions are present in more than half the patients with an aberrant left pulmonary artery (Clarkson et al., 1967).

Edwards (1953) proposed that the varieties of malformations of the great vessels could be predicted from a hypothetic structure of a double aortic arch with a ductus arteriosus on each side and the descending aorta in a neutral position. From each arch the subclavian and common carotid arteries arise separately. Abnormal persistence or obliteration of portions of such a hypothetical structure account for the malformations which he observed pathologically. The most common malformation in his experience was an aberrant right subclavian artery, the first portion of which can be thought of as the dorsal portion of the right aortic arch.

The incidence of symptomatic vascular rings is not known, although in our experience they are a very rare cause of respiratory difficulty in the newborn period.

Clinical Features. Infants with a completely encircling vascular ring have similar symptoms. The outstanding clinical observation is the tendency of the infant to keep his head extended, and sometimes his back as well, so that he assumes the opisthotonic position. In this position the trachea is elongated and thrust forward. Presumably, the anterior cartilaginous portion of the trachea can displace vessels that compress it, whereas the membranous posterior portion is more compliant. If the head is forcibly flexed by the examiner, the infant objects and may even become apneic. Respirations are usually audible, with an inspiratory "crow" and often an expiratory wheeze. Hesitation in swallowing may be evident if the esophagus is also compressed by the anomalous vessels. Regurgitation and vomiting can also occur, and the respiratory distress may be aggravated during and after feedings. Less severe degrees of obstruction may be manifested only during a cry, when a prolonged, wheezing expiration should suggest the diagnosis.

Infants with aberrant subclavian arteries are more likely to have compression of the esophagus than the trachea. Hesitation in swallowing is common, and often the infant appears to be hungry but cannot take more than an occasional swallow. The symptoms are likely to become more prominent when solid foods are started.

Radiologic Diagnosis

The aortic arch is difficult to visualize directly on plain roentgenograms in small infants, and the position of the aortic arch is determined by observing the direction of deviation of the upper mediastinal portion of the tracheal air shadow. Opacification of the esophagus with barium is an additional aid because of its close posterior relationship to the trachea. These structures are gently deviated to the right by the normal left aortic arch. Contrast studies of the trachea do not usually add significant information and may further compromise an already partially obstructed airway. Angiography is only occasionally necessary to establish the diagnosis.

Vascular Rings

This group of anomalies is, with rare exceptions, associated with a right-sided or double aortic arch. Right aortic arch is common in congenital heart disease, especially in tetralogy of Fallot and truncus arteriosus, and causes deviation of the tracheal air shadow to the left. This type of aortic arch is a mirror image of the normal and would not be expected to produce symptoms. Felson and Palayew (1963) have shown that when a right aortic arch exists as an isolated anomaly, a posterior indentation of the esophagus results. This posteriorly placed arch, in association with a remnant of the left aortic arch (diverticulum of Kommerell) and left ligamentum arteriosum, may form a ring around the esophagus and trachea. Constriction is presumably enhanced by traction exerted by the left subclavian artery (Shuford et al., 1970). The combination of a posterior esophageal and anterior tracheal defect will be seen on lateral chest radiographs (Berdon and Baker, 1972) (Fig. 8–5).

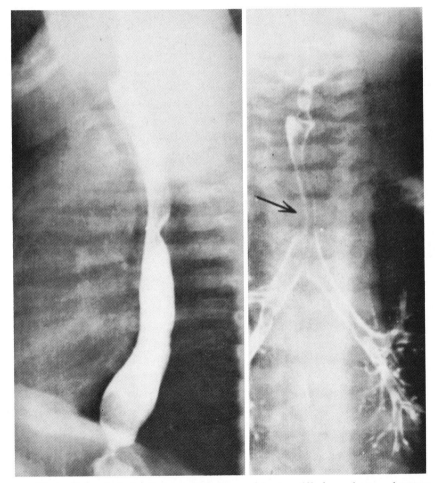

Figure 8–5. A, Lateral view of trachea and barium-filled esophagus, showing anterior tracheal and posterior esophageal compression associated with a right aortic arch. B, Same patient as in A, with demonstration of tracheal compression in AP projection.

A double aortic arch also produces a large posterior defect of the esophagus accompanied by an anterior tracheal defect. On radiographs obtained in frontal projection, the finding of indentations of either side of the esophagus may establish the diagnosis (Stewart, Kincaid, and Edwards, 1964) but frequently this anomaly cannot be differentiated on plain films from a vascular ring associated with a single right aortic arch.

A vascular ring may also be produced by the rare anomaly of a cervical aortic arch (Sheppard et al., 1969). The cervical arch is usually right-sided; it may cause a large posterior esophageal indentation, and it displaces the trachea forward (Chang et al., 1971). Angiography is necessary for exact diagnosis which can be suspected clinically by the presence of a pulsating mass in the neck.

"Anomalous" Innominate Artery

An innominate artery which arises too far to the left of an otherwise normal aortic arch may cause symptoms similar to those caused by a vascular ring. Since the artery must cross the trachea anteriorly, it is recognizable on lateral radiographs by the finding of a constant anterior concavity of the trachea midway between the carina and sternal notch (Berdon et al., 1969). Surgical treatment consisting of attachment of the innominate artery to the sternum has been carried out in some cases (Fearson and Shortread, 1963), but it is likely that improvement may occur spontaneously as "crowding" of the mediastinum lessens with growth.

An anomalous left common carotid artery may similarly compress the trachea as it courses upward into the neck from an origin which is further to the right than normal (Gross, 1967).

The most common vascular anomaly is aberrant subclavian artery which almost always passes posterior to the esophagus (Beaubout et al., 1964) and causes a defect which is readily seen on a lateral film as a posterior oblique indentation at about the level of the third or fourth thoracic vertebra. In this position, the vessel should not cause respiratory symptoms.

Aberrant Pulmonary Artery

This anomaly, also referred to as a vascular "sling," consists of a left pulmonary artery which arises from the main pulmonary artery, courses over the proximal portion of the right main bronchus or trachea, and then travels posteriorly and to the left between the trachea and esophagus (Fig. 8–6A). It, therefore, is capable of compressing the posterior wall of the trachea. Associated cardiac or pulmonary lesions are found in more than half of the patients with this anomaly (Clarkson, 1967).

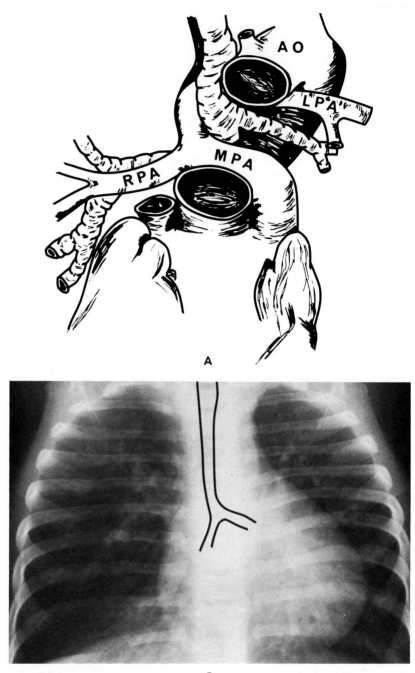

A

B

Figure 8–6.   Diagnosis of aberrant left pulmonary artery made at age 15 months by barium esophagram in infant with wheezing and cough thought to be due to bronchiolitis and pneumonia which had been present since a few months of age. *A,* Diagrammatic representation of course of aberrant left pulmonary artery between esophagus and trachea (ascending aorta has been cut away). (Redrawn from Murphy, D. R. et al.: Surg. Gynec. Obstet. *118*:572, 1964.)

B, Outline of trachea and main bronchi shows indentation and displacement on the right. Also note overinflation of right lung.

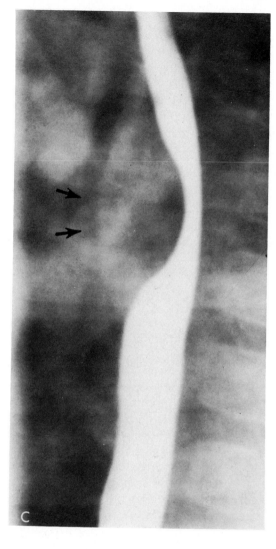

Figure 8–6 Continued.
C, With esophagus filled with
barium, lateral projection
shows separation and compression of trachea (arrows) and
esophagus due to aberrant
course of left pulmonary
artery.

The plain film findings are quite characteristic (Capitanio et al.,
1971). Compression of the bronchus causes alteration of aeration, usually obstructive emphysema of the right lung. The right main bronchus may be anteriorly bowed, and since the aberrant vessel courses
obliquely downward and to the left, the left hilum will be low in
position. An impression on the right side of the trachea, just above the
carina, is usually seen where it is traversed by the posteriorly positioned left pulmonary artery (Dunbar, 1970) (Fig. 8–6B). We have also
noted diminished pulmonary vasculature on the left, presumably due
to decreased blood flow in the aberrant vessel. Fluoroscopy with a
direct lateral x-ray beam will show a pulsating mass between the trachea and esophagus at the level of the carina compressing both
structures (Fig. 8–6C). Angiocardiography has not been necessary for

diagnosis in the patients successfully treated surgically by Murphy et al. (1964), and we have found the sling difficult to visualize by this method. Congenital anomalies of the trachea and bronchi have been discovered on bronchography by Capitanio et al. (1971), but this procedure should probably be reserved for patients with localized abnormalities of lung aeration. The bronchoscopist may be able to see the effects of external compression of the trachea, as illustrated in the cases reported by Holinger et al. (1948).

Absence of a Pulmonary Artery

Hypoplasia or absence of a pulmonary artery may be discovered incidentally in asymptomatic individuals. Usually the ipsilateral lung is a little smaller, and vessels less prominent than in the perfused lung. The hilar shadow is absent on the affected side (Sherrick et al., 1962). If not associated with other malformations, the prognosis is good. Stenosis of the branches of the pulmonary artery is a recognized complication of the congenital rubella syndrome (Rowe, 1963; McCue et al., 1965).

Diagnosis depends on angiography or lung scans. Aeborelius et al. (1971) reported on the use of Xe^{133} radiospirometry for evaluation of congenital malformations of pulmonary arteries in a group of patients aged 10 to 19 years. They pointed out the subtle changes on chest films and the nearly normal lung volumes in several patients, confirming the asymptomatic nature of a unilateral pulmonary atresia. In one patient with multiple stenoses, pulmonary artery hypertension was present. Radiospirometry and lung scans showed that the defects in regional perfusion corresponded to central arterial constrictions that could be approached operatively.

Treatment. Prompt operative correction is indicated if a vascular ring compresses either the trachea or the esophagus sufficiently to cause symptoms. Occasionally, airway obstructive symptoms persist for some weeks postoperatively, since the trachea does not always assume its normal caliber as soon as the vessel compressing it is ligated. Hence, tracheotomy is sometimes indicated (Blumenthal and Ravitch, 1957).

TUMORS AND CYSTS

Tumors

Neoplasms in the airway of the newborn infant occur so rarely that they constitute curiosities. Nonetheless, they have been reported and should be considered in the differential diagnosis of unexplained respiratory distress.

At least one case of a teratoma of the tonsil was described in which asphyxia at birth was followed by labored respirations. The lesion was seen during resuscitative procedures, but an attempt to remove it was unsuccessful (Baugh and O'Donoghue, 1955).

Nasopharyngeal teratomas and pharyngeal dermoids have been successfully removed in the newborn period (Kesson, 1954; Berger et al., 1965; Loeb and Smith, 1967). They may or may not project externally. When attached by a thin pedicle, they can be removed with a snare. This treatment should, however, be approached with caution, since some nasopharyngeal teratomas may extend intracranially (Partlow and Taybi, 1971). Demonstration of the mass can be accomplished by means of a lateral radiograph of the nasopharynx. Its exact outline can be visualized by instilling dionosil through the nostrils. In one such patient reported by Ingram and Poznanski (1969), the airway obstruction could be relieved by placing the patient head down, since a pedicle allowed mobility of the mass away from the hypopharynx in that position. Of 83 cases of teratoma of the neck reviewed by Stone et al. (1967), 32 were in newborn infants. These tumors frequently caused respiratory problems. On roentgenograms, the cervical esophagus and trachea were often deviated, and calcifications were found in the tumor mass.

Congenital subglottic hemangiomas are fairly common, at least 19 cases having been reported in the literature. Four of the reported infants were symptomatic at birth, and all four died (Campbell et al., 1958). Stridor, wheezing, retractions, and cyanosis may be present. Subglottic hemangiomas are usually associated with hemangiomas elsewhere. The diagnosis is probable if high kilovoltage films of the upper airway show a narrowing or irregularity in that region (Fig. 8–7). The lesions may regress on steroid therapy. Prednisone in a dose of 3 mg./kg./day for about a week sometimes relieves the symptoms. The dose may then be reduced to the amount needed to sustain the effect. If there is no response to prednisone, a tracheostomy is essential.

Other tumors in the nasopharynx include hemangiopericytoma. One such lesion presented by causing obstruction to nasal breathing at birth. Difficulty with intubation and observation of a mass in the posterior pharynx necessitated tracheostomy. Roentgenograms demonstrated a large, calcium-containing retrotracheal mass (Fig. 8–8). Supportive care until such lesions regress appears to be all that can be done at this time (Baden et al., 1972).

A similar roentgen appearance would be expected in a cervical neuroblastoma. There is a relatively high cure rate in this and other extra-adrenal neuroblastomas with radiotherapy (Young et al., 1970).

Neurofibromas may involve the larynx, usually in association with other manifestations of neurofibromatosis, such as café-au-lait spots and subcutaneous nodules (Pleasure and Geller, 1967).

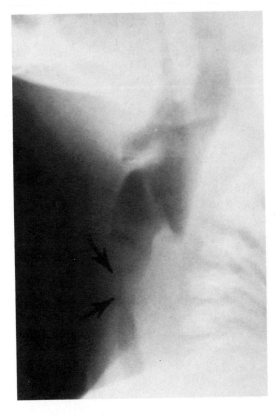

Figure 8-7. A subglottic hemangioma is demonstrated on this lateral view of the neck as a soft tissue mass causing posterior compression of the tracheal lumen (arrows).

Congenital goiters occur most frequently in infants of mothers who continue thyroid suppressant medication or excess iodides throughout pregnancy. The thyroid gland is usually palpable.

Sometimes tracheal compression occurs with a barely palpable gland if it is retrosternal. The use of thyroxin or derivatives to suppress the infant's goiter is indicated, and improvement usually occurs within four or five days. If the tracheal compression is severe, tracheostomy may be necessary (Beaudoing et al., 1964; Galina et al., 1963) (Fig. 8-9).

Thymic tissue may persist in the neck if the thymic primordia fail to descend. It most commonly lies anteriorly and to the left of the midline. The mass infrequently causes respiratory embarrassment (Lewis, 1962).

Cysts

Normal ectopic thyroid tissue is usually located in or near the midline, in the inferior retropharyngeal area, or is retrosternal in position. In contrast, a thyroglossal duct cyst is in the midline and at the base of the tongue (Dunbar, 1970). Lingual cysts can increase in size after birth and may cause significant respiratory distress (Lofgren, 1963).

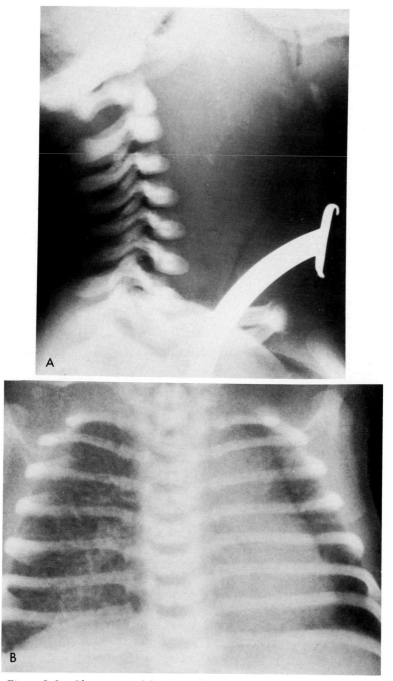

Figure 8–8.   Obstruction of the cervical airway due to a large mass necessitated tracheostomy immediately after birth. On the lateral view of the neck (*A*) the pharynx and trachea are compressed and anteriorly deviated by large mass containing faint, amorphous calcifications. *B*, The pulmonary edema, which apparently resulted from airway obstruction, subsided after tracheostomy. (From Baden, M., et al.: Canada Med. Ass. J. *107*:1202, 1972.)

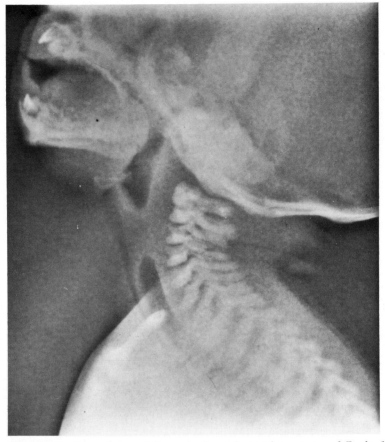

Figure 8–9. Lateral view of the neck of an infant with inspiratory difficulty from birth. The thyroid gland was enlarged and compressed the trachea, seen as a narrow lumen anterior to the esophagus.

Congenital cysts of the larynx may be symptomatic from birth (Holinger et al., 1954). Shackelford and McAlister (1972) described two infants with congenital laryngeal cysts. Both were evident roentgenographically. Direct laryngoscopy confirmed the diagnosis. Needle aspiration of 2 to 3 ml. of clear yellow liquid led to immediate and permanant relief. Radiologic examination showed elevation of the aryepiglottic folds.

External compression of the trachea may also result from lymphangiomas and branchial cleft cysts (Diab and Abu-Jaudeh, 1957). (See page 142.)

AIRWAY OBSTRUCTION ASSOCIATED
WITH OTHER DISORDERS

In the Pierre Robin syndrome (micrognathia and glossoptosis), the tongue may obstruct the nasopharynx and oropharynx when it is

displaced posteriorly. Treatment of the airway obstruction may neces-
sitate tracheostomy (Jeresaty et al., 1969) or prolonged nasoesophageal
intubation (Stern et al., 1972).

Similarly, several patients with the Beckwith-Wiedemann syndrome (exomphalos-macroglossia-gigantism) have been noted to be
cyanotic or apneic (Cohen et al., 1972; MacNamara et al., 1972) presumably because of airway obstruction due to macroglossia (Fig.
8–10).

CONGENITAL LOBAR EMPHYSEMA

Overdistention of one or more lobes of the lung, usually the upper
or right middle lobe, may be noted soon after birth and in some instances presents as acute respiratory distress. More commonly,
respiratory distress is of somewhat later onset, often in the wake of a
mild infection at one or two months of age.

It is implied in emphysema of any sort that there is a defect in the
ability of the lung to deflate normally. Conditions that may contribute
to inadequate deflation are alterations in the elasticity of the lung,
structural defects in the airways which cause them to close when
surrounded by positive pleural pressures, and partial obstruction of
the airway by external compression or intraluminal masses which can
act as a check-valve mechanism. It has not been possible in each case
of congenital lobar emphysema to assign a particular mechanism.
However, there are enough illustrations of several types of mechanisms to establish that lobar emphysema can be traced to different
causes and should be considered a symptom-complex rather than a
disease.

Congenital Deficiency of Bronchial Cartilage

While it is surprising that a deficiency of bronchial cartilage can
be restricted to one lobe, the possibility is clearly demonstrated in a
number of cases. Binet et al. (1962) found mention of abnormal cartilage in 32 of 68 cases reported in the literature. A patient of Holzel's
(1956) was "wheezy" from birth, but became acutely short of breath at
age 11 weeks. Radiographs showed gross overdistention of the left
upper lobe, herniation across the mediastinum to the right, and compression of the left lower lobe. The left upper lobe was resected; on
examination, no cartilage was seen in the medium-sized bronchi, and
only small patches of cartilage were found in the large bronchi (Fig.
8–11). Postoperatively, the infant recovered uneventfully. Other instances of deficient cartilage in a single lobe have been reported by
Nelson (1957), Fischer et al. (1952), and Binet et al. (1962). Lincoln et
al. (1971) found deficient cartilage in 22 of 28 infants in whom lobes
were resected.

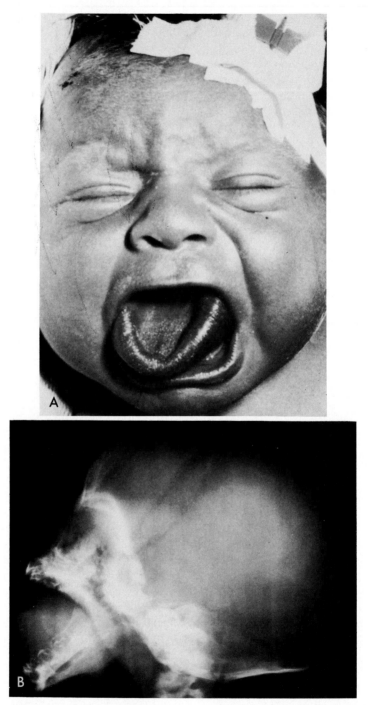

Figure 8–10. Beckwith-Wiedemann syndrome. *A,* Note severe macroglossia. *B,* The tongue is seen radiographically as an anterior soft tissue mass which is obstructing the oropharynx. This patient also had nephromegaly and a large ventral hernia. (Courtesy of Dr. Gilles Perreault, Hôpital Ste. Justine, Montreal.)

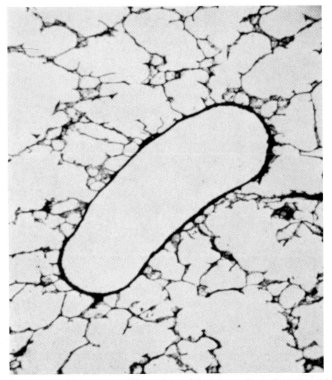

Figure 8–11. Histology of a lobe resected because of emphysema. There is no bronchial cartilage present. (From Holzel et al.: Arch. Dis. Child. *31*:216, 1956.)

Congenital deficiency of bronchial cartilage need not be restricted to one lobe, as is illustrated by the cases of Williams and Campbell (1960). Generalized deficiency of bronchial cartilage in their patients was associated with bronchiectasis as well as emphysema.

Lobar Emphysema from Partial Intraluminal Bronchial Obstruction

Inflammatory exudate or aspirated mucus in a bronchus may act as a check valve that permits air entry when the bronchi are enlarged by subatmospheric pleural pressure but obstructs the egress of air when pleural pressures are higher during expiration. Several such cases were reported by Thomson and Forfar (1958). Two of their infants were symptomatic at birth, one at four weeks of age and the other at 11 weeks. The diagnosis may be suspected if the infant has excessive mucus at birth, or if the symptoms follow an episode of vomiting. Bronchoscopic aspiration of the foreign material may be followed by immediate improvement. Occasionally, symptoms regress spontaneously.

Extraluminal Bronchial Obstruction

Extraluminal compression of a bronchus may also produce partial obstruction with overdistention of one lobe or lung. Figure 8–12 illustrates the marked obstructive emphysema of the left lung in a newborn infant. Death occurred at 24 hours of age, and a large bronchogenic cyst partially compressed the left main bronchus.

Other mediastinal tumors can compress the trachea or bronchi. Teratomas in the anterior mediastinum, neuroblastomas, and mediastinal cysts in the posterior mediastinum have been described in newborn infants, although such tumors are extremely rare (Schaffer, 1960).

The association of lobar emphysema with congenital heart disease was noted by Lincoln et al. (1971) and by Strunge (1972). Only rarely is there anatomical evidence of compression of the bronchus by a vessel. It is uncommon for cardiomegaly in early infancy to be of

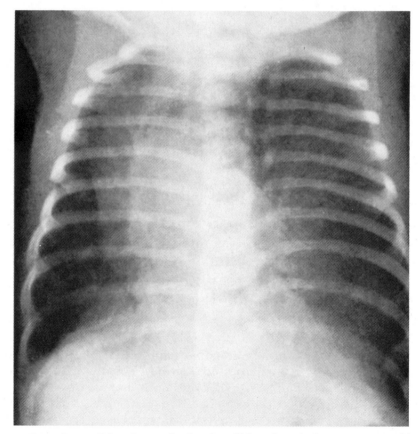

Figure 8–12. Film taken on the first day of life with marked overexpansion of the left lung and shift of the mediastinum to the right. The left upper lobe is overexpanded. Its faint opacity may be attributable to retention of fetal lung liquid. Breath sounds were decreased on the left and normal on the right. The infant died at 24 hours of age from respiratory difficulty owing to extrinsic compression of the left main bronchus by a bronchogenic cyst. (Courtesy of S. Lumpkin, Johns Hopkins Hospital.)

sufficient degree to compress a bronchus and produce a lobar emphysema. Thomson and Forfar (1958) reported an infant of nine months of age in whom there was emphysema of the right middle and lower lobes. The left lower lobe was collapsed by the enlarged heart, and it seems probable that the emphysema on the right was compensatory and not the result of partial obstruction of the bronchi; however, the precise mechanism in this case is unclear. Fischer (1952) reported an infant six and one-half months of age in whom an anomalous pulmonary artery and ductus arteriosus compressed the left bronchus with resultant left upper lobe emphysema. Leape et al. (1970) observed the development of emphysema of the right middle lobe acquired in a patient with patent ductus arteriosus. The cause may have been compression of the middle lobe bronchus by a dilated right pulmonary artery.

Diagnosis. Once suspected, the diagnosis is straightforward. As would be anticipated, the severity of symptoms depends on the degree of overinflation of the affected lobe. Wheezing is characteristic, and in severe cases cyanosis and retractions are present. Breath sounds may be decreased over the affected lobe, and hyperresonance may be evident, although neither sign need be demonstrable in the newborn infant. Displacement of the mediastinum to the contralateral side is usual when marked overdistention is present. The location of the point of maximal impulse of the heart is important as a guide to the possibility of acute changes in the degree of emphysema.

The chest film will show the radiolucent lobe, occasionally herniated across the mediastinum and often compressing the lower lobe on the ipsilateral side. Lobar emphysema cannot always be distinguished radiographically from large cysts. Linear and alveolar densities may be seen in the overexpanded lobe, as in the case of Allen et al. (1966). Histologic examination of that lobe revealed dilated lymphatics and the accumulation of blood in some alveoli. Occasionally the overdistended lobe may be hazy instead of radiolucent and may contain liquid on gross examination (Frankert and Buehl, 1966). Similarly, opaque, rather than aerated, lobes were found in two patients observed by Griscom et al. (1969) who had bronchial obstruction due to bronchogenic cyst and bronchial atresia. Distention of the lobes was due to retained fetal lung liquid.

The need to distinguish between lobar emphysema and associated congenital heart disease may on occasion make angiography desirable. Neches et al. (1972) described one such infant in whom the pulmonary vessels to the emphysematous lobe were dilated and tortuous and delayed the passage of contrast medium. Their infant was one week old at the time of the study, and the affected lobe was not thought to be fully inflated. Staple et al. (1966) described infants with hyperinflated lobes who, on angiography, had stretched, attenuated vessels with little filling of peripheral vessels.

Treatment. No time should be lost in establishing the diagnosis and undertaking treatment if the infant is cyanotic and respirations are labored. Bronchoscopy should be done without delay. Rarely, aspirated mucus or vomitus can be removed to give immediate relief. Excision of the affected lobe is indicated if the infant is not improved by bronchoscopy. It would seem advisable to proceed directly with operation in a symptomatic infant, since it is now clear that defective bronchial cartilage is not uncommon. The operative mortality cited by Fischer et al. (1958) was one in 33 cases, and there were no operative deaths in the 21 cases reported by Leape and Longino (1964). During the same time interval, three infants who were symptomatic in the neonatal period and were not treated by lobectomy died. Occasionally, some wheezing and recurrent infections persist after resection (Sloan, 1953). In the series of Lincoln et al. (1971) from Great Ormand Street during 1954 to 1969, 28 infants were operated on, from ages of a few days to 15 months. Six of this group died, three from their associated congenital heart disease. The authors comment that the follow-up of the treated infants from two months to 14 years shows "surprisingly good" results.

In an asymptomatic infant whose lobar emphysema is discovered, bronchoscopy should be done in the hope of finding a removable obstruction. Lobectomy may be deferred. Some patients may proceed to recovery without therapy, as is illustrated by the patient whose chest film is shown in Figure 8–13. The overdistention of the left upper lobe became less obvious in time, and she has remained asymptomatic.

The long-term prognosis has been thought to be excellent, although very few studies have been published to document that impression. Six patients studied five to 14 years after resection showed a reduction in vital capacity and in diffusion capacity proportional to the amount of lung resected, and an increase in functional residual capacity. Two children had evidence of residual disease, indicated by mild symptoms in one and a significant reduction in the mid-expiratory flow rates of both. These findings suggest that the disease is not always limited to the lobe or lobes most obviously involved in infancy (DeMuth and Sloan, 1966). The ability of previously collapsed lobes to re-expand, however, was demonstrated in a patient who had been followed since infancy and had an emphysematous right upper lobe removed at age 30 years (Ledesma and Girdany, 1972). Roghair (1972) noted the spontaneous return to normal of the chest radiographs of two patients who had lobar emphysema as infants and who were re-examined at ages 16 and 20 years. At the time of follow-up, both were asymptomatic.

ANOMALIES OF THE TRACHEOBRONCHIAL TREE

A wide variety of airway anomalies may be present at birth and may present as stridor or wheezing. If the larynx is involved, the cry

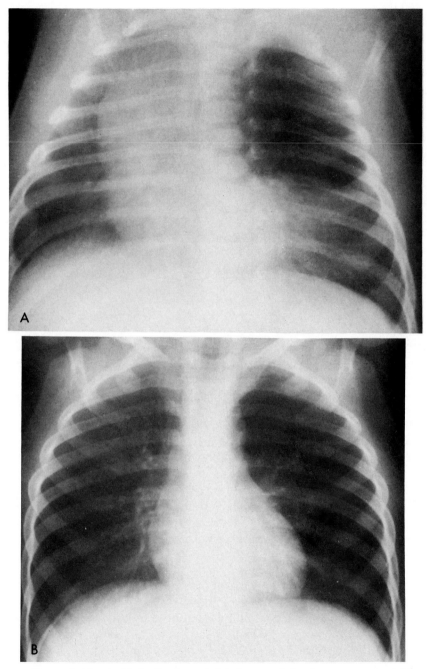

Figure 8–13. A, Markedly distended left upper lobe due to congenital lobar emphysema at three weeks of life. Note displacement of mediastinum to the right. B, At age two and one-half years. There has been relative diminution in amount of air trapped in the left upper lobe, and the patient is asymptomatic.

may be weak or inaudible. This subject has been reviewed by Holinger (1964).

Absence or Deformity of Cartilages

The association of the absence of tracheal or bronchial rings at the site of compression by an aberrant vessel has long been recognized and may account for persistent respiratory symptoms after division of the vessel. Deficiencies or deformities of tracheal cartilage are most often encountered in the cervical segment of the trachea or close to the carina. Occasionally bronchial cartilages are involved, causing lobar or segmental atelectasis. The diagnosis can be suspected from cinefluoroscopy, which may show expansion and collapse of the flaccid trachea, but the marked variations in normal tracheal diameter in different phases of respiration should be kept in mind (Wittenborg et al., 1967). Congenital stenoses of the bronchial cartilages have been noted, presenting as recurrent pneumonia and atelectasis in the first months of life (Litt et al., 1963).

Tracheal Stenosis or Aplasia

Absence of a portion of the trachea is fortunately extremely rare. In a review of this anomaly, Witzleben (1963) noted that the defect was usually associated with a broncho- or tracheoesophageal fistula and, in his case, with multiple anomalies. Even total tracheopulmonary agenesis can occur (Devi and More, 1965) (Fig. 8–14).

The affected infants are usually liveborn; they may gasp but cannot introduce air into the lungs. The longest reported survivor was a patient of Sandison (1955), who lived four hours and 42 minutes and had some air exchange through the fistula which communicated with the esophagus. Intragastric oxygen given to this child probably prolonged life.

As in most congenital malformations, the etiology of the lesion is not known. The major bronchi and the lungs may be normal, and the alveoli may be distended with fluid. The atretic or aplastic portion of the trachea in Witzleben's patient extended from the level of the cricoid cartilage to the carina. No tracheal cartilage or lumen was present. The major bronchi joined in midline, at which point there was communication with the esophagus.

No infants have survived long enough to permit attempts to correct the lesion operatively. Since the lungs are usually normal, it would appear feasible to open the chest and intubate at the distal end of the trachea. The lesion should be suspected when inspiratory efforts fail to move air, and when, on laryngoscopy, the trachea is not visualized below the larynx. Intragastric oxygen is indicated in the hope of prolonging life by flow of air through a fistula long enough for

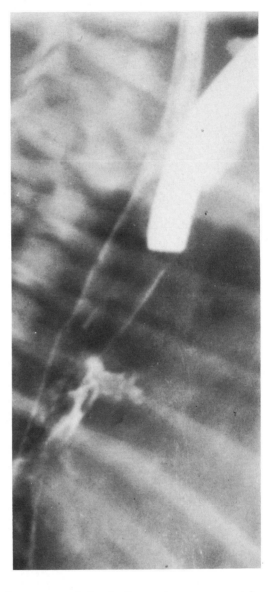

Figure 8-14. Congenital absence of trachea. A nasogastric tube and tracheostomy tube enter the same lumen. Small bronchi are seen arising from the midesophagus.

operative intervention to be accomplished. Operation presumably should be carried out within the first minutes of life to permit survival. Even with intragastric oxygen, most infants do not survive long enough to permit radiologic studies.

Bronchial Atresia

Atresia of a bronchus may be initiated by an intrauterine disturbance of bronchial arterial blood supply (Reid, 1967). In older children and adults it results in a hyperlucent, avascular area of lung, usually in the left upper lobe, associated with a collection of mucus at the site of stenosis. In spite of the apparent congenital nature of this abnormality, this radiologic presentation has not been reported in infants (Genereux, 1971). The expected appearance in the newborn would be a liquid-filled lung distal to the obstruction (see p. 25).

TRACHEOESOPHAGEAL FISTULA

Incidence and Types. Tracheoesophageal fistula is one of the more common congenital anomalies that may cause respiratory symptoms in the newborn period. In a series of infants at Presbyterian Hospital in New York, the incidence of esophageal atresia with and without tracheal fistula was one in 3000 births (Humphreys et al., 1956). Tracheoesophageal fistula is rarely familial. Associated anomalies are common, particularly congenital heart disease (Gross, 1953).

There are at least seven types of related abnormalities, shown schematically in Figure 8–15. The one shown in the upper left corner

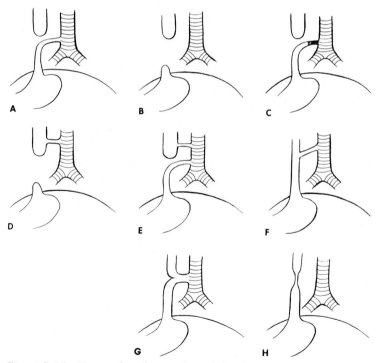

Figure 8–15. Types of tracheoesophageal fistulas. The type labeled A is overwhelmingly the most common, accounting for over 85 per cent of esophageal malformations. B is next most common, and can be distinguished from A by the absence of air in the intestinal tract on roentgenogram. All of the other types have been noted sporadically.

(A) of the diagram is overwhelmingly the most common; it accounted for about 85 per cent of the types observed by Waterston et al. (1963). That in the center top row (B) is next most common, and the others are very rare. The H-type fistula, unassociated with esophageal atresia, accounts for 1.8 to 4 per cent of all tracheoesophageal fistulas.

Clinical Manifestations and Diagnosis. The anomaly should be considered in the presence of maternal hydramnios (Taussig, 1927; Lloyd and Clatworthy, 1958; Waterston et al., 1963). Hydramnios is most common in esophageal atresia in the absence of a fistula, since the amniotic fluid cannot circulate through the fetal gut. Waterston et al. (1963) noted hydramnios in 85 per cent of mothers of infants who had no fistula, and in 32 per cent of mothers of infants with fistulas. Gross (1953) found a high incidence of prematurity among his infants with esophageal atresia. The anomaly is most frequently detected after the first feeding of glucose water, which the infant usually regurgitates immediately and sometimes aspirates with choking and gagging. Abundant oral secretions are common. These symptoms are so characteristic, and recognition of them is so important, that all nursery personnel should be alerted to their significance. With small fistulas, the amount aspirated may be insignificant, but more often there is roentgenographic evidence of pneumonia.

The first diagnostic maneuver is to attempt to pass a catheter into the stomach. In the presence of esophageal atresia, the catheter will meet an obstruction. Since the catheter may curl inside the esophageal pouch, it is useful to inject a little air and listen over the stomach for the expected gurgling. A routine chest film usually confirms the diagnosis. Air in the upper pouch is usually an adequate contrast medium to delineate its blind end (Fig. 8–16A). The presence of a proximal fistula can be excluded by injecting a few drops of bronchographic contrast medium (Fig. 8–16B). If esophageal atresia is present, and there is air in the stomach or intestine, a tracheoesophageal fistula is present (Fig. 8–16C). The absence of air in the stomach, however, does not rule out a small fistula.

The H-type tracheoesophageal fistula poses problems in diagnosis. The classic presentation is severe coughing and choking with feeding, often followed by cyanosis. Bile may be mixed with the bronchial secretions and is noted on suctioning. Another manifestation is abdominal distention caused by air passing from trachea to esophagus. Occasionally infants are not suspected of having H-type fistulas until some months after birth, when the diagnosis is suspected on the basis of recurrent pneumonias. A method of radiographic diagnosis as described by Kappelman et al. (1969) involves the use of a radiopaque catheter introduced through the nose until the tip is in the distal esophagus. A few drops of oily propyliodone (Dionosil) is injected to slightly distend the esophagus. Following this, a thin

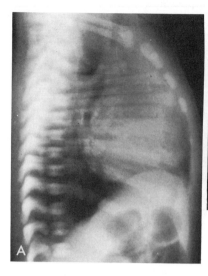

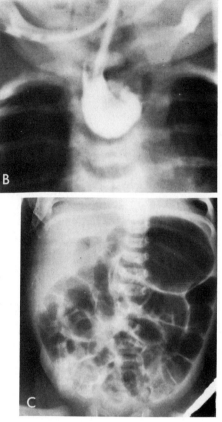

Figure 8–16. A, The distended upper esophageal segment proximal to the
esophageal atresia is outlined with air. *B,*
A small amount of contrast medium demonstrated limits of upper esophageal
pouch. *C,* Generalized gastrointestinal
distention indicates connection between
distal esophageal segment and trachea.
This may also be a presenting finding in
H-type of tracheoesophageal fistula without atresia.

barium suspension may be injected. In lateral projection, a high-
speed cine study will demonstrate the fistula (Fig. 8–17). The fistula
is usually located above the apex of the pleural cavity, making a trans-
cervical operative approach possible. While fistulas without atresia
are rare, they probably constitute 3 to 4 per cent of the anomalies of
the upper esophagus (Haight, 1948) and about 2 per cent of all tracheoesophageal anomalies (Waterston et al., 1963).

Surgical repair should be undertaken as soon as the condition is
recognized and the infant can tolerate the procedure. Gross (1953)
recommends deferring operation for a period of some hours if the infant requires hydration or the associated aspiration pneumonia is extensive. While more than one-half the infants survive operation, recurrent stenosis is common. Obstruction to the passage of swallowed food
above the anastomotic site may present a problem. Persistent abnormal peristaltic activity distal to the anastomosis can lead to reverse
flow with recurrent aspiration (Kirkpatrick et al., 1961).

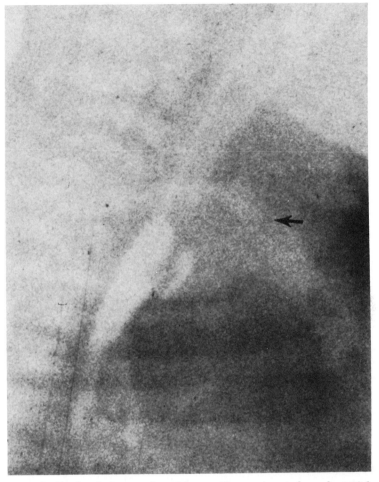

Figure 8–17. Single frame selected from a 16 mm. cine study made at 60 frames per second in direct lateral projection during injection of barium into esophagus shows a connection between esophagus posteriorly and trachea anteriorly. Arrow indicates the approximate level of the clavicles.

LARYNGOTRACHEOESOPHAGEAL CLEFTS

A lesion which presents the same symptoms as those associated with a H-type tracheoesophageal fistula, although much rarer, is a cleft in the posterior wall of the larynx. The defect appears to result from an arrest in the rostral advancement of the tracheoesophageal septum, and from failure of dorsal fusion of the cricoid cartilages, presumably about the 35th gestational day.

The affected infants, only 12 of whom were reported in the literature as of 1965, were symptomatic on the first day of life. Stridor and a

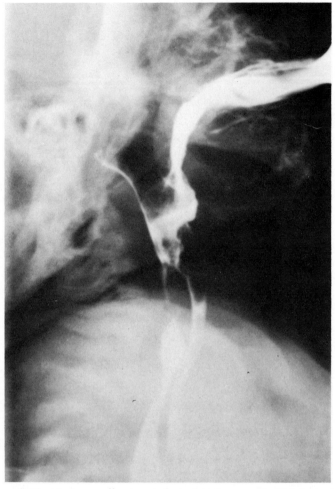

Figure 8–18. A cine-swallowing study in this three-week-old infant with symptoms of recurrent aspiration revealed the communication between trachea and esophagus at the level of the larynx. Vocalization was normal in this infant. He was fed by nasogastric tube for three months and thereafter with thickened oral feedings without further symptoms.

hoarse or feeble cry are usually but not always present, depending on the extent of the defect. Aspiration with feedings occurs regularly. The diagnosis can be established by endoscopy, or cineradiography (Blumberg et al., 1965).

Felman and Talbert (1972) suggest that radiologic examination can be more safely carried out by injection of contrast medium through a catheter with an endotracheal tube in place, so that ventilation and suction can be easily instituted. Unlike H-type tracheoesophageal fistulas, a septum cannot be demonstrated above the communication (Fig. 8–18). Prompt recognition of the problem is essential to

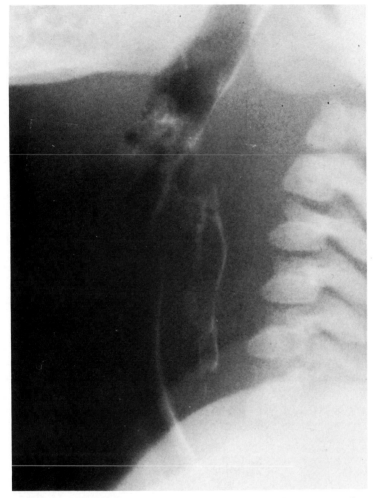

Figure 8–19. A traumatic diverticulum extending from the posterior pharyngeal wall is outlined with barium posterior to the esophagus in this one-month-old infant.

management. Tube feeding or gastrotomy is indicated, and occasionally tracheostomy may be necessary. The tendency to aspirate becomes less as the infant grows, and oral feedings may be well tolerated after the first few months of life. Petterson (1955) reported the first survivor of operative repair of the cleft. Since then, there have been at least five other successful corrections (Geiger et al., 1970).

Persistent esophagotrachea which results from failure of division of the trachea and esophagus as far inferiorly as the carina is "the most severe degree of laryngoesophageal cleft" (Griscom, 1960). This severe malformation is not compatible with life.

TRAUMATIC ESOPHAGEAL PSEUDODIVERTICULA

Pseudodiverticula of the pharynx may produce symptoms similar to those of esophageal atresia and can impede the passage of an
esophageal catheter. Eklof et al. (1969) and Girdany et al. (1969) have
proposed that the lesion is traumatic in etiology, resulting from the
passage of a nasogastric tube or possibly the insertion of the obstetrician's finger into the infant's mouth during delivery of the after-
coming head in a breech presentation.

The pseudodiverticula can be readily visualized radiologically on
contrast examination. They extend from the posterior aspect of the
pharynx or esophagus for a variable distance inferiorly into the neck
and mediastinum (Fig. 8–19). The esophagus is patent, but if there is
associated cricopharyngeal spasm, the opaque material may not enter
the true esophagus, thus confusing the diagnosis (Ducharme et al.,
1971). Unlike traumatic pseudodiverticula, congenital duplications of
the esophagus arise anteriorly (Sidaway, 1964) and frequently present
as a mediastinal mass.

Spontaneous healing of traumatic pseudodiverticula has occurred
(Eklof, 1969) so that surgical intervention may not be necessary.

Chapter Nine

INTRATHORACIC
LESIONS

In addition to lesions that become apparent largely because of their effects on the airways, as discussed in the preceding chapter, the newborn infant may have a number of lesions in the mediastinum or lungs that compromise respiration largely because they occupy space or contain vascular anomalies that adversely affect the circulation.

MEDIASTINAL MASSES

A congenital malformation is the most likely explanation for a mediastinal mass, other than the thymus, in infancy. Although rare, enteric cysts are responsible for most mediastinal masses in the first months of life, and more than 100 have been reported.

Neurenteric Cysts

Cysts of enteric origin, often lined with gastric mucosa, are located in the posterior mediastinum. The symptoms vary with the size and location of the lesion and may relate to the gastrointestinal tract or the upper airway. Occasionally cysts are asymptomatic. Connections may exist with the stomach or small intestine but rarely with the esophagus. Associated anomalies have been reported, most commonly fusion of vertebrae, hemivertebrae, and spina bifida. The preferred treatment is excision, since ulceration with hemorrhage has been noted (Spock et al., 1966).

141

Teratomas

Usually anterior in position, teratomas are among the more common masses found in infants. Occasionally amorphous masses of calcium are evident radiologically; more commonly the diagnosis is made on thoracotomy. Malignant degeneration can occur (Ellis et al., 1955).

Neurogenic Tumors

Posterior mediastinal masses may be described by neurogenic origin and lie in the superior, mid-, or inferior mediastinum. Histologically they can be ganglioneuromas, neurofibromas, or neuroblastomas (Fig. 9–1).

Cystic Hygromas

These comparatively rare lesions are usually found in the neck, but they may extend into the superior mediastinum and produce respiratory distress (Bratu et al., 1970; Schapiro and Evans, 1972).

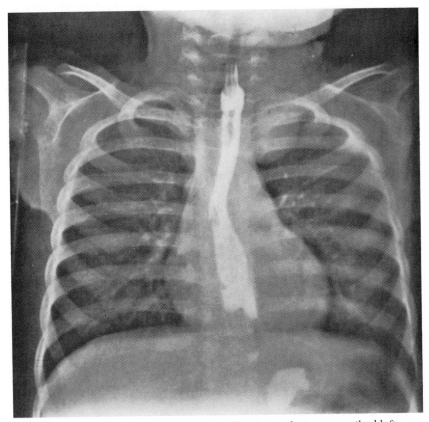

Figure 9–1. Chest film of a 16-month-old infant with a circumscribed left upper lobe mass, which was found to be a neuroblastoma when resected.

Bronchogenic Cysts

The symptoms of bronchogenic cysts are usually periodic episodes of wheezing and stridor, often aggravated by crying. Recurrent infection is common with fever, cough, and infiltration of the lung.

Not infrequently, the cyst itself may not be visible on a chest radiograph. Opsahl and Berman (1962), in their review of bronchogenic mediastinal cysts, noted that the lesion was demonstrable on the chest film in only 14 of 25 symptomatic cases. However, because of their position in the middle mediastinum, bronchogenic cysts may cause severe airway obstruction, with emphysema or atelectasis, independent of their size. When the mass is not visualized on plain films it can be suspected on a lateral esophagram if posterior displacement of the esophagus and anterior displacement of the trachea is seen at the level of the carina (Eraklis et al., 1969). This closely resembles the deformity caused by a pulmonary artery sling (see also page 118).

Other Tumors

Hemangiomas and angiosarcomas have been located at any position in the mediastinum. Occasionally hemangiomas are disseminated through lungs, mediastinum, viscera, and central nervous system. At least 8 infants with diffuse neonatal hemangiomatosis have been reported as of 1970 (Holden and Alexander). Mediastinal goiters and thymomas can occur, although very rarely. In the series of Ellis et al. (1955), which included infants and children, nine of 45 mediastinal tumors were malignant. Exploratory thoracotomy is thus indicated only when a diagnosis cannot otherwise be made. Other rare intrathoracic tumors are mesenchymomas which are large calcium-containing masses which cause erosion of the ribs (Blumenthal et al., 1972) and intrathoracic lipomas which may be recognized because of the relative radiolucency due to their high fat content (Shawker et al., 1972).

PULMONARY ARTERIOVENOUS FISTULA

A life-threatening but potentially curable cause of persistent cyanosis is an arteriovenous fistula in the lungs. Abnormal communications between pulmonary arteries and veins may be single or multiple, are located most commonly but not necessarily in the lower lobes, and are associated with hemangiomas of the skin in about half the reported cases (Kafka et al., 1961).

The disorder has rarely been recognized in newborn infants. The infant reported by Hall et al. in 1965 was in severe respiratory distress at birth, with grunting, cyanosis, and tachycardia. A harsh systolic murmur heard at birth had become continuous by five hours of age.

Evidence of left ventricular preponderance was seen on ECG. The chest film showed an ill-defined density at the base of the left lung, which was proved to be a vascular malformation with angiography. Resection of the left lower lobe resulted in prompt relief of all symptoms.

LUNG CYSTS

Cysts in the lungs of stillborn and newborn infants are not common, but they can be symptomatic in the newborn period and are, on occasion, operable. The classifications of lung cysts are almost as numerous as the authors who write them. For example, they have been classified as symptomatic or asymptomatic (Brunner et al., 1960); as derived from airspaces, lymphatics, or pleural elements (Moffat, 1960); as congenital or acquired, with multiple subclassifications (Spencer, 1962); or as multiple or solitary (Potter, 1961).

It would seem to be of central importance to recognize that cysts of many sorts may be present as congenital malformations; to distinguish acquired from congenital cysts; to inquire of the natural history of each sort; to know which may be familial; and to search for the pathogenesis of acquired cysts.

Congenital Cysts

Caffey (1953) pointed out the rarity of congenital lung cysts. He reported 13 cases demonstrated before the age of six months, and he followed them roentgenographically. Ultimate disappearance of the cysts in eight infants suggested that the cysts were not the result of a congenital malformation but that they represented acquired pneumatoceles. No cysts were found in a series of 500 chest films from unselected newborn infants. Only one lung cyst was seen in a stillborn infant, and none were found in neonates over a 22-year period at Babies Hospital in New York. Caffey challenged the belief that cysts in the lungs of young infants were always congenital and, by implication, irreversible.

It is often very difficult to decide whether a cyst which is first noted after the newborn period is congenital or acquired. The histologic finding of a lining of ciliated columnar epithelium has been cited as evidence for the congenital origin of a cyst. However, the studies of Pryce (1948) cast doubt on this assumption. He found resected cavities lined by ciliated columnar epithelium in two patients whose lungs had previously been normal on roentgenogram. Conway's suggestion (1951) seems pertinent. He said, "A congenital etiology is obvious when cysts are found in stillborn or newly delivered infants, but in any other age group definite malformation must be observed which could not have arisen from an acquired pathology."

Etiology. While it is difficult to assign an etiologic agent or event in the pathogenesis of congenital lung cysts, as it is in the most congenital malformations, it is generally true that lung cysts are not associated with cystic lesions in other organs or with any other single malformation elsewhere. They are sometimes associated with bronchostenosis or abnormalities of the pulmonary artery (Spencer, 1962). The lesion is not familial, nor is it restricted to one sex.

A peculiarly high frequency of cystic changes in the lung has been noted in Israel, especially among peoples from Yemen and Iraq, which suggests an ethnic association. The pathologic changes were more consistent with a congenital defect than an acquired one, although further study of these patients is needed (Baum et al., 1966).

The more common type of congenital cyst is in the lung periphery and probably represents a disorder of bronchial growth at a later stage in fetal life than the more central bronchogenic cysts. The peripheral cysts may or may not communicate with the bronchi. Their walls contain some irregular plates of cartilage and elastic tissue, but are rarely muscular. They may be solitary or multiple, and sometimes honeycomb the lungs. A patient of Clark et al. (1956) showed diffuse involvement of one lung with multiple cysts that contained air and displaced the mediastinum to the opposite side. Pneumonectomy on the ninth day of life was followed by adequate expansion of the normal lung and recovery.

Cysts arising from the major bronchi may partially obstruct the bronchus and present as lobar emphysema. Not infrequently, the cyst itself may not be visible on a chest film. Opsahl and Berman (1962), in their review of bronchiogenic mediastinal cysts, noted that the lesion was demonstrable on the chest film in only 14 of 25 symptomatic cases.

The symptoms of bronchiogenic cysts are usually periodic episodes of wheezing and stridor, often aggravated by crying. Recurrent infection is common with fever, cough, and infiltration of the lung. When the diagnosis is suspected, a swallow of contrast media may show displacement of the esophagus. Bronchograms will delineate the cyst if it communicates with the bronchus or will reveal narrowing of the bronchus by compression. The cysts may change in size, and hence produce changes in the radiograph as a function of the degree of bronchial obstruction. Complete obstruction will result in resorption atelectasis, partial obstruction in overdistention of the affected lobe.

Acquired Cysts in Infancy

Many patients previously reported as having congenital cysts of the lung which became infected probably had pneumatoceles in the wake of staphylococcal pneumonia. The sudden appearance of a radiolucent area in the lung of an infant with fever and cough is well known in staphylococcal pneumonia, and occasionally in pneumococ-

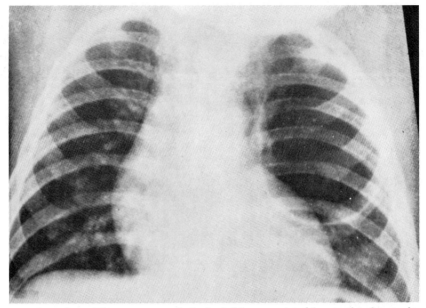

Figure 9-2. This pneumatocele in the left lung persisted for months after staphylococcal pneumonia, but eventually disappeared. The patient had no chest problems over the subsequent four years of follow-up.

cal, *E. coli,* or streptococcal pneumonias. While it is the rule for such cyst-like distortions of the lung to change in size during the disease, and often to regress completely, some become infected and pus-containing and may persist for weeks until adequately drained. Some of the patients reported by Ravitch and Hardy (1949) doubtless belong in the group of patients with staphylococcal pneumonia. The youngest patient in their series was 13 weeks of age, the oldest 13 years; it is impossible to rule out initial infection in many of them. Those with a trilobed left lung or aberrant vessels probably had congenital cysts, on the basis of the likely coexistence of combined pulmonary abnormalities.

Schenck's review (1936) of 232 cases of lung cysts revealed 38 with other malformations, 17 of which were accessory lobes of the lung. It is not possible to distinguish congenital from acquired cysts in the remainder of this series.

It seems probable that acquired cysts are more common than congenital ones, at least in localities where staphylococcal disease is prevalent. The importance of recognizing the etiology of the cyst is apparent from the difference in their natural courses. Figure 9-2 illustrates the radiographic appearance of a pneumatocele acquired in the course of staphylococcal pneumonia. Its persistence for weeks after the infant became asymptomatic would have raised the possibility of a congenital etiology, but it ultimately disappeared. By con-

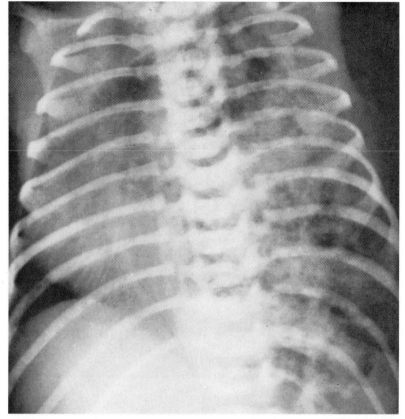

Figure 9–3. This term infant was cyanotic and tachypneic at birth. The film at 30 hours of age showed the extensive cystic malformation of the left lung, which was mistakenly diagnosed in a small community hospital as diaphragmatic hernia. At operation at 48 hours of age, the nature of the malformation was appreciated, and the chest was closed.

trast, Figure 9–3 illustrates the appearance of an extensive congenital cystic malformation of the left lung. This infant underwent operation for suspected diaphragmatic hernia in the newborn period, only to reveal a grossly malformed lung. The lung was not resected, so it has been possible to follow the course of the disease. Figure 9–4 shows the diminution in relative size of the cysts, but nevertheless their persistence for nine years as the remainder of the lung has grown. This child has remained asymptomatic and has had no pulmonary infections.

Treatment. Resection is indicated if the infant is symptomatic at birth from the presence of a space-occupying mass in the lungs. Otherwise, potentially normal portions of the lung cannot be adequately ventilated, and death from hypoventilation may occur. If a cyst is present and in communication with the airway, the probability of infection is sufficiently great that resection is indicated. The prog-

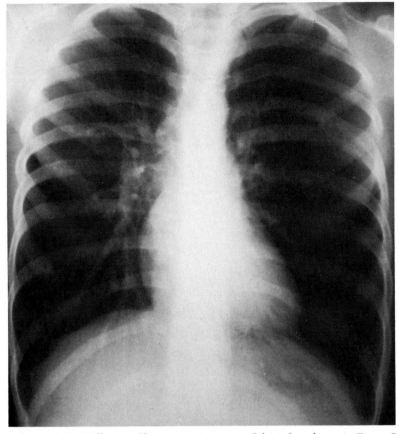

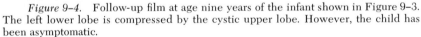

Figure 9–4. Follow-up film at age nine years of the infant shown in Figure 9–3. The left lower lobe is compressed by the cystic upper lobe. However, the child has been asymptomatic.

nosis of infants is better if they are treated operatively for bronchogenic mediastinal cysts (Opsahl and Berman, 1962). The treatment of infants with asymptomatic cysts not in communication with the airway is more debatable. It has been our feeling that operation is indicated, on the basis of our lack of knowledge of the natural course of such lesions and the possibility of enlargement or compression of normal lung.

In summary, then, operative resection of cysts is urgent if the infant is acutely symptomatic; it is desirable and carries a better prognosis than medical management if the infant is symptomatic in any way at all; it is probably advisable if the cyst communicates with the airway because of the risk of infection; and resection is done for asymptomatic cysts not communicating with the airway because of the compromise to expansion of normal lung and the remote risk of its being a solid tumor.

CONGENITAL CYSTIC ADENOMATOID
MALFORMATION OF THE LUNG

Stoerk in 1897 first reported a rare form of congenital cystic disease of the lung, characterized by a mass of cysts lined by proliferating bronchial or cuboidal epithelium and interposed between normal portions of lung. At least 35 cases have been described since then with at least seven survivors (Spector et al., 1960; Kwitten and Reiner, 1962; Belanger et al., 1964; Holder and Christy, 1964).

Onset and Symptoms. The affected infants are often born prematurely, with the onset of symptoms in the reported cases usually at birth or in the first weeks of life. The disorder has occurred in all lobes of the lung, although it has rarely been bilateral in a given patient. In one infant of 1.55 kg., the opposite lung was hypoplastic (Spector et al., 1960). There is no suggestion of a familial predisposition to this malformation, and both males and females are affected.

The symptoms are those of acute respiratory distress with tachypnea, cyanosis, and sometimes labored breathing. Displacement of the mediastinum may be present. Nearly half of the reported patients have had anasarca, and hydramnios was present in seven. However, infants with associated anasarca have usually been stillborn (Ch'In and Tang, 1949).

Radiographic Features. An intrapulmonary mass is evident, often with scattered radiolucent areas. The involved lung frequently herniates to the opposite side (Fig. 9–5).

Pathology. The affected lobe is greatly increased in size and weight, and the usual lobular septation is lacking. There is a polypoid proliferation of respiratory epithelium, an absence of cartilage plates in the bronchioles, and, sometimes, communication of a portion of the deformed lung with the airway. Aberrant vessels to the malformed lung are not a feature of this syndrome as they are in a sequestered lobe, such aberration being presumably the result of an insult at an earlier embryonic period (Kwitten, 1962). In some cases, there is an excess of elastic tissue in the walls of the cyst. A single case of hamartoma of the lung in a premature infant who died at one hour of age was reported by Jones (1949).

Therapy. Prompt resection is indicated to prevent further compression of normal lung if the infant shows symptoms (Craig et al., 1956).

CONGENITAL PULMONARY LYMPHANGIECTASIS

A condition only recently brought to the attention of pediatricians as unusual but not extremely rare is a congenital dilatation of the lymphatic vessels of the lungs. The lesions may be restricted to the

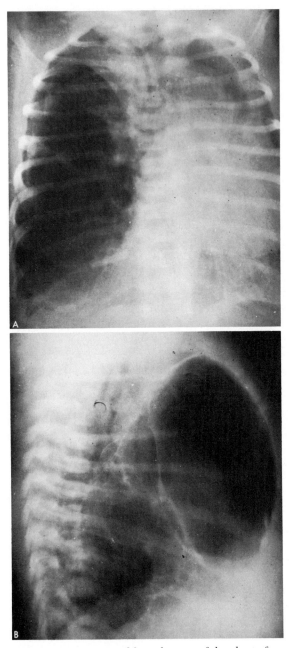

Figure 9–5. Anteroposterior and lateral views of the chest of a one-week-old infant with respiratory distress from birth. The cystic adenomatoid malformation in the right lower lobe was removed at operation, with recovery of the infant. (Courtesy of Dr. E. Ide Smith; Children's Mercy Hospital, Kansas City, Mo.)

lungs or may be associated with lymphedema of other portions of the body and intestinal lymphangiectasis. In over half the cases coming to autopsy, congenital malformations of the heart have been found (Laurence, 1959; Giammalvo, 1955).

The probability that abnormal dilatation of the lung lymphatics may exist in several different conditions was supported by Noonan et al. (1970). In a very careful study of three patients, they found two with obstructed total anomalous venous return and a ventricular septal defect in the third. After a review of 45 patients described in the literature, they concluded that pulmonary lymphangiectasis may occur as part of a generalized lymphangiectasis, secondary to pulmonary venous obstruction, or as a primary developmental defect of the lung. Absence of other lesions was the case in 30 of the 45 patients reviewed.

Symptoms. All of the 13 infants who were studied at autopsy by Laurence had respiratory distress with cyanosis at birth or shortly after. Most of them were at term, and both males and females were affected. The longest survival among Laurence's patients was eight days.

Two of the three patients described by Le Tan Vinh et al. in 1964 were cyanotic from the time of birth and died shortly thereafter. The third lived for three months, and had associated congenital heart disease, including a single ventricle and anomalous venous return. At least one child, in whom the diagnosis was confirmed by lung biopsy, was alive at age nine months, although subject to episodic wheezing and cough (Javett et al., 1963). Several children with intestinal lymphangiectasis have been found to have radiographically evident pulmonary lymphangiectasis in the absence of signs or symptoms of lung dysfunction.

Radiologic Findings. The radiologic features are somewhat variable, possibly depending on the presence of associated pulmonary or cardiovascular abnormalities. The lungs are frequently hyperaerated and may present a "ground-glass" appearance (Noonan et al., 1970). Carter (1961) described fine, diffuse granular densities representing dilated lymphatics. A reticular pattern of prominent interstitial markings correlates with the pathologic findings of dilated lymphatic channels (Theros, 1967).

Pathology. The lungs are bulky, with pronounced lobulation (Fig. 9–6). The subpleural lymphatics are prominent, and on cut section cystic dilatation of the lymphatics is apparent. Serous fluid may ooze from the cut surface. The interlobular septa are thickened and simulate fibrosis. On histologic examination it is evident from the distribution of the cystic spaces close to blood vessels and bronchi that they are dilated lymphatic vessels (Fig. 9–7). The diffuse nature of the lesion distinguishes it from the even rarer intrapulmonary lymphangioma. Chylothorax has not been described in association with

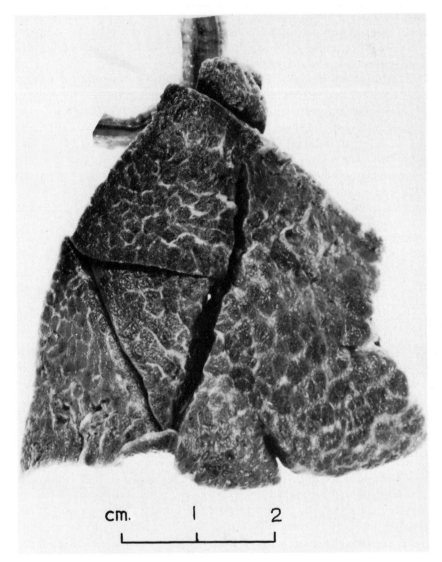

Figure 9-6. Lung of an infant with congenital lymphangiectasis. Note the marked dilatation of the subpleural lymphatics. (From Laurence, K. M.: J. Clin. Path. 12:62, 1959.)

lymphangiectasis, although it might be expected in association with disordered lymphatic drainage (see page 263).

Etiology. Laurence (1959) suggested that the disturbance in development was the failure or cessation of growth of the lymphatic trunks in the septa. The tissue elements in the lungs of these infants at term have approximately the same relationships as are found at 16 weeks' gestation, except for more alveolar proliferation than would be found at 16 weeks. Since the lymphatics originate as discrete spaces in the mesenchyme and later fuse to form endothelium-lined channels,

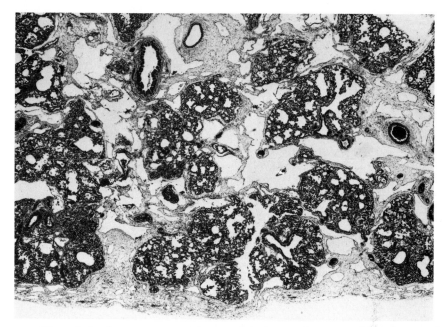

Figure 9–7. Low-power magnification of the lung with congenital lymphangiectasis. (From Laurence, K. M.: J. Clin. Path. *12*:62, 1959.)

it seems possible that an arrest in development could produce the cystic changes as suggested by Giammalvo (1955). The lesion is surely present at birth in most, if not all, instances and has been described in a stillborn infant who also had dilated lymphatics in other organs and generalized edema (Frank and Piper, 1959). The disorder is not known to be familial.

AGENESIS AND HYPOPLASIA

Primary Agenesis

The whole of one or both lungs may be absent; a rudimentary bronchus may exist with no pulmonary or vascular tissue around it; or there may be a poorly developed bronchus in a mass of ill-defined pulmonary tissue.

Bilateral agenesis of the lung is extremely rare, fortunately, and is not known to be familial. Claireaux and Ferreira (1958) described a term male infant who lived 15 minutes and made gasping efforts. At autopsy, the trachea was seen to end blindly, and no pulmonary tissue was present. The pulmonary artery joined the aorta. No pulmonary veins or bronchial arteries were present. The gasping efforts which this infant made prove that the absence of stretch receptors from the lung does not interfere with the stimuli for the first breath.

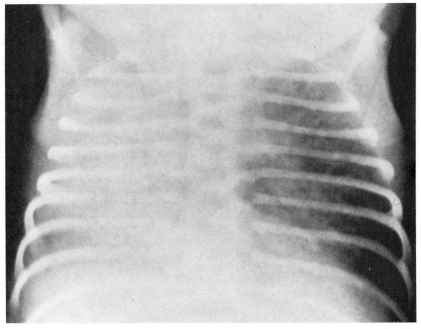

Figure 9–8. This infant has absence of the right lung with displacement of the mediastinal structures to the right.

Unilateral agenesis of the lung is much more frequent and may be familial. In a review of 85 cases, Wexels (1951) noted that nearly half of the patients had associated congenital anomalies (Fig. 9–8).

The left lung is more frequently absent than the right. In cases studied at autopsy, the trachea appears to continue directly into a main bronchus. The remaining lung is larger than normal and often herniates into the contralateral chest.

The diagnosis of unilateral agenesis of the lung should be suspected when a patient with a symmetric or nearly symmetric chest has a marked deviation of the trachea to one side, with rotation of the mediastinal contents. Breath sounds may be heard over the portions of the affected side into which the remaining lung was herniated, although they are usually absent in the subaxillary area. Smart (1946) found no abnormalities in the spirograms or pleural pressures in his patients, which suggests that the enlargement of the remaining lung was not associated with emphysematous changes but, rather, was the result of hypertrophy. If the lung is absent altogether, cyanosis will not be present.

Agenesis of a lobe of the lung is very rare and may be asymptomatic. The patient of Storey and Marrangoni (1954) with congenital absence of the left lower lobe was 19 years old before he developed symptoms of bronchiectasis in the left upper lobe. The oldest patient cited by Oyamada et al. in their review was 72 years (1953).

Hypoplastic Lungs

Hypoplastic lungs are most often associated with other congenital malformations, chief among which is diaphragmatic hernia. Presumably, the upward displacement of a hemidiaphragm by abdominal viscera, or herniation of the viscera into the chest, interferes with lung growth on the affected side. The incidence of the association of hypoplastic lung in diaphragmatic herniation is not established, although the report of 10 instances in a series of 24 infants operated on by Roe and Stephens (1956) suggests that it is not unusual (Sabga et al., 1961). The degree of hypoplasia depends on the degree of reduction in thoracic size (Potter, 1961). With a moderate degree of herniation, the lung may be normal histologically although it is under the expected weight. Retardation in pulmonary differentiation is apparent with more severe restriction in thoracic size. The number of bronchial branchings is reduced, although each bronchus may lead to a normal number of alveoli (Areechon and Reid, 1963).

deLorimier et al. (1967) produced diaphragmatic hernias surgically in fetal lambs. At term, the animals had hypoplastic lungs with low lung weights, diminished distensibility, and immature pressure-volume characteristics.

In a follow-up study of 14 children whose hernias had been repaired in infancy, Chatrath et al. (1971) noted normal static lung volumes, but a reduction in the forced expiratory volumes. These data suggest a persistent ventilatory defect consistent with lower airway obstructive disease and compensatory overdistention of airspaces.

Another malformation associated with hypoplastic lungs is renal agenesis, first described by Potter (1946), and often referred to as Potter's syndrome. The alveoli may be almost absent, and the lung poorly vascularized. About three-fourths of the affected infants are males, and have, in addition to the lethal renal and pulmonary malformations, large low-set ears. Oligohydramnios is regularly associated with this syndrome. Other anomalies may coexist, especially in the genital system. The facies is characteristic, with an expression of old age and with prominent epicanthic folds, flattened nose, and low-set floppy ears. The placenta characteristically has multiple nodules or plaques on the fetal surface. A right-to-left shunt exists with arterial unsaturation and cyanosis when hypoplastic lungs are perfused but not ventilated (Oyamada et al., 1953). Such patients not infrequently also have malformations of the heart (Ferencz, 1961), so that without angiography cyanosis should not be ascribed to the intrapulmonary shunt. If the shunt is restricted to the lung, the patients will be benefited by resection of the vestigial lung. Resection may be indicated in the presence of congenital heart disease, although the outlook depends on the nature of the cardiac malformation.

An unusual variety of hypoplastic lung with systemic arterial supply and venous drainage into the inferior vena cava—the "scimitar syndrome"—was reported in a father and daughter by Neill et al.

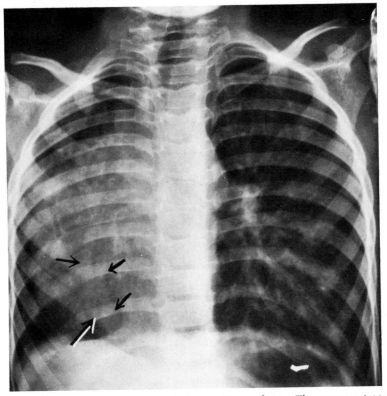

Figure 9–9.   Film of a patient with the scimitar syndrome. The arrows point to the scimitar-like anomalous trunk (this area retouched slightly) that empties into the inferior vena cava. The right lung is hypoplastic.

(1960). The father was asymptomatic, but the daughter had marked dextroposition of the heart and pulmonary hypertension and died after a pneumonectomy. The syndrome may be suspected from the chest roentgenogram, which shows a "scimitar"-shaped shadow of an anomalous pulmonary vein along the right border of the heart, with a shift of the heart to the right (Fig. 9–9). Associated cardiac malformations were present in eight of 22 cases in children reviewed by Jue et al. (1966). The lower lobe of the hypoplastic right lung may be perfused by an aberrant artery from the subdiaphragmatic portion of the aorta.

About 150 cases of this syndrome had been reported by 1971, mostly in adults without symptoms. The condition has rarely been diagnosed in infancy, although Park in 1912 described the condition at autopsy in a two-and-one-half-month old infant. Mortensson and Lundstrom's patient was an infant in whom heart failure was evident by nine days of age. The right atrium and ventricle were enlarged. The heart was dextropositioned and the left pulmonary vessels were

Table 9–1.   Differences between Accessory and Sequestered Lobes

	Intralobar Sequestration	*Accessory Lobe*
Arterial supply	Large vessels from aorta	Small and variable vessels
Venous drainage	To pulmonary vein	To azygous vein
Connection with foregut	None	Sometimes
Side	60 per cent left	90 per cent left
Diagnosis at neonatal autopsy	None	Frequent
Anatomical relations	Constant and intralobar	Variable
Associated anomaly	None	Frequent

prominent. At angiography, there was no right pulmonary artery. The right lung was perfused by arteries that arose from the abdominal aorta, and drained into the inferior vena cava. Since the infant did not respond to medical management, a right pneumonectomy was performed. It was noted that most of the lung was adherent to the thoracic wall. She did well until one year of age when she died of aspiration. No other lesions were noted at autopsy.

ACCESSORY AND SEQUESTERED LOBES

The distinction between accessory lobes (extralobar sequestrations) and sequestered lobes (intralobar sequestrations) is useful. Spencer (1962) considers accessory lobes to consist of pulmonary tissue that is separated from the rest of the lung by a pleural investment, although such lobes may communicate with the major bronchi, the trachea, or portions of the gut. Sequestered lobes, on the other hand, are considered separately as portions of pulmonary tissue which do not have the usual relations to the rest of the lung but which may be intralobar. Smith (1956) suggested that intralobar sequestrations originated from a disturbance of the blood supply to a portion of the lung, whereas accessory lobes represented an earlier defect in lung development. His argument was based on differences in the two conditions as shown in Table 9–1. Gerle et al. (1968) however, suggest that intralobar and extralobar sequestration have a common embryogenesis and should be collectively termed congenital bronchopulmonary foregut malformations. One type of accessory lobe is a lower lobe, sometimes called a diaphragmatic lobe, because it usually is a smooth, rounded mass lying above the dome of the diaphragm and below the inferior surface of the lung. It is not attached to the lung and derives its blood supply from an artery from the aorta. Histologically, it shows bronchi, alveoli, and bits of cartilage, although the architecture is distorted. Usually diagnosed on chest film, these lobes are characteristically asymptomatic. They have been resected as mediastinal

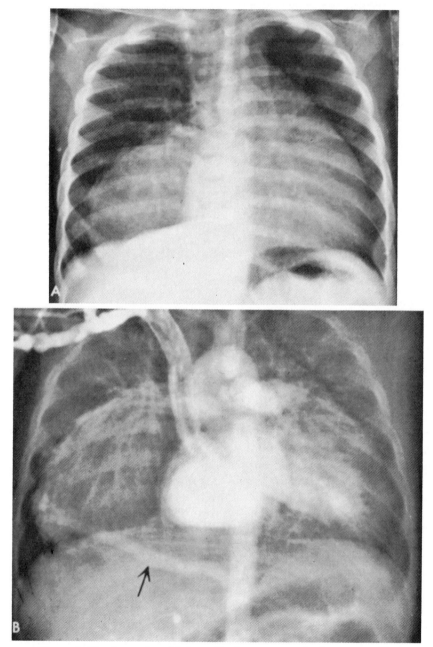

Figure 9–10. Sequestered lobe with aberrant vessels from aorta. The arrow points to the anomalous artery.

tumors because of the uncertainty as to their identity (DeBakey et al., 1950).

Other accessory lobes may have bronchial or gut attachments. Occasionally, an extra bronchus leads to pulmonary tissue, which is usually malformed, resembling a hamartoma, as in the case of Thomas (1949). An accessory right bronchus from the trachea was noted by Cotton et al. (1952). In this case, the bronchus led to an accessory lung, with three lobes and a pleural covering. The remaining lung on the same side had only two lobes, but after resection it filled the right hemithorax. Accessory pulmonary tissue may arise from portions of the foregut, just as the primitive lung does in embryogenesis. Scheidegger (1936) found an accessory lobe of lung connected to the stomach by a tube lined with gastric mucosa which passed through the diaphragm. Others have noted aberrant lung tissue attached to the esophagus (Gans and Potts, 1951). Lane et al. (1971) demonstrated a bronchopulmonary foregut malformation on an esophagram which showed a partially intrathoracic stomach communicating with a pulmonary sequestration above the left diaphragmatic dome.

The most common form of sequestration is a portion of lung incorporated in a lower lobe of an otherwise normal lung. The sequestered portion is not in communication with the bronchi and has an independent blood supply from one or more vessels arising from the aorta (Fig. 9–10). The atelectatic mass of lung may be replaced by a collection of cysts; thus, many cases have been reported under the heading of congenital cystic disease of the lung. Kergin (1952) reported a series of adults with intralobar sequestrations that had undergone cystic changes. His patients were not symptomatic in childhood.

Rarely respiratory distress in the newborn may result from a sequestered lobe that impairs ventilation of normal lung. Klein (1970) reported an infant who was symptomatic from birth and in whom a sequestered left lower lobe was resected at 36 hours of age. The arterial supply of this lobe arose from the celiac axis below the diaphragm. The infant recovered completely after the resection. Severe symptoms in the first days of life necessitated exploration for a presumed eventration of the diaphragm in the case of Pearl (1972). In addition to the eventration, an extralobar mass, perfused by vessels from the aorta, was found occupying more than 80 per cent of the left hemithorax.

Chapter Ten

ABNORMALITIES OF
THE DIAPHRAGM
AND CHEST WALL

Lesions of the diaphragm, rib cage, intercostal muscles, or other muscles of respiration can be present at birth and cause respiratory distress. Although usually in the category of congenital malformations, they include infectious processes and metabolic derangements. The diagnosis of a "chest wall" problem is often evident on inspection, as in the case of a bifid sternum or a chondrodystrophy. A prominent chest and a scaphoid abdomen should support displacement of abdominal contents into the thoracic cage, as in diaphragmatic hernia. The diagnosis of muscle weakness is not as straightforward but should be suspected when the infant is unable to make strenuous respiratory efforts on stimulation. In such an event, either central nervous system depression or muscle weakness must be present. They can be distinguished on the basis of history and assessment of the alertness of the infant.

CONGENITAL EVENTRATION OF THE DIAPHRAGM

In this condition, one leaf of the diaphragm has defective musculature and balloons as a thin aponeurotic sheet high in the chest. All degrees of involvement exist, so that some patients are asymptomatic throughout life, whereas others die shortly after birth. In the latter group, pulmonary hypoplasia is probably a major problem, as it is in congenital diaphragmatic hernia.

The diagnosis is established on roentgenographic examination (Fig. 10–1). Synchronous motion is present in at least half of these pa-

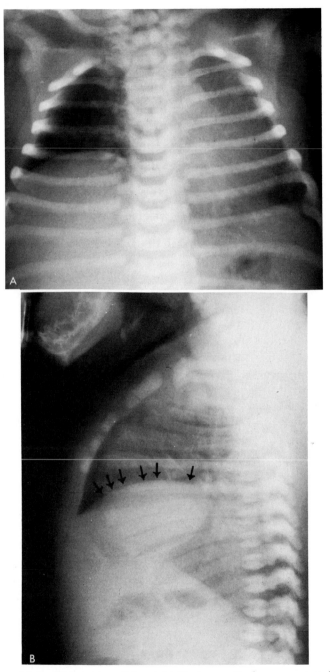

Figure 10–1. Eventration of the right diaphragmatic dome, causing shift of the mediastinal structures to the left (A). On the lateral view (B), the arrows point to the elevated dome.

tients (Laxdal et al., 1954). In those in whom paradoxical movement is present, differentiation from phrenic nerve paralysis cannot be made.

The evidence supporting the concept that defective diaphragmatic musculature is a congenital defect is that it can occur in the fetus and that it is frequently associated with other congenital anomalies.

Treatment is rarely necessary. Plication can be done if there is atelectasis or respiratory embarrassment.

ACCESSORY DIAPHRAGM

A muscular and tendinous membrane that partitions a hemithorax is an extremely rare anomaly. Hashida and Sherman (1961) reported an infant who was in respiratory distress at birth and died shortly thereafter. At autopsy, an accessory diaphragm was found to separate the right upper lobe from the middle and lower lobes. Their patient was the only one reported as symptomatic at birth.

In the eight other cases reviewed by Davis and Allen (1968), hypoplasia of a lobe or anomalous vascular supply was present in three. The roentgen features included displacement of the mediastinal structures to the affected side (usually right) with loss of definition of the ipsilateral border of the heart. On lateral projection, a sharply defined density was seen parallel to the sternum in the anterior chest which was due to areolar tissue. Except for two patients in whom the accessory diaphragm was said to have been directly visualized, the plain film findings appeared to be identical to those described by Felson (1972) in lobar agenesis or aplasia wherein the extrapleural areolar tissue which replaces the lobe is visible on the lateral radiograph (Fig. 10–2).

PHRENIC NERVE PARALYSIS

An unusual but well-known cause of respiratory distress with onset at birth is paralysis of the phrenic nerve. It is usually associated with a brachial paralysis, but can occur independently of brachial involvement (Blattner, 1942; Bingham, 1954). Paralysis of an arm alone, however, is much more common than phrenic involvement.

In a review of 64 cases, with 10 new ones added, Richard et al. (1957) found these lesions to be most common in large infants and clearly related to dystocia. Paralysis occurred on the right side in 58 cases, and on the left in only 16 cases, unlike congenital eventration which was more common on the left. Horner's syndrome was also present in four infants, and a right vocal cord palsy was present in one.

Etiology.   Trauma at the time of delivery is usually incriminated in the etiology of phrenic paralysis. The occasional demonstration at

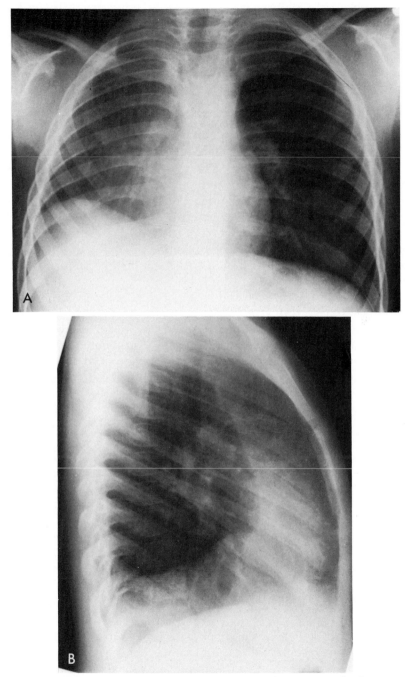

Figure 10-2. Hypoplastic right lung with possible accessory diaphragm in a seven-year-old child. Note the small volume of the right lung and elevation of the right hemidiaphragm on frontal view (A). On lateral projection (B), the curved retrosternal density most likely represents areolar tissue. These findings had been present since birth.

autopsy of avulsion of the nerves testifies to this etiology. In the patient reported by Blattner (1942), there was increased cellularity with fewer axons in the phrenic nerve, but no evidence of rupture at least to the level of the cord. He postulated that there was a compression of the nerve between the head and shoulder of the fetus in utero. Such a mechanism is unproved, and it must be much rarer than trauma, if it does occur.

Symptoms. The symptoms of phrenic nerve paralysis are nonspecific. Cyanosis, tachypnea, feeble cry, and apneic spells may occur in the event of a severe injury. Minor degrees of injury may be present without overt clinical findings. The practice of taking routine chest films or, preferably, of fluoroscopy in infants with Erb's palsy will uncover unsuspected cases of diaphragmatic paralysis.

Careful inspection of the chest wall, especially during a cry, will usually show a decrease in movement of the affected side. The roentgenographic signs are an elevated hemidiaphragm with paradoxical movement and a mediastinal shift with each breath. Atelectasis may occur on the affected side.

Prognosis. Death occurred in 15 of the 74 cases reviewed by Richard et al. (1957). Most of the deaths were associated with infection in the atelectatic lung and occurred before the infants were three months of age. None occurred after the age of six months. If the lesion is an avulsion of the cervical nerves at their origin from the cord, as in one patient studied at autopsy by Turner and Bakst (1948), no recovery would be possible. Tension or edema at the nerve roots is potentially reversible. Very prompt recovery from a brachial palsy may occur within a few days, or the recovery may be slower, over a period of several months.

Treatment. Plication of the diaphragm may be lifesaving in the severely symptomatic infant (Bingham, 1954; Bishop and Koop, 1958). Milder degrees of impairment rapidly regress, and no treatment is indicated. Antibiotics are indicated, of course, in the presence of infection. The patient described by Smith (1972) had only mild respiratory distress even with paradoxical movements of the right hemidiaphragm. By 18 days of age, he had recovered completely.

DIAPHRAGMATIC HERNIA

Congenital defects in the diaphragm may be associated with the displacement of abdominal viscera into the chest of the fetus so that the initiation of respiration is impaired. Occasionally, the viscera can move freely through the defect, so that they are sometimes in the thoracic cavity, especially when the infant is horizontal, or in the abdominal cavity, when the infant is upright.

Site of Defect. By far the most common site for a defect is the posterolateral portion of the diaphragm or the foramen of Bochdalek.

Herniation through the left portion of the diaphragm was about five times more common than herniation through the right in Gross's series (1953). Bilateral Bochdalek hernias occur very rarely (Levy et al., 1969).

Clinical Findings. Some diaphragmatic hernias are associated with no symptoms at all, so that they may be detected first on a chest film taken for other reasons in childhood. The degree of symptomatology depends on the amount of abdominal viscera in the chest. Some infants have so little space for lung expansion that they fail to initiate respiration. The frequency of this lethal form of the disease was noted by Butler and Claireaux (1962), who found in a mass survey of perinatal deaths that deaths from diaphragmatic hernias were more frequent than was reported by pediatric centers to which infants were referred for operative repair of the hernia. Presumably, many infants die before the diagnosis is made. Infants who succeed in establishing respiration may have labored breathing and cyanosis, which can be quite indistinguishable from other forms of neonatal respiratory distress. The abdomen will be scaphoid if there has been a shift of much bowel into the chest. Examination of the chest may reveal a decrease in breath sounds on the ipsilateral side. The presence of dullness to percussion should suggest the diagnosis, but the absence of dullness does not rule it out if the bowel contains air. The heart is usually shifted to the opposite side. The diagnosis should be suspected if bowel sounds are clearly heard in the thorax; however, bowel sounds may be absent in the chest even with the bowel herniated into it. A chest film is the most helpful diagnostic aid (Fig. 10–3). Sometimes it is hard to distinguish the pneumatoceles of staphylococcal pneumonia, or the cysts of congenital cystic disease of the lung, from bowel in the chest. On close inspection, typical bowel markings might be seen. A diminution in the amount of bowel below the diaphragm is also a helpful sign. Contrast studies are indicated only if doubt of the diagnosis exists (Fig. 10–4).

Treatment. In contrast to eventration of the diaphragm, immediate operation is indicated once the diagnosis of diaphragmatic hernia is established. Infants tolerate operation well in the first 48 hours of life when very little anesthesia and added fluids are required. It is a dangerous policy to defer operation, since the displacement of the abdominal viscera may become worse, and intestinal obstruction is possible when oral feedings are begun. Gross (1953) discussed the operative approach to the different types of diaphragmatic hernia.

MORGAGNI HERNIA

Rarely viscera herniate through the foramen of Morgagni which is a defect in the diaphragm on either side of the sternum (Comer and

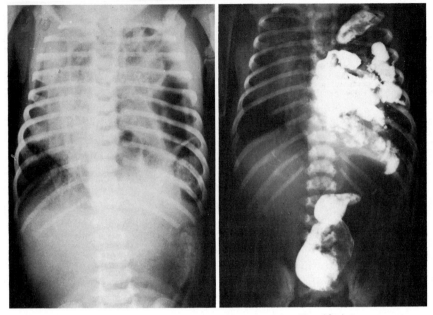

Fig. 10–3   Fig. 10–4

Figure 10–3. Film of the chest and abdomen of a two-week-old infant with herniation of the bowel into the left hemithorax. Note the cyst-like radiolucencies in the chest and the lack of abdominal bowel pattern.

Figure 10–4. Same infant as in Figure 10–3, after a gastrointestinal series.

Clagett, 1966). The liver and intestine are most commonly involved and the herniation is usually right-sided, producing a mass in the anterior mediastinum, contiguous to the heart (Fig. 10–5). This condition may be apparent early in life or may be acquired later and is often asymptomatic. Contrast examination of the gastrointestinal tract may be helpful and the presence of intrathoracic hepatic tissue can be demonstrated by isotope studies (Spencer et al., 1971). The diagnosis can be confirmed by means of an intraperitoneal injection of a "negative" contrast medium such as carbon dioxide.

Anterior diaphragmatic defects are associated with defects of the anterior abdominal wall and distal sternum. (Cantrell et al., 1958; Toyoma, 1972). The defective diaphragm and pericardium may allow herniation of intestine into the pericardial sac.

Occasionally, abdominal viscera may herniate through the esophageal hiatus.

CHEST WALL DEFORMITIES

Abnormalities of bone and muscle may prove to be such a mechanical hindrance that ventilation of portions of the lung is impaired.

Although congenital abnormalities of the bony structure of the thorax are rare, they are immediately recognizable and are sometimes amenable to operative correction (Ravitch in Benson, 1962).

Thoracic-Pelvic-Phalangeal Dystrophy

This rare disorder, described by Jeune et al. (1954) and named by him "asphyxiating thoracic dystrophy of the newborn," is part of a generalized chondrodystrophy. The hallmarks of this disease are a relatively small thorax, tachypnea, depression of the diaphragm so that liver and spleen are readily palpable, and radiographic abnormalities of the extremities. Renal involvement, hypotonia, and recurrent respiratory infections are frequent. Of the forty odd cases described to date, death has usually occurred from respiratory difficulties in the first year of life. Reduction in number of alveoli has been found in one such infant who died 12 hours after birth (Feingold et al., 1971). The disorder is familial, occurring in one of four siblings. No minor cases have been recognized, thus no parent-child occurrence has been noted (Fig. 10–6).

Radiologically this disorder is characterized by a small thorax in which the ribs appear shortened and the costochondral junctions are flared and irregular. The clavicles, which are unaffected, appear relatively long. The thorax assumes a bell-shaped configuration. The pelvis may be abnormal and show flaring of the iliac crests with inferior bony protrusions involving the greater sciatic notch and lateral aspect of the roof of the acetabulum (Langer, 1968). When polydactyly is present, the roentgen picture may be indistinguishable from the Ellis–van Creveld syndrome (chondroectodermal dysplasia). Kohler and Babbitt (1970) have emphasized the variety of disorders of endochondral bone formation which can result in chondrodystrophic thoraces and respiratory distress.

Unlike the patients with thoracic-pelvic-phalangeal dystrophy who may live beyond the newborn period, there are several disorders related to achondroplasia which are more immediately lethal because of severe thoracic dystrophy and respiratory failure. The most notable of these are thanatophoric (death-bringing) dwarfism, achondrogenesis, and homozygous achondroplasia. These conditions, however, can be differentiated radiologically from thoracic-pelvic-phalangeal dystrophy by their more marked micromelia and poorly ossified vertebral bodies (Langer et al., 1969).

Other Thoracic Wall Abnormalities

Absence or separation of ribs is often associated with hemivertebrae and scoliosis and may require surgical intervention (Ravitch, 1966). Multiple anomalies of the ribs and spine (spondylocostal

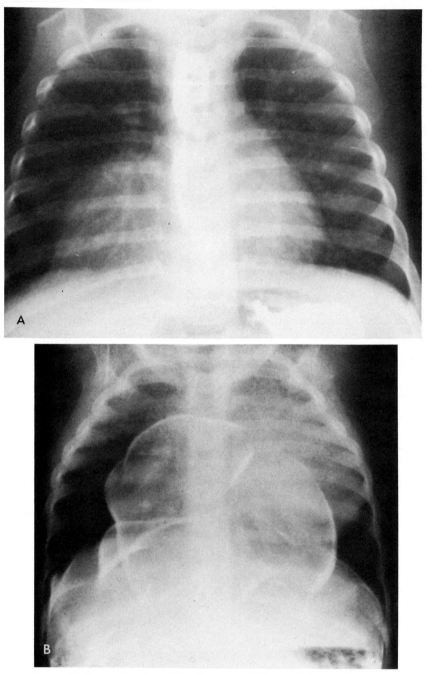

Figure 10–5. A, Hernias of the foramen of Morgagni frequently present as a mass, contiguous to the right border of the heart, as in this patient. *B,* In another patient, a large Morgagni hernia was outlined after introduction of water-soluble contrast medium into the peritoneal cavity. Similarly, carbon dioxide can be used instead of an opaque contrast medium. (From Oh, K. S., et al.: Radiology, *108*:647, 1973.)

(Illustration continued on opposite page.)

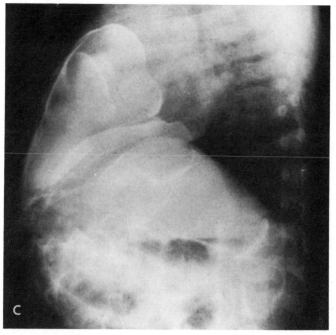

Figure 10–5 Continued. C, Note the anterior position of the hernia on the lateral view.

dysplasia) may be inherited by individuals who have no respiratory symptoms (Rimoin et al., 1968). However, the deformities can be severe enough to result in death from respiratory causes during infancy (Pochaczevsky et al., 1971).

Infants with a Pierre Robin–like syndrome may occasionally exhibit defective ossification of ribs ("rib-gap defects") which may contribute to a respiratory death (Miller et al., 1972). Although rib abnormalities are frequent in Poland's syndrome (absence of pectoralis major muscle and syndactyly), surgery is usually necessary only for cosmetic reasons and when lung herniation is present (Brooksaler and Graivier, 1971).

Occasionally, stress fractures are seen on chest radiographs of newborn infants who have had prolonged respiratory distress (Burnard et al., 1965); they do not appear to be related to metabolic bone disease or specific trauma and are most likely analogous to "cough fractures" of later life (Fig. 10–7).

FAILURE OF STERNAL FUSION

Partial or complete defects of fusion of the sternum are probably due to failure of midline fusion of the paired sternal bands. Complete

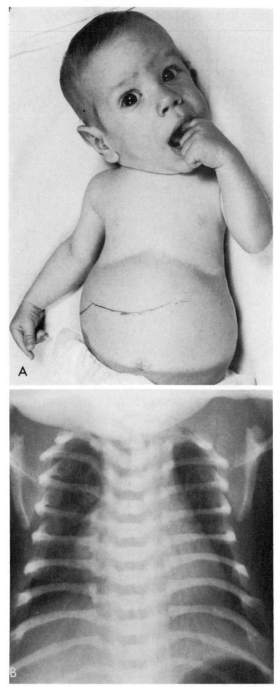

Figure 10–6. Thoracic-pelvic-phalangeal dystrophy in a three-month-old infant who has evidence of a small thoracic circumference as compared to the abdominal circumference. *A,* The liver and spleen are displaced downward but are of normal consistency. (Courtesy of Dr. Pamela Fitzhardinge.) The radiographs made in the newborn period show shortened, anteriorly flared ribs seen on AP *(B)* and lateral *(C)* projections. The thoracic cage is narrowed in its transverse diameter.

(Illustration continued on opposite page.)

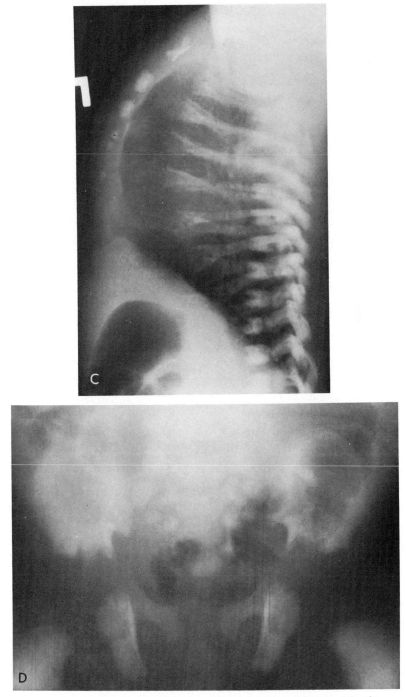

Figure 10–6 Continued. D, The film of the pelvis shows flaring of the iliac crests and irregular ossification of the triradiate cartilage with typical bony protrusions.

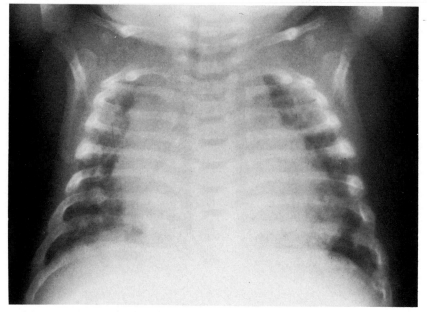

Figure 10-7. Multiple, bilateral, healing rib fractures in infant with severe hyaline membrane disease who was managed on long-term respirator therapy.

separation allows protrusion of the cardiovascular structures and has been reported as ectopia cordis. There are usually associated lethal malformations of the heart. However, Maier and Bortone (1949) reported successful closure of a complete sternal cleft.

Upper sternal clefts are more common. The pulsations of the great vessels are easily felt. Early operation is advised to shield the underlying structures from injury and because of the greater ease in approximating the separated parts of the sternum in the first days of life than at later ages (Longino and Jewett, 1955; Sabiston, 1958) (Fig. 10–8).

The chest roentgenograms of patients with congenital bifid sternum and partial ectopic cords are striking (Chang and Davis, 1961). The medial ends of the clavicles are more widely separated than usual, and the normal shadow of the manubrium is absent. Characteristically, there is also superior mediastinal widening.

Distal sternal clefts are usually associated with other anomalies, such as defects in the abdominal wall, diaphragm, and heart (Cantrell et al., 1958).

The most common sternal defects are in the group of depression deformities, usually designated as pectus excavatum. The sternum dips toward the vertebral column and is maximally depressed just above the xiphoid. The condition may be evident at birth, although it usually becomes noticeable when the infant is several months of age. Occasionally, sternal depressions at birth become less marked in time, particularly if they develop in the course of respiratory distress.

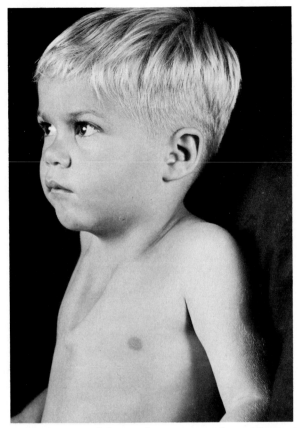

Figure 10–8. There is a defect in the sternum with partial ectopia cordis. The two sides of the chest are connected anteriorly by a small bridge at the xiphoid process. (From Sabiston, D.: J. Thorac. Surg. 35:118, 1958.)

While pectus excavatum is often sporadic in occurrence, it may be familial. It is usually an isolated deformity, but can be associated with the Marfan syndrome. It is useful to document the degree of abnormality with serial photographs, which are preferable to serial chest films because they show the deformity better and avoid unnecessary irradiation. The indications for operative correction are shortness of breath, rotation of the mediastinal structures as manifested by electrocardiography, and progressive deformity with its attendant psychological disturbances. Ravitch reported the results of 135 patients treated operatively at the ages of two months to 40 years, with one death. Symptoms have always been relieved, although one patient required a second operation (Benson et al., 1962).

Protrusion deformities of the sternum, often called pigeon breast, are less common than depression deformities. They may become more marked in time, but operative correction has been advised only for cosmetic reasons.

Chapter Eleven

INFECTIONS

PNEUMONIA

The most common serious infection in newborn infants is pneumonia, which can be acquired in utero or in the early neonatal period. In the British perinatal mortality survey, pulmonary infection was considered the cause of death in 5.5 per cent of stillbirths and neonatal deaths (Butler and Bonham, 1963). Pneumonia, however, accounts for about 90 per cent of deaths from infection. (Claireaux in Holzel and Tizard, 1958). Since it may be prevented in some instances or treated successfully with prompt recognition of its presence, the predisposing conditions and clinical features are of importance to anyone responsible for the care of infants.

Incidence. The incidence of pneumonia at autopsy will vary widely, just as does the incidence of most infections (Schaffer et al., 1955). Even in hospitals with the best facilities and staff, however, pneumonia continues to be seen in recent years as a principal cause of death. Anderson et al. (1962) found evidence of pneumonia at autopsy in 2.7 per cent of all stillbirths in whom death occurred more than 48 hours before delivery, and in 17.4 per cent of stillbirths nearer the time of delivery. Pneumonia was found in 9.1 per cent of all infants who died after 48 hours of age. At the Boston Lying-In Hospital pneumonia was present in 22 per cent of 337 unselected autopsies of newborn infants, and in 6 per cent of 224 autopsies of stillborn infants (Benirschke, 1960). Schaffer (1955) stated that one of 12 perinatal deaths is caused by pneumonia. In a consecutive series of 1044 autopsies of stillborn and newborn infants from Babies Hospital, New York, Naeye et al. (1971) found congenital pneumonia in 23 per cent.

Predisposing Conditions and Pathogenesis. Factors that favor

174

the penetration of organisms from the vagina into the uterine cavity, and thus ascending infection, are (1) prolonged rupture of the membranes, especially with a delay before the onset of labor, (2) prolonged labor even with intact membranes, and (3) excessive obstetrical manipulation.

The extensive studies of Gosselin (1945), on the presence of bacteria in amniotic fluid and fetal blood with relation to the duration of rupture of membranes and labor, show the greater importance of the duration of labor than that of membrane rupture per se with respect to the numbers of positive cultures (Table 11–1). Recovery of pathogenic bacteria from the maternal reproductive tract and urinary tract is significantly associated with congenital pneumonia. The organism present in the infant's post-mortem lung culture often is the same pathogen. Naeye et al. (1971) also noted that 37 per cent of the infants with congenital pneumonia had no pathogenic organisms identified at autopsy.

The risk of fetal or neonatal death was about 25 per cent greater with premature rupture of the membranes in the series of Flowers et al., and 32 per cent of the deaths were due to antepartum or intrapartum infection (1958). In another study of 179 parturient mothers with rupture of the membranes six or more hours before delivery, sepsis was proven in 8 per cent of the infants. Death occurred in 4 per cent of the infants, but was attributed to pneumonia in only one stillborn infant (Pryles et al., 1963). If placentitis is used as an index of infection, its incidence rises from 1 per cent if membranes are ruptured less than 35 hours to 52 per cent if they are ruptured over 35 hours (Anderson et al., 1962).

The overwhelming importance of the ascending route of infection was stressed by Benirschke (1960) on the basis of the similarity of bacteria in the vagina and in the infant's respiratory passage, the progression of inflammatory changes from the membranes near the vagina, and his study of 170 consecutive twin placentas in which the twin nearer the cervical os was infected 17 times, both twins six times, and the second twin was never the only one infected. Penetration of intact fetal membranes by organisms can probably occur, as suggested by

Table 11–1. Relationship between Duration of Labor after Rupture of Membranes and Positive Amniotic Fluid and Blood Cultures*

Duration of Labor in Hours	Bacteria in Amniotic Fluid	Bacteria in Blood
0 to 6	5%	2%
6 to 24	51%	47%
More than 24	90%	80%

* This high incidence of fetal bacteremia does not imply an equal incidence of fetal infection, since many infants have adequate defenses against bacteremia and are not clinically disturbed. (From Gosselin, O., 1945.)

the case of congenital systemic candidiasis reported by Dvorak and Gavaller (1966). The infant was delivered by cesarean section without known prior rupture of the membranes. There was no maternal septicemia, and only the amniotic surface of the placenta was involved. *C. albicans* was recovered from the mother's vagina, infant's blood, lung, gastric aspirate, stool, and urine.

Hematogenous placentofetal infection is also possible in the presence of maternal infection. Toxoplasmosis, cytomegalic inclusion disease, and Coxsackie and Listeria infection may occur and be associated with pneumonia in the newborn, although other organ systems are usually more seriously involved (Flamm, 1959). Careful examination and culture of the placenta may indicate the etiologic diagnosis, as demonstrated in the case of infection from *Listeria monocytogenes* reported by Driscoll et al. (1962). Bacteria are rarely found in transplacental infection, although *E. coli*, staphylococci, streptococci, and pneumococci, as well as congenital tuberculosis and syphilis, have occurred (Blanc, 1961). In some infections such as tuberculosis, the placenta itself is infected and discharges organisms into the amniotic sac, which the fetus may then aspirate. In others, such as some viral infections, the placenta may appear to be normal, suggesting that the viruses can cross intact villi (Blanc, 1961).

Infection can be acquired during passage through the vagina. Herpes simplex and varicella zoster are examples of such infections. In a series of 15 infants born to mothers with varicella before delivery, four had lesions at nine to 20 days, consistent with intrauterine infection in some, or acquisition at delivery in others. (Abler, 1964). The clinical course is usually benign, although fatalities have been described (Oppenheimer, 1944). Herpes simplex, usually acquired at delivery, can also be congenital, as noted by Sieber et al. (1966). One infant of 965 gm. expired at 71 hours of age with extensive skin and cerebral lesions. The other infant of 1960 gm. was delivered by cesarean section and died at 11 days with interstitial pneumonia, skin lesions, and liver and cerebral involvement.

Premature infants appear to be more at risk than term infants from either hematogenous or ascending infections, with three times the incidence of placental inflammation (Blanc, 1959). In a review of 55 fatal cases of pneumonia, nearly half of the infants were premature (Bernstein and Wang, 1961). Negro and Puerto Rican infants had more infection than Caucasian infants; this is thought to be related in part to socioeconomic factors (Naeye et al., 1971; Naeye and Blanc, 1970).

Organisms.   Staphylococci, *E. coli*, and streptococci dominate in most series of cultures of organisms in amniotic fluid or at autopsy of infants with pneumonia (Anderson et al., 1962; Blanc, 1961; Olding, 1966).

Diagnosis.   Leukocytic infiltration of the cord seen on frozen section has been used to demonstrate the presence of amnionitis, and this infection may be associated with fetal pneumonia (Benirschke and

Clifford, 1959). In a total of 253 autopsies of stillborn and liveborn infants, Blanc found inflammation of the membranes in 98 instances, and pneumonia in 14. Of 155 infants without amnionitis, only one had pneumonia at autopsy (1959). The presence of amnionitis does not always denote disease in the infant, nor does the lack of it assure the absence of infection in the infant. Nonetheless the correlations are fairly good, and in some instances this factor is a useful diagnostic aid. In some infants, a stain of aspirated gastric fluid will reveal polymorphonuclear leukocytes which suggest the presence of amnionitis (Blanc, 1953).

When there is roentgenographic evidence of localization of pneumonia, a lung aspirate may be helpful. The procedure should be restricted to those instances in which there is poor resolution of the pneumonia and the organism is unknown. The major complication is pneumothorax, which occurs after 5 to 10 per cent of aspirations. The likelihood of pneumothorax is lessened if a number 20 needle is used and the procedure done quickly.

Symptoms. The infant may be stillborn, or desperately ill at birth in the event of intrauterine infection. The onset of respiration may be delayed, and, once initiated, labored and inadequate. The infants are usually hypothermic for longer periods than expected, especially if they are premature; if they survive for some hours they may have fever, which is rarely over 102°F. Fever is more common in term infants than in premature ones. Rales may or may not be present. Occasionally, heart failure ensues terminally, with a descent of the liver and pulmonary edema. The white blood cell count may be elevated, but it is not consistently so.

The onset of symptoms will occur later in infants who acquire their infection at or shortly after birth. Cyanosis, irregular respiration with apneic spells of over 10 seconds, retractions, tachypnea, and tachycardia may be present, but are neither pathognomonic of pneumonia nor always present. There are no consistent changes in white count, but either a depression below 5000 ml. or above 15,000 ml. is suggestive of infection. Hypothermia is the rule in very small infants. If the environmental temperature is constant, a slight increase in temperature may occur and suggest the presence of infection, even if the body temperature is lower than normal.

Radiographic Findings. The chest roentgenogram is the most useful diagnostic tool. Bilateral, occasionally unilateral, central, ill-defined streaky densities are the most frequent radiographic manifestations of pneumonia in the first days of life. The densities show a varying degree of an exudative component which results in confluent mottled opacities in more advanced cases. Peribronchial thickening as a part of the bronchopneumonic process will appear as tiny ring-like densities in the perihilar areas when the bronchi are seen on end. Air bronchograms may also be seen as the air-filled bronchi are contrasted against the airless alveoli (Figs. 11–1, 11–7, 11–8, 11–9).

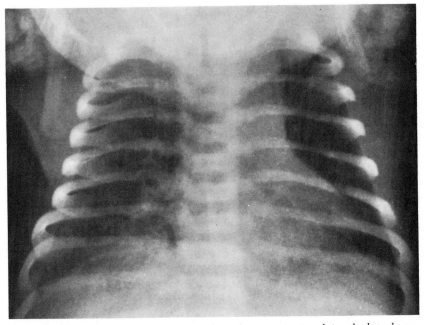

Figure 11–1.   Film of an infant with bilateral pneumonia involving the lung bases.

Pathology. Fatal pneumonia in the first days of life is almost always a diffuse process. The diagnosis cannot be established grossly except in the rare case in which pleuritis is apparent. The lungs are usually congested and heavy, and often indistinguishable from pulmonary hemorrhage, or from atelectasis with or without hyaline membranes. On histological examination, almost all cases in larger premature and term infants show some squamous cells indicative of aspirated amniotic sac debris. A marked polymorphonuclear response characterizes most cases of pneumonia, even in infants of a few hundred grams (Fig. 11–3). Bernstein and Wang pointed out the frequent association of bronchitis and bronchiolitis in association with alveolar inflammation, and the rarity of isolated bronchitis or bronchiolitis (1961). They noted vascular lesions only in association with *Pseudomonas* infections. Widespread alveolar hemorrhage is frequently associated with a polymorphonuclear response, so that the question which was first is not always answerable. Microabscess formation may occur in association with staphylococcal infection, but is unusual with other organisms (Bernstein and Wang, 1961).

Treatment of Pneumonia in the Newborn. Antibiotics should be administered in the presence of any clinical or roentgenographic evidence of pneumonia as soon as cultures are obtained, preferably within an hour of birth. When symptoms are not present, but there is gross inflammation of the placenta or a history of labor of more than 24 hours

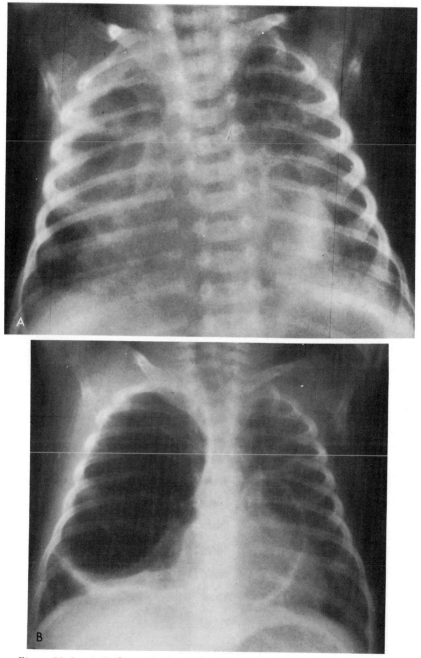

Figure 11–2. A, Radiograph of a 10-day-old infant with extensive pneumonia due to *Klebsiella* infection. B, The same infant has a large pneumatocele at age two and one-half months. It slowly increased in size, and at age seven months tube drainage was necessary. The involved lung was later resected.

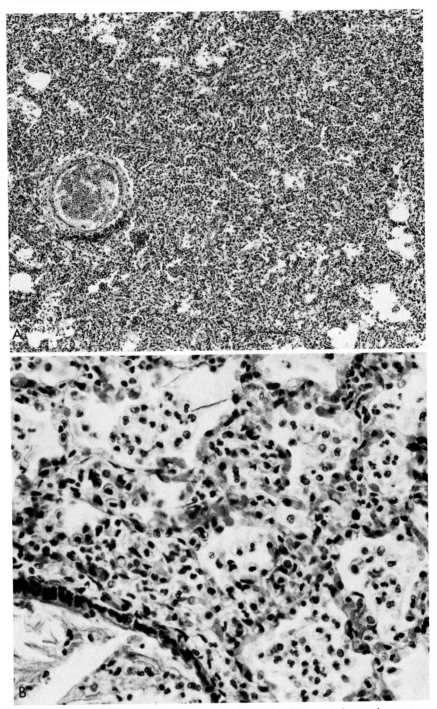

Figure 11–3.   A, Low-power view of the lung of an 800-gm. infant with an extensive inflammatory response. × 100. B, Section of the lung of an infant with intrauterine pneumonia with many polymorphonuclear cells. × 400.

with prior rupture of the membranes, the risk of pneumonia seems great enough to warrant obtaining cultures of the infant's nose, throat, and blood and promptly initiating antibiotic therapy. In the absence of symptoms, and with a shorter interval of rupture of the membranes and labor, differences of opinion exist as to the management of the infant. In one controlled trial, no benefit was found from routine use of penicillin and streptomycin in infants born after membranes had been ruptured for six hours (Pryles, 1963). If the evidence for exposure to infection is inflammation of the cord on frozen section, antibiotics could perhaps be deferred if the infant is vigorous. Nonetheless, cultures are always indicated if there is any possibility of exposure of the infant to infection.

There is no agreement on the antibiotics of choice in the prophylaxis of pneumonia or sepsis in the absence of knowledge of the bacteria. Statistical evidence of the likelihood that the infant will harbor the same organisms as are in the maternal vagina is sufficiently strong to warrant the use of an antibiotic or combination of antibiotics to cover both gram-positive and gram-negative organisms. One of the principal problems in the selection of antibiotics for use in the newborn infant is to be certain that there will be no untoward side effects which may occur if the systems for detoxification and excretion are not fully developed. At this time, it appears that aqueous penicillin, 40,000 to 60,000 units/kg./day, administered intramuscularly in two divided doses, is safe and effective in newborn infants. Significant improvement in the treatment of septicemia in premature infants has been reported when combinations of antibiotics include kanamycin, 7 to 15 mg./kg./day (Buetow et al., 1965). It should be used on the basis of in vitro sensitivities and it is bactericidal against *E. coli* and some strains of *Staph. aureus* (Gluck et al., 1966). Nephrotoxicity is uncommon in newborn infants. Ototoxicity is a potential hazard, but is apparently rare in the absence of renal disease or with dosages of 10 mg./kg./day (Yow and Tengg, 1961; Yow et al., 1961). In nurseries where *Klebsiella*, enteric bacilli, and *Pseudomonas* infections are frequent or *E. coli* is resistant to kanamycin, gentamicin is the drug of choice. In the first week of life the dose is 5 mg./kg./day in two divided doses. After the first week, it should be 7.5 mg./kg./day in three divided doses. (McCracken and Jones, 1970; McCracken, 1971). Methicillin and ampicillin appear safe, and are occasionally indicated.

SYPHILIS

Congenital syphilis is very rarely seen in this country, hence it infrequently enters the differential diagnosis of respiratory difficulty at birth. As of 1963, the last case indexed in the autopsy files of The Johns Hopkins Hospital occurred in 1947. A resurgence in recent

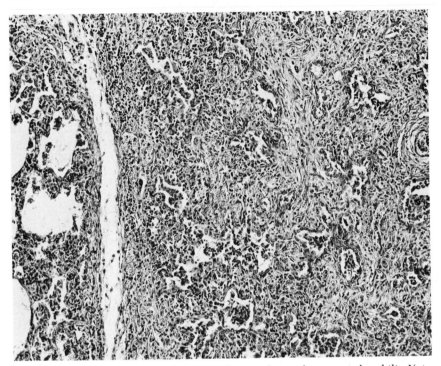

Figure 11–4. Section of a lung of a stillborn infant with congenital syphilis. Note the marked interstitial scarring with a few chronic inflammatory cells. The few remaining airspaces are lined with cuboidal epithelium. × 100.

years has necessitated a new look at an old problem. Pneumonia is a well-known lesion of intrauterine syphilitic infection. Affected infants are usually stillborn, or die shortly after birth. The lungs are firm and heavy, and a uniform yellow-pink—hence the name, pneumonia alba. There is an increase in connective tissue, distention of alveoli with macrophages, and a dense infiltration of mononuclear cells (Potter, 1961) (Fig. 11–4). The diagnosis should be suspected when other signs of congenital syphilis are present such as desquamation of the extremities, snuffles, ascites, and pseudoparalyses. Other manifestations of congenital syphilis are more common, including bone lesions, liver involvement, pancreatic lesions, and skin lesions. The persistence of spirochetes in some tissues even after the usual two-week course of treatment with penicillin suggests therapy should at times be extended (Hardy et al., 1970; Oppenheimer and Hardy, 1971).

TUBERCULOSIS

Intrauterine infection from tuberculosis is extremely rare in parts of the world where antenatal care and tuberculosis control programs are widely distributed; moreover, it is unusual even if the mother has active tuberculosis. Nonetheless, the vulnerability of the infant to tuberculosis is so great that vigilance is indicated to detect this potentially curable illness. One hundred thirty-three proved cases were found in a review of the literature by Corner and Brown in 1955.

There are three potential routes of fetal infection. One is hematogenous transplacental infection, in which case the primary complex is usually in the liver and adjacent lymph nodes. Occasionally when the organisms bypass the liver they may settle in the lung. Another route is ingestion of infected amniotic liquid with intestinal and mesenteric node involvement. Third, the infant may aspirate infected amniotic liquid with widespread tuberculous pneumonia the consequence. When pneumonia is associated with tuberculous endometritis in the mother, aspiration of infected liquid seems the likely route of fetal infection (Voyce and Hunt, 1966). The disease may be localized to the site of primary involvement, or disseminated through most of the organs of the body. Hepatosplenomegaly, generalized lymphadenopathy, and skin nodules have been noted. Extensive tuberculosis in the infant, acquired after birth, has been thoroughly documented (Grady and Zuelzer, 1955). In many instances in which the infant was not separated from the mother at delivery, the time of acquisition of the infection cannot be established.

Management

Congenital Tuberculosis. If the mother has miliary disease, the infant deserves intensive investigation, including gastric aspirate for smear and culture, CSF smear and culture, chest film, and urinalysis. The tuberculin test may not become positive for three to five weeks in such an infant, and if the infant has overwhelming infection, he may be anergic. Separation of the infant from the mother is self-evident, and institution of INH 10 mg./kg./day is appropriate in the absence of manifest disease. INH blood levels should be obtained since newborn infants may metabolize the drug slowly. With manifest disease, a second drug should be added, depending on sensitivities.

Infant of a Mother on Therapy for Pulmonary Tuberculosis. It seems appropriate to separate the infant from the mother as long as she is sputum-positive. After she is negative, she may care for the infant, although it should be noted that such an infant is still at risk of acquiring infection. Close follow-up of the infant, such as monthly visits, is in order.

Infant of a Mother with a Past History of Tuberculosis. The possibility of maternal relapse is greatest if she has been off therapy for less than five years. A postpartum chest film is indicated, and close follow-up of both mother and infant are indicated.

Role of BCG. The freeze-dried preparations now available are stable and effective; they are manufactured by Glaxo Laboratories,

Ltd., Middlesex, England and are distributed by Eli Lilly & Co., Indianapolis, Ind. The dose is 0.1 ml. by intradermal injection, and the likelihood of tuberculin conversion in two to three months is nearly 90 per cent. Extensive studies with this preparation show a marked reduction in the complications of primary tuberculosis. In areas of high prevalence of disease, or cases in which follow-up with serial chest films or tuberculin testing is inappropriate, BCG is indicated. When the infant can be followed, the loss of the tuberculin test as an indicator of infection after BCG administration may reduce the desirability of BCG.

PNEUMOCYSTIS CARINII

Pneumonia caused by infection with an agent presumed to be a protozoan parasite, *Pneumocystis carinii*, is uncommon in premature infants in this country, but lately has been widely recognized as a secondary invader in chronic illness at any age. It has been noted especially in association with hypogammaglobulinemia (McKay and Richardson, 1959; Sheldon, 1962; Hendry and Patrick, 1962). However, *Pneumocystis carinii* is recognized frequently among premature infants in Europe, especially in crowded nurseries. Over 700 cases were reported in Switzerland between 1941 and 1948, and 191 cases in Hamburg, Germany, from 1950 to 1954. The European literature has been thoroughly reviewed with the finding that the disease occurs in all countries in which a search for it has been undertaken. (Gajdusek, 1957; Goetz, 1960; Robbins, 1967.)

Etiology. The organism found in the lungs of premature infants at autopsy, and considered to be causative of the interstitial plasma cell pneumonia, was first described by Chagas (1909), and named for Carinii (1910) who studied the parasite in lungs of rats infected with *Trypanosoma cruzi.*

The parasite has an oval free form with a single nucleus within a mucoid envelope. It is assumed to multiply by binary fission, so that two, four, six, or eight nuclei may be found within a cyst. The intracystic bodies, 1.0 to 1.5 μ in diameter, are surrounded by a three-layered membrane and contain organelles resembling endoplasmic reticulum and mitochondria (Barton and Campbell, 1967). The cytoplasm is pale blue with Giemsa stain, and the nuclear mass a dark violet. A delicate capsule surrounds the cytoplasm, and the encysted parasite is 4 to 10 μ in diameter. The reproductive cycle has been deduced from observations on histologic preparations, since no one has been successful in growing the organism and since reports of transmission of the disease to suckling animals are complicated by the coexistence of other infections (Simon, 1953). In human infection, too,

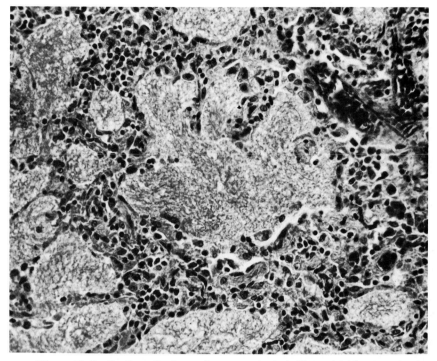

Figure 11–5. Section of a lung of a two-and-one-half-month-old premature infant with interstitial pneumonia associated with *Pneumocystis carinii.* Note the spongy exudate in the airspaces. × 300.

other agents such as the virus of cytomegalic inclusion disease are often present. On histologic examination, the alveoli are dilated and contain a spongy exudate in the midst of which the organism can be found. There is usually a mononuclear infiltration in the septa, which some workers have considered plasma cells, others, histiocytes (Figs. 11–5 and 11–6).

Epidemiology. *P. carinii* infection is widespread in animals, including rats, mice, rabbits, guinea pigs, dogs, cats, sheep, goats, and monkeys (Gajdusek, 1957). The mode of transmission of the organism is unknown. Outbreaks in premature nurseries in Europe suggest that the organism can be transmitted from human to human, although it is not clear whether an asymptomatic adult carrier is involved in the nursery epidemics. Positive complement fixation tests have been found in pregnant women, raising the possibility of intrauterine infection (Bárta et al., 1955). There is at least one recorded case of congenital pneumocystic infection in a stillborn baby (Pavlica, 1962). Three full-term siblings were reported by Bazaz et al. (1970) to be symptomatic in the immediate neonatal period. They were born in 1962, 1964, and 1967 of an asymptomatic mother. Repeated smears of maternal cervical secretions were negative for the organism. The

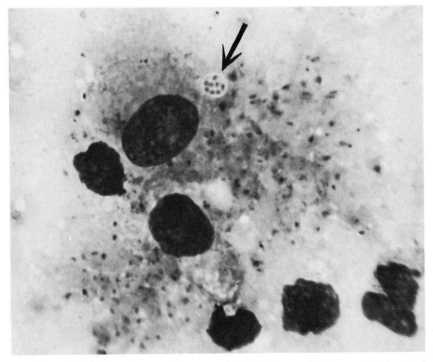

Figure 11–6. Lung smear. The arrow points to the encysted organism identified as *Pneumocystis carinii.* × 1500. Giemsa stain. (Courtesy of W. H. Sheldon, Johns Hopkins Hospital.)

possibility of transplacental infection seems likely, although unproved, in these infants.

Clinical and Laboratory Features. The illness in infants is most commonly recognized between the ninth and sixteenth weeks. Tachypnea, perioral or periorbital cyanosis, cough, and retractions are the outstanding physical findings. The lungs may be clear to auscultation, or fine crepitant rales and bronchial breath sounds may be present. The white blood cell count is usually normal, with mild to marked eosinophilia on differential count. Low-grade fever may be present. The roentgenographic appearance, although not specific for pneumocystis infection, is similar in the reported cases. Usually the hilar regions are involved first, with progression of a fine, granular density throughout the parenchyma. The lungs may be overinflated, with interstitial emphysema and pneumothorax complicating the illness. The radiographic appearance may resemble alveolar proteinosis. Areas of consolidation and atelectasis may appear (Fig. 11–7). The process usually lasts four to six weeks, with a mortality estimated at 20 to 50 per cent (Capitanio and Kirkpatrick, 1966; Ebel and Fendel, 1967).

Treatment. Definite clinical improvement has been noted in some patients with the use of pentamidine isethionate, 4 mg./kg./day

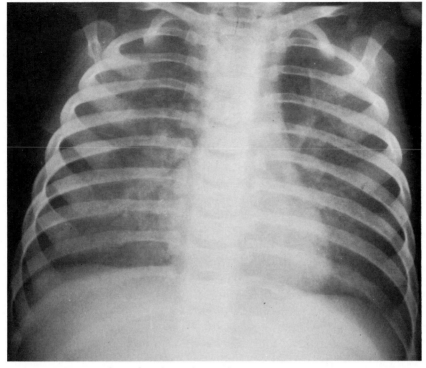

Figure 11-7. Chest film of an infant with pneumocystic carinii pneumonia. Note the overinflated lungs, with a fine granular density most marked in the hilar regions, but extending throughout the parenchyma. (Courtesy of Dr. John Kirkpatrick.)

intramuscularly (Patterson et al., 1966). This agent is effective against some protozoan diseases and may act as a folic acid antagonist. Few side effects other than megaloblastic changes in the bone marrow have been noted. Corticosteroids are not effective and may be dangerous in that they depress host resistance.

VIRAL PNEUMONIA

The possibility of a viral pneumonia of congenital origin was raised by Adams (1948) on the basis of his finding of cytoplasmic inclusion bodies in the pharyngeal epithelium of two mothers and their infants. In one case, the mother had mild respiratory symptoms, and the infant had rapid respirations from the first day of life, with an increase in bronchovascular markings on chest film. Rales and cyanosis appeared by the fifth day of life, and the infant's temperature rose to 103.4°F. He subsequently recovered. Other infants reported by Adams showed infiltrations in the lung fields on radiographs, and a similar clinical course. The illness may occur in epidemics and may be lethal (Adams, 1941). Histologic features are a proliferation of bronchial epithelium, with peribronchial mononuclear cell infiltration.

Typical cytoplasmic inclusion bodies 3 to 6 μ in diameter, which stain with Giemsa stain, are present in the epithelium. Adams recommends treatment with gamma globulin, 2 ml. intramuscularly, every few days.

Neonatal herpes simplex is usually acquired during vaginal delivery from the genital type or HSV type 2 infection. Disseminated disease is the usual pattern in the infant, although occasionally only skin or central nervous system involvement occur (Sieber et al., 1966).

The age of appearance of symptoms is from birth to 16 days. One infant described by Pettay et al. (1972) had vesicles on both arms at birth. They noted peripheral eosinophilia in several infants. Placenta lesions, similar to the visceral ones, were found by Witzleben and Driscoll (1965) in one infant delivered by cesarean section who had no contact with the mother after birth.

Although skin and nervous system involvement is most likely, hepatomegaly, jaundice, and pulmonary infiltrates may occur. Treatment with intravenous iododeoxyuridine, 60 mg./kg./day, has been encouraging (Nahmias et al., 1970). In older infants and in adults, Itryniuk et al. (1972) found a good response to the antileukemic agent cytarabine (cytosine arabinoside). Further studies are needed to evaluate this agent in neonatal herpes.

Intrauterine infection with rubella may produce an interstitial pneumonia that can be fatal. Phelan and Campbell (1969) described seven such infants, six of whom died from their pulmonary complications. The virus was isolated from the lungs post-mortem in four of the infants. The onset of respiratory symptoms, notably breathlessness, was usually after several weeks or months of life, and death occurred between three months and one year. Radiographically the lung showed a diffuse interstitial process (Fig. 11–8). Retractions and scattered crepitations were noted. Pathologically, the lesions resembled hyaline membrane disease in the florid cases, or an interstitial pneumonia with septal cell metaplasia in others. The one survivor in the Australian series recovered completely, as did the patient of Williams and Carey (1966).

An outbreak of pneumonitis occurred in full-term infants in Sendai, Japan, in 1952. The infants were febrile and had a leukocytosis of 15,000 to 40,000 cells, 60 to 80 per cent of which were polymorphonuclear leukocytes. Ten of the 17 afflicted infants died of the disease. A virus was recovered which has been called the Sendai virus, and is classified as a parainfluenza type I virus. The chest roentgenograms revealed diffuse shadows, more dense in the fatal cases, in one or both lungs (Sano et al., 1953; Kuroya and Ishida, 1953).

Parainfluenza type III virus was isolated from throat swabs of premature infants with stuffy noses, half of whom also had pneumonia, in an outbreak in Denver in January and February, 1960. All of those infants whose symptoms were restricted to the upper respiratory tract recovered, and there was only one death among the 13 infants with pneumonia (Moscovici et al., 1961).

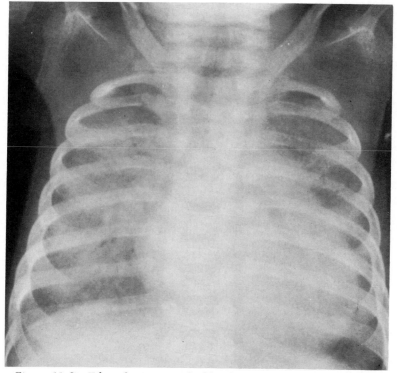

Figure 11–8. Film of a one-month-old infant exposed to maternal rubella in utero. Note the extensive bilateral infiltrates.

Respiratory syncytial virus infection may occur in epidemic form in premature nurseries. The initial symptoms are coryza, followed by cough and dyspnea one to eight days later. Chest films may vary from minimal bronchopneumonia to consolidation. The infants are usually afebrile, in contrast to those with Sendai viral pneumonia. Virus isolation and a rise in neutralizing and complement-fixing antibody titers were reported by Berkovich in 1964. A high attack rate in Eskimo infants was noted during an outbreak of RS virus. Death occurred in three infants, and two others required artificial respiration for several days.

Chany et al. (1958) reported adenovirus in association with pneumonitis in infants and children, but noted the rarity of this virus in pneumonia in the first six months of life. Of 92 cases of pneumonia studied in infants under six months of age, only one was associated with adenovirus. The youngest patient with virus pneumonia in the series of Goodpasture et al. (1939) was two weeks old at the time of diagnosis, although symptoms of poor feeding, lethargy, and episodic cyanosis were present from birth. This infant had a necrotizing inflammatory process of the tracheobronchial tree and alveolar walls, with intranuclear inclusions in the epithelial cells. Adenovirus 7

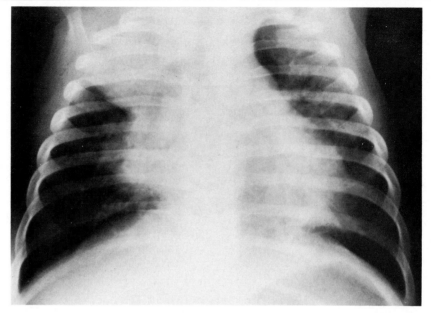

Figure 11-9. An 11-month male infant with chronic pneumonia proved to be due to adenovirus on lung aspiration. Chest film taken one month following onset shows air-space consolidation and collapse of right upper lobe with obliteration of right and left borders of the heart, indicating consolidation of right middle lobe and lingular segment of left upper lobe, respectively. Right lower lobe is overinflated. Slow improvement was noted but significant disease was still present on chest radiograph nine months later.

pneumonia was reported in eight patients under one year of age by Brown et al. (1973) (Fig. 11-9). In these patients, wheezing was a common feature. In some infants, the necrotizing bronchiolitis associated with adenoviral pneumonia may result in unilateral hyperlucent lung syndrome (Cumming et al., 1971).

The scarcity of reports of proved viral pneumonia in the newborn period does not mean that the infection is unusual, since probably it has not been searched for very diligently. However, lethal viral pneumonia must be uncommon, since the inclusions should have been noted at autopsy.

Viral Upper Respiratory Tract Illness

Viral upper respiratory tract disease must be common, although it has seldom been carefully studied or well documented in premature infants. Bauer et al. (1972) reported three infants with upper respiratory tract symptoms, a mild elevation in leukocyte count, fever, and a benign course of about four days. Influenza A/Hong Kong/1/68 (H3N2) was isolated from throat swabs or nasopharyngeal swabs in two of the three infants, all of whom were sick at the same time during an outbreak of Hong Kong influenza in Montreal.

Chapter Twelve

HYALINE MEMBRANE DISEASE

No condition in recent years has excited the interest of individuals concerned with newborn infants to quite the extent that hyaline membrane disease has. It is not a new disease. More than half a century has elapsed since the original description of Hochheim (1903) of a peculiar membrane in the lungs of two infants who died shortly after birth.

In 1925 Johnson and Meyer described the histologic findings in eight cases, and in 1931 Farber and Sweet added 18 more cases, although they considered the membranes to be aspirated vernix. Confusion about etiology led to confusion of terminology. De and Anderson, in their extensive review of the literature in 1953, list the following terms used to describe the same histologic findings:

1. Myelin formation in lungs
2. Congenital aspiration pneumonia
3. Asphyxial membrane
4. Desquamative anaerosis
5. Congenital alveolar dysplasia
6. Vernix membrane
7. Hyaline membrane
8. Hyaline-like membrane
9. Hyaline atelectasis

The ensuing years have seen a tremendous interest in this subject, but perhaps no less confusion as to etiology and terminology. At an international symposium on this subject in 1959, a group of pediatricians and pathologists found it difficult to agree on clinical diagnostic criteria, pathologic findings, and, finally, on even a suitable name. The final vote was between idiopathic respiratory distress of the newborn, pulmonary syndrome of the newborn, and hyaline membrane syndrome, with the former the victor (Rudolph and Smith, 1960). Subsequently other names have been suggested, usually by those who favor a particular theory of pathogenesis. The pulmonary hypoperfusion syndrome was proposed by Chu et al. in a preliminary paper (1965), only later to be changed by the same authors to neonatal pulmonary ischemia (1967). Gluck in 1972 proposed the name developmental respiratory distress consistent with his theory that the disorder is not a disease, but a developmental problem with respect to surfactant production. In practice, many speak of the respiratory distress syndrome (RDS); others prefer to use the name hyaline membrane disease (HMD) in deference to historical precedent.

It is pertinent to ask why there is so much interest in this subject. Dick and Pund (1949) noted the high incidence of what they considered to be the "vernix membrane" in autopsies of liveborn infants, and its absence in lungs of stillborn infants. That same year, 1949, Miller and Hamilton first questioned the concept of aspiration of vernix as the cause of the lesion, and highlighted the condition as an entity that deserved serious investigation because of its frequency and uncertain pathogenesis. They stated: "The failure to identify the hyaline-like material in the lungs of stillborn infants, whose likelihood to aspirate as the result of asphyxia was greater than that of most of the liveborn premature infants whose lungs contained this material, suggested that the aspiration theory might not be correct. This dis-

Table 12–1. Primary Necropsy Diagnosis in Perinatal Deaths
(Queen Charlotte's Maternity Hospital 1963–1970)

	Rate per 1000 Total Births
Congenital malformations	3.7
Antepartum deaths (no major lesion)	3.4
Intrapartum anoxia	3.0
Iso-immunization	2.2
Antepartum anoxia	2.0
Hyaline membrane disease	2.0
Intraventricular hemorrhage	1.5
Early neonatal death (no histopathology)	1.5
No necropsy	1.0
Miscellaneous	0.9
Massive pulmonary hemorrhage	0.6
Intrapartum anoxia + cerebral trauma	0.5
Pneumonia	0.5
Cerebral trauma	0.4
Average perinatal mortality rate 1963–1970	23.2 per 1000

Total babies delivered, 31,090; total stillbirths, 409; total early neonatal (first week) deaths, 313; total perinatal deaths, 722.
Data of Pryse-Davies (1972).

crepancy between the postmortem findings and the currently held theory of 'vernix membrane' formation has led to a re-examination of the facts on which the theory is based. From an appraisal of these facts it is suggested that the hyaline-like membrane or 'vernix membrane' is not aspirated vernix but represents a tissue reaction to injury of the bronchioles, alveolar ducts, and alveoli." The following year, 1950, Miller and Jennison reported the finding of atelectasis with hyaline membranes in 68 per cent of liveborn infants weighing between 1 and 2 kg. who were autopsied.

Blystad et al. (1951) concurred in the high incidence of the lesion in premature infants and evaluated the clinical aspects of the illness which soon became known in the literature as hyaline membrane disease.

Gregg and Bernstein (1961) have written an extensive review of studies on hyaline membrane disease up to that year. More recent reviews are those of Gairdner (1965), Keuth (1965), Rudolph et al. (1966), Sinclair (1966), Nelson (1970), Reynolds (1970), Lauweryns (1970), and Stern (1972).

INCIDENCE OF ATELECTASIS AND MEMBRANES

In all parts of the world in which careful studies have been conducted, hyaline membrane disease does occur. The per cent of deaths from this cause does differ just as the incidence of other causes of death differs, but the per cent of deaths from hyaline membrane disease, per numbers of infants born, varies very little. Any careful comparison of the incidence will be difficult as long as pathologic criteria differ; some pathologists recognize membranes in nearly every high power field before they will make the diagnosis, others consider the typical pattern of atelectasis with only a few membranes sufficient, and others suspect the disease if the atelectasis is present, whether or not membranes are evident (Gruenwald, 1952; Briggs and Hogg, 1958). Different investigators who study the same case material may disagree in their final calculation of incidence (Avery and Oppenheimer, 1960). Despite these limitations, investigators in many parts of the world consider hyaline membrane disease to be a leading cause of death of liveborn premature infants (Table 12–2).

Note that these authors subdivide infants by different weight groups. Since the risk of the disease is not the same in all weight groups, the numbers are not directly comparable. They serve to show the world-wide occurrence of the disease. It is estimated that about 300,000 premature infants are born each year in the United States. If the death rate from hyaline membrane disease is 3.8 per cent of live premature births, then about 12,000 infants die of hyaline membrane

Table 12–2. Incidence of Hyaline Membrane Disease

	Birth Weight	Nos.	HMD/100 Births	HMD/100 Deaths
Baltimore	1.0–1.5 kg.	27	17.8	36.5
1954–1958	1.5–2.0 kg.	19	6.2	38.8
(Avery and Oppenheimer, 1960)	2.0–2.5 kg.	10	0.97	45.4
Total > 1 kg.— < 2.5 kg.			3.8	38.8
Lebanon	Infants	35		38.4
(Younozai, 1962)	< 2.5 kg.			
Singapore	0.5–1.0 kg.	13		29.5
(Sivanesan, 1961)	1.0–1.5 kg.	45		45.0
	1.5–2.0 kg.	41		38.3
	2.0–2.5 kg.	17		32.7
	2.5–3.0 kg.	3		10.7
Total > 0.5 kg.— < 2.5 kg.				32.9
New York	< 1 kg.	19	16.4	23.7
(Silverman and Silverman, 1958)	1.0–1.5 kg.	35	16.2	61.4
	1.5–2.0 kg.	32	8.9	74.4
India	Total		7–9.9	46.4
(Webb et al., 1962)	< 2.5 kg.			
London, England	Total		3.9	
(Barrie, 1962)	< 2.5 kg.		4.7	

disease each year. Since some infants weighing more than 2.5 kg. at birth—particularly infants of diabetic mothers—also die of the disease, and others die of atelectasis without membrane formation (which may be the same process), the total deaths from the disease are probably nearer 25,000 per year in this country.

The review of autopsies performed at the Boston Lying-In Hospital from 1955 to 1960 shows the frequency in which pulmonary disorders are found, and specifically the central importance of hyaline membrane disease (Table 12–3).

PATHOLOGY OF HYALINE MEMBRANE DISEASE

At autopsy the lungs are airless, red-purple, and liver-like. They are not significantly heavier than lungs of most infants at autopsy; however, control data of lung weight of infants who succumbed to nonpulmonary diseases are lacking. The process is uniform throughout the lungs. On histologic examination the striking finding is atelectasis, so that individual alveoli are rarely distinguishable (Figs. 12–1 and 12–2). Membranes are rarely present in infants who live less than a few hours; those who live longer show the eosinophilic membrane adjacent to the aerated portions of the lung, usually the terminal bronchiole and alveolar ducts. The dilated bronchioles contain a pro-

Table 12-3.   Pulmonary Disorders as Major Cause
of Neonatal Death[*]

Diagnosis	Body Weight				
	≤ *1000* gm.	*1001–1500* gm.	*1501–2000* gm.	*2001–2500* gm.	> *2500* gm.
Hyaline membrane with atelectasis	33	41	42	32	14
Pneumonia	5	14	7	4	8
Massive aspiration	0	2	0	1	5
Idiopathic pulmonary hemorrhage	3	1	5	1	3
"Structural immaturity"	46	0	0	0	0
Totals	87	58	54	38	30

[*] Boston Lying-In Hospital, 422 neonatal autopsies, July 1, 1955, through June 30, 1960. From Driscoll, S. G., and Smith, C. A.: Pediat. Clin. N. Am., 9:325, 1962.

teinaceous coagulum, which is best demonstrated when the lung is fixed in Helly's fluid or Bouin's fluid (Shanklin, 1964). Dilated lymphatics are also regularly present, sometimes to an extreme degree (Lauweryns et al., 1965, 1968). Leukocytes are rarely seen in infants who die in less than 24 hours; after that time they are usually present. When infants die on the third day of life, the membrane may be fragmented and partially ingested by macrophages (Potter, 1953; Driscoll and Smith, 1962). Epithelial cells from the body surface are rarely seen in the airways with this disease. After seven to 10 days, infants who have had hyaline membrane disease, but who succumb to other causes, may have small remnants of membrane while lung architecture is normal. Vascular engorgement and frank hemorrhage may be associated lesions, but are not invariably present (Driscoll and Smith, 1962).

Epithelial necrosis in the terminal bronchioles at sites underlying the membrane suggests that a reaction to injury takes place (Barter and Maddison, 1960). Buckingham and Sommers (1960) noted hypersecretory changes in the cells that line the terminal bronchioles and alveoli. Reparative phenomena, characterized by cellular proliferation, are almost always present in infants who survive more than 48 hours (Boss and Craig, 1962).

Under the electron microscope, the membrane is composed of a matrix with the periodicity of fibrin, and cellular debris. The alveolar lining layer is disrupted in places underlying the membrane, with discontinuities of the basement membrane of the alveolar cells (Van Breeman et al., 1961; Campiche et al., 1961). Groniowski and Biczyskowa (1963) noted vesicles in the capillary endothelium suggestive of pinocytosis.

Lauweryns (1970) points out the variability in the appearance of the epithelial cells. The granular pneumocytes (type II cells) usually contain an impressive number of osmiophilic inclusions, as noted

Fig. 12–1

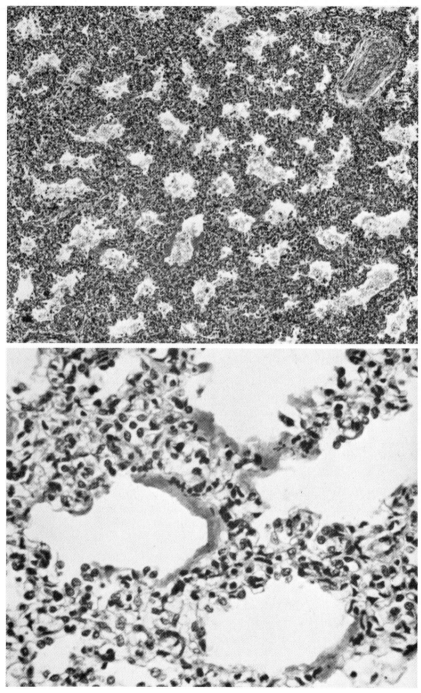

Fig. 12–2

Figure 12–1. Section from a lung with atelectasis and hyaline membranes. The membrane lines some of the aerated spaces. × 100.

Figure 12–2. High-power view of the homogeneous, eosinophilic hyaline membrane. × 400.

also by Balis et al. (1966). Since the osmiophilic inclusions are thought to relate to the pulmonary surfactant, which is deficient in hyaline membrane disease, many questions arise. Are they present in greater number the longer the infant lives and hence represent a phase in recovery? Are they normal in all respects? Or is there a problem in surfactant release, assuming surfactant is stored in the inclusions?

Histochemical studies of the membrane itself establish the presence of materials from the blood. The membrane stains positive for iron-containing compounds, and a hemoglobin-like compound that gives a positive benzidine and Nadi reaction is present (Lynch and Mellor, 1956). Under ultraviolet light with a Woods filter, the membrane fluoresces, and the fluorescence is enhanced after staining with auramine (Duran-Jorda et al., 1956). Gitlin and Craig (1956) confirmed the presence of fibrin by using fluorescin-stained antibodies. Berezin doubts the importance of fibrin because of the absence of reactivity for tryptophan. He was impressed by the presence of a glycoprotein containing tyrosine and arginine (1969).

The cumulative electronmicroscopic and histochemical evidence leaves little doubt that the membrane itself is derived from substances in the circulation and injured epithelium, and is not exogenous in origin.

OTHER CONDITIONS ASSOCIATED WITH HYALINE MEMBRANES

Before we consider in more detail the features of hyaline membrane disease in infants, it is worthwhile noting other conditions in which a similar eosinophilic membrane is found in lungs. While the profound diffuse atelectasis with hyaline membranes seems restricted to the premature infants, there are numerous conditions that occur at other times of life in which membranes are present with variable degrees of atelectasis and edema. It may be that recognition of their common features will elucidate the disease in infancy.

Poison Gases

Aschoff in 1916 described hyaline degeneration of the respiratory tract from inhalation of war gases. Phosgene poisoning characteristically results in edema and membrane formation (Groll, 1921). The inhalation of mercury vapor produces a lesion indistinguishable from hyaline membrane disease histologically, although this gas, as well as others, is more likely to produce patchy disease than the widespread sort seen in infancy (Matthes et al., 1958).

Aspiration

Hyaline membranes may be present after aspiration of milk (Bovet-DuBois, 1951) or kerosene (Barter, 1962).

Viral Pneumonias

Influenza pneumonia is characterized by atelectasis and membrane formation very similar to that seen in infants. Opie studied this lesion in 1928, Farber and Wilson further described it in 1932, and extensive studies on patients who died in the Asian influenza A epidemic in 1957 and 1958 further clarified this lesion (Martin et al., 1959). Destruction of the alveolar lining by the influenza virus in mice was shown by Hers et al. (1962).

Rheumatic Pneumonitis

Many workers have described the pulmonary lesion of the rheumatic state as a fibrinous exudate in alveolar ducts and alveoli, with necrosis of the alveolar walls. This lesion is more exudative than that usually seen in infancy, but it does bear a close resemblance to hyaline membrane disease (Goldring et al., 1958).

Other Diseases

Capers reported 18 severe cases of pulmonary hyaline membranes in adults who died of 16 disease processes, including bronchogenic carcinoma, hepatic insufficiency, and Hodgkin's disease (1961). The lesion in these individuals was not diffuse and therefore bears little resemblance to hyaline membrane disease of infancy. Nonetheless, the nonspecific character of membrane formation is illustrated by this study.

Oxygen and Carbon Dioxide Poisoning

Prolonged use of pure oxygen delivered by respirators is associated with a significant incidence of hyaline membranes in the lungs examined post-mortem (Cederberg et al., 1965). It has been known for years that exposure of animals to 100 per cent oxygen for three to four days will result in pulmonary death, with edema, atelectasis, and membrane formation. These studies, recently reviewed and extended by Berfenstam et al. (1958), have led to the suggestion that oxygen poisoning may play a role in the disease of infants. It is not clear from the oxygen studies whether the lesion is from the high oxygen tension in the airways or the associated high carbon dioxide tension in the blood, which in itself can produce membranes in animals (Sehlkopf and von Werz, 1948; Niemoeller and Schaefer, 1962).

Irradiation from X-rays

Studies of the effects of radiation on human and animal lungs show swelling and distortion of the alveolar lining cells, some desquamation of them, and a hyaline-like membrane adherent to the alveolar walls. This reaction requires high doses of irradiation, and does not appear to be very significant clinically. Fibrosis is the more characteristic lesion from chronic irradiation given on therapeutic indication (Warren and Gates, 1940).

After Cardiopulmonary Bypass

Patients undergoing open-heart surgery may have progressive pulmonary dysfunction in the postoperative period. Atelectasis edema and some hyaline membranes are often found in these patients (Tooley et al., 1961).

CLINICAL MANIFESTATIONS

Infants at Risk

The infants at risk are mainly those born prematurely and of appropriate size for gestational age. In general, birth weight of 1 to 1.5 kg. is most common, and the incidence in infants of over 2.5 kg. is of the order of one in 6000 births, if infants of diabetic mothers are excluded. In a review of 2001 premature infants, Cohen et al. (1960) analyzed the complications of pregnancy and route of delivery in an attempt to isolate predisposing factors. Hyaline membrane disease was 8.9 times greater among infants delivered by cesarean section than among those delivered vaginally. However, if a history of maternal bleeding was taken into consideration, it was apparent that the correlation of hyaline membranes with maternal hemorrhage was most important. For those pregnancies with a history of bleeding, no statistically significant differences were noted between the two methods of delivery. These data confirm those of Strang et al. (1957) that elective cesarean section per se does not increase the risk of hyaline membrane disease. In a review of 571 consecutive cesarean sections. Hess concluded that section, in itself, should not add to fetal mortality (1958). However, Usher's review of the experience at The Royal Victoria Hospital in Montreal showed that cesarean section per se did predispose to the respiratory distress syndrome in infants of less than 270 days gestational age (1964). The risk of death from respiratory distress in infants delivered by section was 40 per cent at 29 to 33 weeks, 10 per cent at 34 to 36 weeks, one per cent at 37 to 38 weeks, and was the same regardless of the indication for which cesarean section was performed. In the comparison of section and vaginal deliveries, the incidence of clinical respiratory distress was three times greater by section at 31 to 33 weeks, and 14 times greater at 37 to 38 weeks. The magnitude of the difference is so great at 37 to 38 weeks as to be well beyond a chance observation. An important observation on the relationship of labor to deaths with hyaline membrane disease was reported by Fedrick and Butler (1972). They noted that the incidence among babies born by cesarean section before the start of labor was four times that found among babies delivered by cesarean section during labor (p < 0.001).

Maternal diabetes appears to predispose infants to hyaline membrane disease, since it was found in 71 of 95 infants of diabetic mothers who were studied post-mortem (Driscoll et al., 1960). It was the major lesion in 49 of these infants. It is difficult to be certain of the role of prematurity in the pathogenesis of the disease in the group of infants who are oversized for gestational age, and hence may be premature by date if not by weight. Even so, it appears that infants of diabetic mothers of 36 to 37 weeks' gestation die of hyaline membrane disease more often than other infants of comparable gestational age. Clear evidence on this point is lacking at this time. In some respects, the infant of a diabetic mother may be thought of as a premature infant seen through a magnifying glass.

The risk of recurrence of respiratory distress in subsequent low birth weight infants is nearly 90 per cent; the risk of occurrence after one normal low birth weight infant is less than 5 per cent (Graven and Misenheimer, 1965).

A history of asphyxia at birth is more common in infants who later succumb from hyaline membrane disease than in those who do not. Likewise the second-born of twins is at greater risk than the first-born, perhaps because of the greater likelihood of asphyxia. (Crosse, 1957; Keuth, 1965; Rokos et al., 1968).

Prenatal Detection

Knowledge of infants at risk allows some possibility of prenatal detection of postnatal respiratory distress. Much improved approaches depend on a measurement of lung maturation, particularly with respect to surfactant synthesis. Since lung liquid enters the amniotic pool, it is possible to search for the phospholipid components of the surfactant in amniotic fluid. Gluck et al. (1971) demonstrated changes in lecithin and sphingomyelin concentrations throughout the last weeks of gestation, with a sharp increase in lecithin from 34 weeks to a peak at 36 weeks. Sphingomyelin tended to peak at 30 to 32 weeks and fell after 35 weeks' gestation. They suggested that checking the ratio of lecithin to sphingomyelin would be a useful way to obviate problems with differing amounts of amniotic fluid, and should be predictive of the respiratory distress syndrome. When the ratio of lecithin to sphingomyelin exceeds 2.0, the infant is unlikely to have respiratory distress; between 1.5 and 1.9, the distress will be mild; and a ratio of 1.0 to 1.49 is predictive of immaturity of the lung and moderate to severe respiratory distress. Whitfield et al. (1972) agree that the determination is predictive of respiratory distress in the infant. Others have questioned the validity of these predictors and suggest that the concentration of lecithin in the amniotic fluid is a better indicator of the likelihood of respiratory distress than is the lecithin/sphingomyelin ratio (Nelson, 1969; Bhagwanani et al., 1972).

A more rapid and more readily available test was described by Clements et al. (1972). Their method depends on the ability of the pulmonary surfactant to generate stable bubbles in the presence of ethanol. By their method, the surfactant becomes detectable in amniotic fluid at about 33 weeks, although it is variable from 25 weeks to term. Equal volumes of 95 per cent ethanol and amniotic fluid are mixed, then further diluted with saline in serial dilutions. The tubes are shaken for 15 seconds and are then allowed to stand. Fifteen minutes later observation of the presence or absence of small stable bubbles allowed an estimate of the presence of surfactant.

These studies are of significance since they permit prediction of which fetuses may be capable of breathing normally after birth. Occasionally delivery can be delayed until lung maturity is established. Unfortunately, not all births can be postponed to the ideal moment, so means of conserving preexisting surfactant or supporting infants without it deserve continued study. (See pages 13–15.)

Onset of Symptoms

One of the most striking and constant features of this disease is the predictability of the early onset of symptoms. If it is certain that an infant has breathed normally in all respects for more than six or eight hours, that infant will not have hyaline membrane disease. Inadequate observation occasionally leads to the impression of a symptom-free interval of hours. As more consistent and careful observations have been made on these infants, it has become clear that most have had some respiratory difficulty in the delivery room, and the rest have shown elevations of the respiratory rate and some retractions by a few hours of age (James, 1959). Latham et al. (1955) reported that nearly 80 per cent of 124 infants who died with hyaline membrane disease were in fair or poor condition at birth. Miller (1962) found that the mothers of half of the severely affected infants had complications capable of producing intrauterine asphyxia, unresponsiveness at birth, and severe respiratory distress from the time of birth. The remainder of the infants in Miller's series were not severely depressed at birth, nonetheless some succumbed from hyaline membrane disease. Auld et al. (1961) mentioned death from hyaline membrane disease in five infants who were in excellent condition at birth. If careful records of respiratory rate and retractions are kept, it will be evident that even these infants who are vigorous at birth are in respiratory difficulty by several hours of age (Miller and Conklin, 1955).

Signs

Infants who subsequently die of hyaline membrane disease, and many others who go on and recover, have an elevated respiratory rate, and retractions of the soft tissues during inspiration. Often the lower portion of the sternum appears to meet the vertebral column, and may even be depressed throughout the respiratory cycle. The upper chest may appear to be overinflated. The abdomen may protrude during inspiration in a sort of "see-saw" pattern with respect to the chest (Miller and Behrle, 1958). A useful system of grading the severity of the retractions has been devised by Silverman and Anderson (1956), Bauman (1959) (Fig. 12–3).

In severely affected infants, expiration is accompanied by a whimper or cry. Apneic periods of more than 10 seconds, interposed by periods of very rapid breathing, are a poor prognostic sign in hyaline membrane disease. Percussion of the chest is of little help in any pulmonary disorder of premature infants, since sounds are so widely transmitted. Auscultation is more useful, as it gives some estimate of the degree of air exchange. Harsh breath sounds are the rule, and occasionally fine rales are present, especially at the end of a deep inspiration that precedes a cry.

The cardiac manifestations of hyaline membrane disease do not appear to be constant. Burnard (1958, 1959) was impressed with the frequency of roentgenographic evidence of cardiomegaly and the

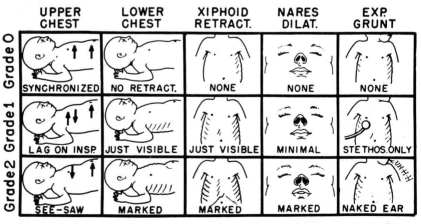

Figure 12–3. Observation of retractions. (From Silverman, W.: Pediatrics 18:614, 1956.)

presence of a systolic murmur. Others have found these signs less commonly (Driscoll and Smith, 1962). The heart rate is not usually outside the wide limits of normal in premature infants, except terminally when bradycardia is the rule. A tendency toward a fixed heart rate of 110 to 120/min. has been noted, as if normal vagal control were deficient. It is a serious sign, present in about one-half of distressed infants, but may be reversible (Burnard, 1959; Rudolph et al., 1965).

Systemic hypotension is now well documented (Neligan and Smith, 1960). The poor peripheral circulation is one of the outstanding clinical features of the disease. The infants may look pale and dusky even with hematocrit values of 60 per cent or greater, and pooling of the circulation is evident in the darker coloration in the dependent areas. Peripheral edema is usually present, as is commonly so in premature infants, but it is more pronounced in hyaline membrane disease (Sutherland et al., 1959).

Cyanosis is always present in severely affected infants. Strang and also Prod'hom demonstrated the persistence of arterial unsaturation even with oxygen breathing in these infants, establishing the presence of right-to-left shunts (Strang and MacLeish, 1961; Prod'hom et al., 1965; Nelson et al., 1963). (See pages 64–65.) Progressive cyanosis is one of the most grave prognostic signs in the disease. Extensive circulatory studies in 168 infants with clinical and radiologic findings typical of hyaline membrane disease were reported in 1972 by Stahlman and her colleagues. Umbilical artery catheters were advanced to the mid-abdominal aorta, and an umbilical venous catheter was guided through the ductus venosus into the left atrium via the inferior vena cava and foramen ovale. Pressure measurements and indicator-dilution curves were carried out. They confirmed the presence of systemic hypotension, and noted that it progressed in the more severely ill infants. A rise in blood pressure was a good prognostic sign.

Both right-to-left and left-to-right shunts may exist during the disease. Stahlman et al. found about half of the infants had large right-to-left shunts at less than 13 hours of age; only 15 per cent had large left-to-right shunts at that age. Over the next 24 hours, only 25 per cent had large right-to-left shunts. The trend was for more prominent left-to-right shunts with recovery.

The site of shunting can change during the disease. Early in life, or in the sickest infants, it can occur through the foramen ovale and occasionally through the ductus arteriosus. The most significant left-to-right shunting was through the ductus after the first 12 hours of life.

Hypothermia is usually present, in an environmental temperature of 88 to 90°F. Persistent body temperatures lower than 95°F when the infant is in a warm environment should alert the physician to serious illness. Incubator temperatures of over 95°F are usually required to raise body temperatures to normal levels.

Course

If death results from uncomplicated hyaline membrane disease, it almost always occurs before 72 hours of age. Death occurs in rare cases at four or five days of age, but in such infants intracranial and pulmonary hemorrhage or pneumonia is usually coexistent (Silverman, 1961). Life may be prolonged in some infants with the use of respirators, and recovery is usually, but not always, complete. Prolonged hypoxemia in most infants with severe hyaline membrane disease was first reported by Adamson et al. (1969). They postulated persistent inequalities of ventilation and perfusion in most infants for about two weeks and in those who required respirators for many weeks. They advocate careful monitoring of arterial oxygen tensions to guide the gradual reduction in inspired oxygen concentrations in these infants. Delayed closure of the ductus arteriosus has been noted in some infants who had recovered from the respiratory distress syndrome (Kitterman et al., 1972). Five of seven such infants went into heart failure but recovered on medical management (Auld et al., 1966). (See page 47.

Radiology of Hyaline Membrane Disease

The demise of the "no-touch" technique in the care of premature infants and the subsequent employment of radiologic diagnostic techniques eventually has led to a high degree of accuracy in the diagnosis of hyaline membrane disease (Fig. 12–4). The radiologic appearance of the lungs in hyaline membrane disease was recognized as a "patchy mottling" (Meschan et al., 1953), and Donald and Steiner (1953) described three distinct stages of the disease with progression from (1) "a fine miliary mottling" of the lungs, to (2) "a more coalescent opacity" through which the bronchial tree was well visualized, and finally to (3) increasing confluence of the density due to consolidation and collapse. The third stage was associated with subsequent death but the possibility of clearing of the lungs and complete recovery of the infant was also recognized (Steiner, 1954). Ellis and Nadelhaft (1957) stressed exaggeration of the normal bronchial air shadows (air bronchogram) associated with a granular pattern. Accuracy of diagnosis based on the typical findings of diffuse mottling or granularity (Singleton, 1967) is probably about 80 per cent (Driscoll and Smith, 1962). This pattern is usually present in the distressed infant within a few hours of birth; in the series of Wolfson et al. (1969), 90 per cent of the radiographs of 75 infants with hyaline membrane disease were positive by five hours of age. However, its appearance may occasionally be delayed (Harris, 1963; Peterson and Pendleton, 1955). Increase in severity may occur within the first 12 to 24 hours (Peterson and Pendleton, 1955). Feinberg and Goldberg (1957) demonstrated abnormal chest radiographs in three infants prior to the onset of respiratory symptoms.

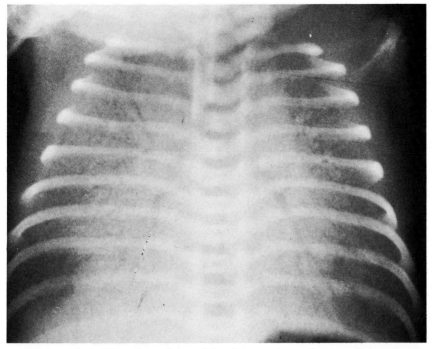

Figure 12–4. Film of an infant with hyaline membrane disease, taken at age two hours. The reticulogranular infiltrates are distributed throughout the lung fields, and the tracheobronchial tree can be seen against the opacified lung, the so-called "air bronchogram." An endotracheal tube has been inserted.

Roentgenologic-Pathologic Correlation. The granular pattern seen roentgenographically is due to alveolar atelectasis interspersed with aerated bronchioles and alveolar ducts (Recavarren et al., 1967) (Fig. 12–5) and is not due primarily to the presence of hyaline membranes. In fact, the infant may die before hyaline membranes have formed (Landing, 1955). According to Lauweryns (1970), the classic radiologic appearance of the post-mortem lung is dependent on re-expansion of the lungs; a long interval between death and autopsy examination produces an uneven pattern of aeration.

Atypical Patterns. In the very premature infant, the lung parenchyma may be completely opaque because of inadequate mechanical forces necessary for alveolar expansion. When better expansion is possible, the production of a diffuse, symmetric granular pattern is the rule but occasionally irregular distribution occurs, sometimes in entire lobes (Rudhe et al., 1970). Superimposed inflammation or hemorrhage may also alter the roentgen appearance. Ablow and Orzalesi (1971) have suggested that limitation of the typical pattern to the lower lung fields in two infants and more rapid clearing of the upper lobes in one patient may reflect earlier maturation of the upper lobes analogous to experimental observations in fetal rabbits and

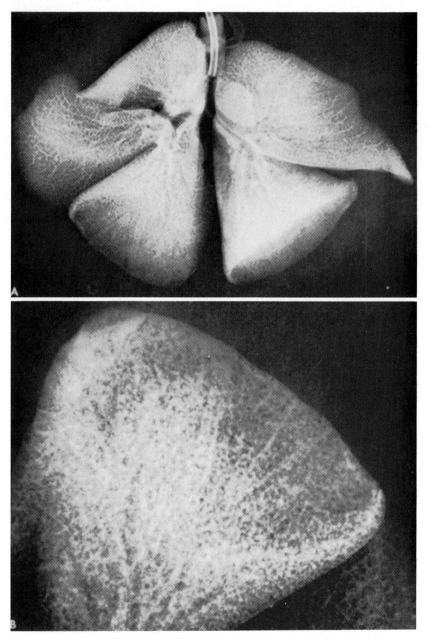

Figure 12–5. Inflated excised lungs from an infant who died with hyaline membrane disease. *A* shows the diffuse and even distribution of the pathologic process.
B is a higher powered view of a portion of one lobe, showing the lack of inflation of the
peripheral air spaces. The granularity seen on the chest films presumably represents the
airless terminal airspaces. (From Recavarren et al.: Seminars Roentgen. *2:*22, 1967.)

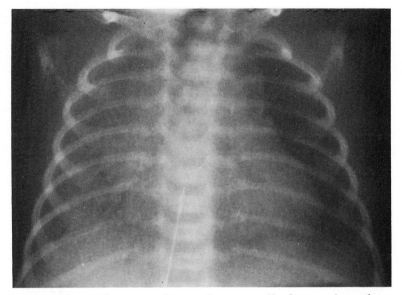

Figure 12–6. In this patient, the granular pattern of hyaline membrane disease is much more marked on the right than the left. (From Tchou, C.-S., et al.: J. Canad. Assoc. Radiol. 1972.)

lambs. Tchou et al. (1972), however, found a surprisingly high incidence (18 of 64 infants) of asymmetric distribution of hyaline membrane disease, usually more severe on the right. This could not be related to technical factors or the presence of superimposed disease (Figs. 12–6 and 12–7).

Prognostic Value of Radiographs. Marked reticulogranularity and reduced volume of the lung fields are associated with a bad prognosis, whereas patients with overexpanded lungs may be expected to recover (Iannaccone et al., 1965). Reduced lung volume even prior to the onset of the typical granular pattern of hyaline membrane is also a poor prognostic sign (Remy et al., 1970). Inability to expand the lungs may be related to central nervous system damage or mechanical weakness of the thorax. Fletcher and Taeusch (1972) have shown a correlation between decreased aeration of post-mortem chest radiographs of newborn lambs and physiologic measurements of pulmonary immaturity associated with diminished amounts of surfactant.

Radiologic Changes Associated with Survival. In the infants who survive, radiologic clearing has been noted to be complete by one week of age (Peterson and Pendleton, 1955). With the advent of assisted ventilation, a decrease in mortality has occurred, and follow-up studies suggest that the disease is not self-limiting but that morphologic abnormalities may persist into later life. A marked delay in clearing of the lungs is frequently observed, and overinflation of the lung with linear densities in the lower lobes were seen in 11 hyaline mem-

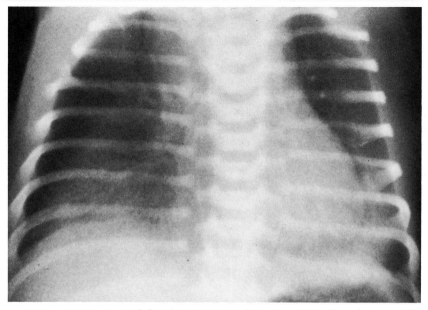

Figure 12–7.   Atypical distribution of granular pattern of hyaline membrane disease, which is confined to the lung bases.

brane disease survivors aged two to five years who had been managed in a negative-pressure respirator (Fletcher et al., 1973) (Fig. 12–8). These findings were similar to those reported by Shepard et al. (1968). The question of whether the abnormalities are a reparative stage of hyaline membrane disease or are due to the effects of assisted ventilation remains open.

Electrocardiogram

There is some dispute about the value of the ECG in evaluation of hyaline membrane disease. Keith et al. (1961) suggested that a tall R wave over the right precordium, indicative of high pulmonary vascular resistance, is associated with a better prognosis than the presence of a deep S wave over the right precordium, indicative of low pulmonary vascular resistance. Others have pointed out prolongation of the P-R and QRS intervals late in the course of the disease, in association with elevated serum potassium concentrations (Usher, 1959). These changes are surely nonspecific, however, and not regularly seen in hyaline membrane disease. Nicolopoulos and Smith (1961) found that clinical severity of the disease was only inconclusively related to the amount of tissue catabolism and not at all to the degree of hyperkalemia.

LABORATORY DETERMINATIONS

Blood Chemical Determinations

There are no consistent changes in the NPN, blood glucose, potassium, sodium, chloride, or total proteins which distinguish premature infants with hyaline membrane disease from others of comparable weight (Nicolopoulos and Smith, 1961). Serum bilirubin levels tend to be higher in infants with respiratory distress than in those of similar weight with normal respiration (Miller and Behrle, 1958). Lactic acid levels are elevated; levels about 45 mg. per cent are associated with a poor prognosis (Stahlman et al., 1962).

Cooke (1960) measured serum protein levels in premature infants with and without respiratory distress, and found that the prognosis was better when serum proteins were over 5 gm. per cent than when they were less than 5 gm. per cent protein. He divided his patients into two groups, one of which he treated with 4 mg./lb. of 25 per cent serum albumin as soon as possible after birth, the other being untreated as a control group. Of 18 treated premature infants, none died from hyaline membrane disease. Six of the 18 untreated control infants died from the disease. This provocative account led to further studies on more infants in whom the favorable results were not confirmed (Fraillon and Kitchen, 1962).

The prognostic value of total serum proteins measured on cord blood was convincingly reaffirmed by Bland et al. (1972). Severe disease was restricted to the group with a level below 4.6 gm. per cent.

Blood Gas Determinations

Arterial oxygen unsaturation and a combined respiratory and metabolic acidosis are regularly found in hyaline membrane disease. The studies of James and of Reardon on acid-base status at birth provide a background for the interpretation of the persistent evidences of asphyxia in infants with pulmonary inadequacy (James et al., 1958; Reardon et al., 1960). Infants at birth have an arterial pH of about 7.25 to 7.30, with PCO_2 of 50 to 70 mm. Hg, and bicarbonates of 18 to 22 mEq./liter. The normal infant depends on the initiation of respiration to blow off carbon dioxide and correct the respiratory acidosis, and by several hours of age has usually retained enough bicarbonate to correct the metabolic component as well (Oliver, 1961). Bruns et al. (1961) found that infants born of mothers whose arterial and intervillous space oxygen tension was low had a more marked respiratory and metabolic acidosis, and subsequently developed hyaline membrane disease. The persistence and aggravation of carbon dioxide retention and acidosis is a measure of ventilatory inadequacy. Infants with se-

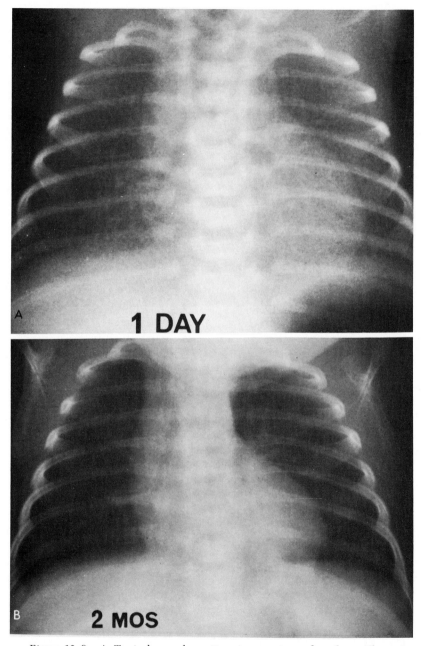

Figure 12–8. A, Typical granular pattern is seen at one day of age. The patient was managed in a negative pressure respirator. B, The lungs had not completely cleared by the time of discharge from the nursery at age two months. Bilateral confluent densities remained in the lower lobes.

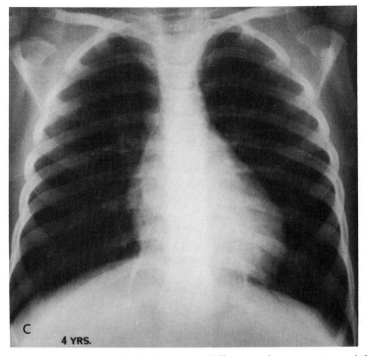

Figure 12–8 Continued. C, Long-term follow-up shows persistent bilateral basilar linear densities, which are still present at age four years. There were no respiratory symptoms. (From Fletcher, B. D., et al.: Ann. Radiol. 1973.)

vere hyaline membrane disease may have an arterial pH of 7.0, PCO_2 of over 60 mm. Hg, and PO_2 of less than 40 mm. Hg, even in 100 per cent oxygen.

Changes of this degree in blood gases are usually lethal. The precise values at which an irreversible stage of hyaline membrane disease has been reached are not yet established (James et al., 1958), although Usher feels that venous pH below 7.15 or PCO_2 of over 70 mm. Hg, and bicarbonate value of less than 18 mEq./liter is usually lethal without therapy (1961). Boston et al. (1966) consider infants at high risk of dying if blood gases before 10 hours of age show a $P_aO_2 \leqq 100$ mm. Hg while breathing 100 per cent oxygen, and pH $\leqq 7.20$. They found serial measurement of P_aO_2 most useful in monitoring the course and severity of the disease.

Measurements of Pulmonary Function

Despite the obvious difficulties in the measurement of pulmonary function in sick premature infants, the functional derangements in hyaline membrane disease are probably as well documented as they are in any pulmonary disease. As noted earlier, the respiratory rate is elevated from an average of 40 to 50 in normal infants to 70 to 120/min. in hyaline membrane disease. Tidal volume is decreased, and minute volume normal or increased. The low tidal volume suggests that the dead space is increased to more than half the tidal volume, and measurements confirm this (Karlberg et al., 1954). Lung distensibility or compliance—the change in volume per unit change in pressure at points of no flow—is reduced to one-fourth or one-fifth the usual value. The functional residual capacity is greatly reduced, and the crying vital capacity likewise restricted. Airway resistance is essentially unchanged, but the decrease in compliance contributes to greatly increased work of breathing (Karlberg et al., 1954; Berglund and Karlberg, 1956; Sutherland and Ratcliff, 1961; Auld et al., 1963).

Nelson et al. (1962) have demonstrated the ventilation-perfusion imbalance present in distressed infants on the basis of a significant arterial-alveolar tension gradient for carbon dioxide. They infer from these findings an increased alveolar dead space owing to poor perfusion of ventilated portions of the lung. The finding of low arterial oxygen tensions even with high inspired oxygen mixtures attests to the right-to-left shunt, some of which may be through the foramen ovale or ductus, but much of which is probably intrapulmonary in that blood may flow past nonventilated portions of the lung parenchyma just as it may bypass ventilated portions. The site of shunting of blood is not yet clearly established (Woodrum et al., 1972).

Normal newborn infants may shunt nearly one-fourth of their cardiac output from right to left in the first few days of life. The magnitude of the right-to-left shunt in infants with respiratory distress is much greater, up to two-thirds of the cardiac output (Nelson, 1963). Strang demonstrated a significant negative correlation between alveolar ventilation and right-to-left shunts—the less the ventilation, the greater the shunt (Strang, 1961). Woodrum et al. (1972) noted a significant alveolar-arterial difference for oxygen tensions in all premature infants, although it was more marked in those with hyaline membrane disease.

Measurements of Cardiovascular Function

Cardiac catheterization studies on the circulation of infants with severe respiratory distress have revealed the ductus arteriosus to be widely patent with a large left-to-right shunt, and, on occasion, right-to-left shunts through it. Both pulmonary arterial and systemic arterial pressures were lower than expected on the basis of a control group of somewhat heavier infants. There was no elevation of left atrial pressure (measured with respect to atmospheric pressure) as is usually found in left ventricular failure (Rudolph et al., 1961). Measurements on infants who subsequently died, and in whom the autopsy diagnosis was hyaline membrane disease, are especially significant in that they establish the fact of vascular hypotension. Systemic pressures ranged from 29/16 mm. Hg to 60/30 mm. Hg, whereas pulmonary artery pressures were from 23/14 to 58/28 mm. Hg. Systemic arterial oxygen saturations in these infants were from 77 to 98 per cent while breathing oxygen.

Limb blood flow is reduced from levels of 10 to 12 ml./100 ml. tissue/min. in normal premature infants to levels of 2 to 7 ml./100 ml. tissue/min. in those with the respiratory distress syndrome. Since systemic arterial pressures were not reduced in these particular infants, the suggestion is that peripheral vascular resistance is increased (Kidd et al., 1966).

Measurements of Renal Function

Impaired urine production is often noted during the severe phases of hyaline membrane disease. A diuresis occasionally heralds recovery. Allen and Usher (1971) found a deficiency in renal acid excretion in sick infants compared to other premature infants. The sick infants failed to excrete appropriate amounts of acid in the face of acidemia; occasionally they aggravated the situation by excreting bicarbonate.

STUDIES ON EXCISED LUNGS

The physical properties of the lungs of infants with hyaline membrane disease, studied after death, are strikingly different from properties of lungs of infants dead from nonpulmonary causes (Gruenwald, 1947; Gribetz et al., 1959; Behrle et al., 1951). They fail to expand as fully as other lungs; static pressures of 35 cm. H_2O, which are sufficient to fully inflate a normal lung, permit only a small volume of air to enter the lung of an infant with hyaline membrane disease, and most of this air is in the bronchioles (Gribetz et al., 1959). Dissection of air into the interstitial spaces is likely to occur at higher pressures. In some lungs with hyaline membranes, however, some alveoli are opened at higher pressures (Gruenwald, 1963). In others, pressures as high as 60 cm. H_2O fail to achieve expansion of the terminal airspaces (Fig. 12–9).

Greater expansion is possible if the excised lungs are made airless, then inflated stepwise with saline at slow enough intervals so that volume equilibrium occurs (Fig. 12–9). This observation, noted by Potter in 1952, establishes the ability of the alveoli to inflate and rules out the possibility of an anomaly of the terminal airspaces. The lungs do not seem to be so readily distensible with more viscous solutions, however. Craig et al. (1958) failed to fill the distal airspaces of lungs with hyaline membrane disease with either gelation-India ink

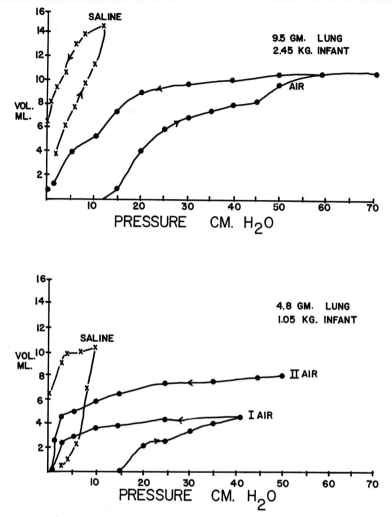

Figure 12-9. The solid line with circles indicates the pressure-volume character-istics of an excised lung of an infant with hyaline membrane, distended with air over a wide range of pressures. The line with crosses illustrates the relationships with saline filling. Note that the lung can be distended with saline, at very low pressures. The differences in pressure across the lung distended to a given volume with air and with saline are an index of the forces of surface tension. (Unpublished data of J. Guinane and M. E. Avery.)

or latex solutions, even though control lungs of infants of comparable weight filled well.

The deflation characteristics of excised lungs are of special in-terest. After distention to a peak distending pressure with air, step-wise deflation results in premature emptying of the gas in the lung (Fig. 12–10). The slope of the deflation curve, plotted as volume versus pressure, which is a measure of the elastic recoil of the lung, is abnor-

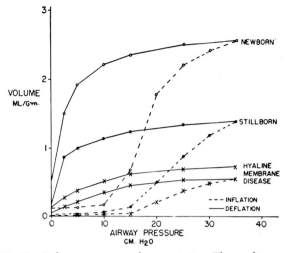

Figure 12–10. Volume-pressure characteristics. The ordinate refers to gas volume in milliliters per gram of tissue; airway pressure on the abscissa is equivalent to transpulmonary pressure. Four of the lungs with hyaline membrane disease were studied only during deflation and are represented by a separate curve. (From Gribetz, et al.: J. Clin. Invest., 38:2168, 1959.)

mal; thus, at pressures that would be the equivalent of end-expiratory pleural pressures, 1 to 2 cm. H_2O, the lungs are nearly airless, whereas control lungs at these pressures contain about 40 per cent of total lung volume. From these observations, Gribetz et al. (1959) calculated that the compliance of the lung during life would be about 0.8 ml./cm. H_2O, whereas measurements made with esophageal pressures used as indices of pleural pressure gave values of 0.7 to 1.3 ml./cm. H_2O. They also deduced that the functional residual capacity would be reduced to about one-fourth, the expected value, which is similar to the data of Berglund and Karlberg (1956), and Auld et al. (1963). Thus, the elastic recoil of the lung appears to be increased.

The means by which the disease affects the elastic behavior of the lungs is not clear. There is no histological evidence that elastic tissue is altered or that fibrosis occurs. It seems probable that the increase in surface tension of the fluid lining the airways contributes to the increased tendency of these lungs to empty. The studies of air filling and liquid filling of the lungs attest to the marked effect of an air-liquid interface on the volume-pressure relationships.

Further studies on the effects of surface tension in these lungs were made on washings from the airways or minced portions of lung parenchyma (Avery and Mead, 1959). It may be assumed that the most surface-active material in the lung will be at the air-liquid interface, not only within the lung, but in vitro. Thus it will seek the surface of a trough and be available for direct measurements of surface tension. (See pages 10–15.)

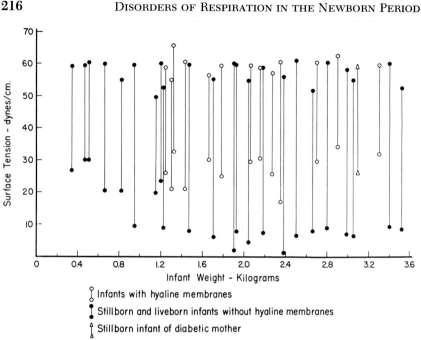

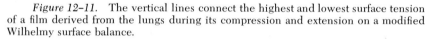

Figure 12–11. The vertical lines connect the highest and lowest surface tension of a film derived from the lungs during its compression and extension on a modified Wilhelmy surface balance.

Material from lungs of infants with hyaline membrane disease differed from that of controls in having a smaller change of surface tension with area and in the failure to achieve a low tension (Fig. 12–11). This observation suggested to Avery and Mead that the disease was associated with the absence or delayed appearance of the substances which in the normal subject render the lung stable at low lung volumes and thus prevent atelectasis.

Further studies on the pressure-volume characteristics of the lungs and surface behavior of extracts from them showed a correspondence between premature closure of alveoli and absence of detectable surface-active material on a trough (Gruenwald et al., 1962). The absence of surface-active material in lung extracts may occur in lungs of infants who were stillborn (Avery and Mead, 1959), and suggests the prenatal origin of whatever insult alters the alveolar lining layer (Gruenwald, 1960).

Studies of fibrinolytic enzyme activity in the lungs of newborn infants with hyaline membrane disease reveal conflicting findings. Lieberman (1959) used bovine fibrin to study plasminogen activator activity in saline homogenates of lung tissue. Deficiencies in this enzyme were noted in seven of 45 control specimens, and in 13 of 16 specimens with hyaline membranes. In many specimens an inhibitor was demonstrated on the basis of failure of fibrinolysis when 0.5 ml.

aliquots of normal lung homogenate were mixed with 0.5 ml. aliquots of abnormal lung. Moreover, saline extracts of placenta were found to have a potent inhibitor effect against the plasminogen activator of lung. By contrast, Ambrus et al. (1963) used human fibrin as a substrate and found abundant plasminogen-activator activity in lungs of infants with hyaline membrane disease. They found no qualitative abnormality of the fibrinolytic system in hyaline membrane lungs. They did find a lack of plasminogen in the serum of premature infants, whether healthy or sick, and a value lower than the adult value in mature infants, which confirms the observations of others (Phillips and Skrodelis, 1958; Samartzis et al., 1960; Quie and Wannamaker, 1960). Samartzis et al. (1960) noted a more marked deficiency in plasma fibrinolytic activity in three infants who died of hyaline membrane disease; but 20 infants with the clinical syndrome who survived had levels comparable with those of normal controls. Serial measurements of fibrinolytic activity with the englobulin fibrinolysis method showed a depression of activity in premature infants, which was most marked in those who died with the respiratory distress syndrome. It is not clear whether the findings relate to hyaline membrane disease, or to all conditions characterized by hypoxia and acidemia (Markarian et al., 1967).

OTHER, POSSIBLY RELATED, PATHOLOGIC FINDINGS

Adrenal Glands

The relationship between adrenal structure and the development of hyaline membrane disease was pursued by Naeye (1972) in the light of the observations of Liggins that fetal glucocorticoid production could promote delivery and lessen the likelihood of respiratory distress. deLemos et al. (1970) had established that fetal glucocorticoid administration could accelerate lung maturation.

Detailed studies of 387 infants of the Babies Hospital series who lived from 7 to 72 hours showed the adrenal glands of infants with hyaline membrane disease were 19 per cent lighter than expected. The smallest adrenals for body size were in infants over 35 weeks' gestation who developed hyaline membrane disease. Naeye suggested that these undersized adrenals produced inadequate corticosteroids to promote lung maturation in utero. No deficiency of corticosteroids has been noted in affected infants after onset of respiratory distress, however. It seems equally probable that the small adrenal is the result of the stress of the disease. Postnatal release of glucocorticoids could explain the failure of hydrocortisone after birth to benefit the infants. (Baden et al., 1972). It could also explain the time of recovery from the disease if two to three days is required for induction of the capability of surfactant synthesis in the human, as it is in the lamb and rabbit.

Lymph Nodes

In a study of the maturation of lymph nodes in relation to birth weight and postnatal survival, Black and Speer (1960) noted a delay and inadequacy in development of the reticuloendothelial cells in infants with hyaline membrane disease. They further noted a prominence in eosinophilic leukocytes in nodes of affected infants. They suggested that immaturity of the reticuloendothelial system could be a factor in increased permeability of capillaries.

Liver

Thrombi in the hepatic sinusoids have been noted to be more common in infants dead from hyaline membrane disease than in infants dead from "other causes." This led Wade-Evans to suspect a disturbance in the circulation to the liver, with consequent anoxia. Fatty metamorphosis of the liver may be seen in infants asphyxiated from many causes (Benitez, 1952), but the thrombi appear to be more commonly associated with hyaline membrane disease in particular (Wade-Evans, 1961).

Bleeding

An association between intracranial hemorrhage and hyaline membrane disease has been noted by several investigators (Blystad et al., 1951; Ambrus et al., 1963; Harrison et al., 1968). In Ambrus's series, 67 per cent of infants autopsied with hyaline membrane disease had cerebral hemorrhage, and 53 per cent had pulmonary or visceral hemorrhage. In a series from Queen Charlotte's Maternity Hospital (1963–1970), 40 per cent of cases of intraventricular hemorrhage also showed hyaline membrane disease (Pryse-Davies, 1972). Several explanations are possible. One, the profound tissue hypoxia before death may be associated with capillary bleeding. Two, clotting factors are depressed in severe hypoxia. And three, the respiratory effort and grunting may be associated with an elevation of cerebral venous pressure. Which one or more of these possibilities is responsible for the lesion in hyaline membrane disease is not clear. In some infants disseminated intravascular coagulation has been noted (Alstatt et al., 1971; Margolis et al., 1973).

Case with Aberrant Vessels to Part of the Lung

A most remarkable experiment of nature, reported by Bozic (1963) occurred in an infant in Lausanne, Switzerland. The infant died of respiratory distress on the third day of life, and at autopsy all of the right lung and the upper portion of the left lung were airless. The inferior portion of the left lower lobe was aerated and emphysematous, but received its blood supply from three aberrant vessels from the aorta. Histologic examination and perfusion studies showed that all of the lung perfused from the pulmonary circulation had classic hyaline membrane disease, and that portion with systemic perfusion was unaffected.

Changes in Costochondral Junctions

Trabecular rarefaction in costochondral junctions occurs in a number of neonatal conditions, but especially in association with hyaline membrane disease, as reported in 11 of 12 autopsies by Robertson and Ivemark (1969). No correlation was noted with birth weight or postnatal age in their total series of 50 consecutive neonatal autopsies. The lesion was noted in a few stillbirths.

Central Nervous System Lesions

No lesions have been described in association with hyaline membrane disease that are not also found in infants who die of asphyxia or after prolonged hyperoxia. However, several reports of the association of intracranial hemorrhage with pulmonary disease have been made (Harrison et al., 1968). Lesions of the dorsal vagal nuclei have been noted (Buckingham et al., 1967), and fibrillary gliosis as well as severe vasoproliferation has been described (Brand et al., 1972). The latter lesions were noted in infants with bronchopulmonary dysplasia and were most prominent after a week or two of age. Brand et al. speculate that the perinatal brain may possess mechanisms for dealing with hypoxia; later this flexibility disappears and adaptive changes intervene. An alternate possibility is that the late changes relate to hyperoxia, which may occur during convalescence from hyaline membrane disease. The prevalence of central nervous system lesions in autopsied infants makes one wonder about neurological sequelae in survivors. Apparently they are no more susceptible than other prematures if careful attention is given to keeping blood gases in balance during the acute phases of the illness. The warning should be that either hypoxia or hyperoxia can be damaging to the brain of premature infants.

PATHOGENESIS

Although some debate exists about pathogenesis, most students of the subject now agree to the central role of immaturity of the lung with respect to its capacity to synthesize or secrete the pulmonary surfactant into the alveolar surface (see also pages 10–15).

The LaPlace relationship between the pressure across a curved surface, surface tension at the air-liquid interface, and radius of curvature of the surface is illustrated in Figure 12–12. Two properties of the material lining the alveoli evidently are essential for alveolar stability (or the prevention of alveolar closure at expiration). One property is to achieve a low surface tension, the other is to have surface elasticity, or change in tension with change in area. A substance with these properties, presumably a phospholipid, lines the terminal airspaces in normal lungs (Clements, 1962). This surface-active substance is not demonstrable by usual methods of detection in lungs of infants who die of hyaline membrane disease (Avery and Mead, 1959; Pattle et al., 1962). Phospholipids are also reduced in quantity in these lungs, with a significant reduction in the saturated fatty acids in the alpha position of lung phosphatidyl choline (Brumley et al., 1967).

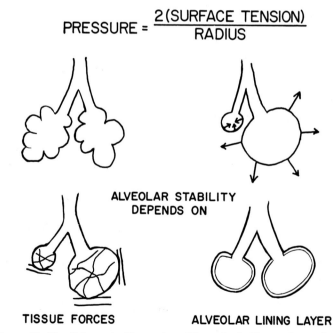

$$\text{PRESSURE} = \frac{2\,(\text{SURFACE TENSION})}{\text{RADIUS}}$$

ALVEOLAR STABILITY
DEPENDS ON

TISSUE FORCES   ALVEOLAR LINING LAYER

Figure 12–12. Schematic illustration of how the LaPlace relationship, between pressure across a curved surface, surface tension at air-liquid interface, and radius of curvature of surface, would promote an unstable equilibrium in the lung. Tissue forces, and particularly the alveolar lining layer, help to stabilize the airspaces.

This finding suggested that the deficiency of the normal alveolar lining layer could explain the profound atelectasis seen early in the disease, as well as in all immature infants in whom lung maturation had not progressed to the stage of alveolar formation. Certain clinical features of hyaline membrane disease are consistent with the delayed appearance, intrauterine inhibition, or destruction of alveolar cell secretions. First, the disease has not been seen in stillborn infants. Surface forces could not operate before the production of an air-fluid interface. Second, symptoms are usually present at birth or very shortly thereafter. Death or recovery ensues in four to 72 hours. Although a normal initial expansion of the lungs would be expected, it would take time for subsequent mechanical difficulties to be evident. The half-life of surfactant is about 16 hours; if an insult were to destroy the ability of the alveolar cells to synthesize it, rather than destroy that which was previously formed, one would expect clinical deterioration after some hours of reasonably normal breathing (Tierney et al., 1967). If "maturation" of the alveolar cells occurred in the first few days of extrauterine life, recovery would be expected. Third, the disease is most frequent in infants who weigh 1.0 to 1.5 kg. at birth. There are several possible reasons for the lack of the full histologic picture in infants under 1.0 kg. birth weight. They rarely survive many hours, and several hours of breathing are usually required before membranes are seen. Also, the distance from capillary to airway lumen is greater in very immature infants, and transudation may be less common. Very small infants who die normally have the type of atelectasis seen in hyaline membrane disease, even if they lack the membrane.

Although it is not clear how a deficiency in the alveolar lining layer can account for the membrane itself, it is tempting to speculate that the same insult that led to inadequate function of the alveolar cells could injure bronchiolar epithelial cells and result in necrosis, exudation, and membrane formation. Alternately, one role of the normal alveolar lining layer may be to protect cells from injury. It is also possible that the altered pressure relationships around capillaries in the lung promote transudation in the aerated portions. The presence of the membrane in the aerated parts of the lung makes this latter hypothesis attractive.

OTHER SUGGESTED ETIOLOGIC CONSIDERATIONS

A number of theories of pathogenesis, proposed in the 1950's and 1960's, may have some bearing on the clinical course in a few infants. In the interests of historical documentation, and because some observations deserve to be remembered, a list of other etiologic considerations follows.

Aspiration

For many years the predominant thought was that the membrane consisted of material that was aspirated, then impacted against bronchiolar and alveolar walls by air breathing. Atelectasis would then occur distal to the obstructive membrane (Dick and Pund, 1949; Bovet-DuBois, 1951; Claireaux, 1953; Campbell, 1959; Snyder, 1961). The advocates of this theory based their conclusion on findings of amorphous debris in the airways, and the ability to produce a similar lesion in animals after the installation of large volumes of amniotic fluid (Blystad et al., 1951). They also cite the association of the disease with intrapartum asphyxia that could induce gasping and aspiration by the fetus. The role of cesarean section in the pathogenesis of the disease is not established, but there are those who feel that infants delivered by this route have greater difficulty. They invoke the lack of the "big squeeze" at birth as failing to empty the lungs of fluid, hence predisposing the infant to hyaline membrane disease.

The possibility that aspiration of amniotic liquid could wash out or otherwise alter the pulmonary surfactant was tested by Johnson and Faridy (1965). Fetal lambs, in which 30 to 76 ml. of their own amniotic liquid was instilled into their tracheas, demonstrated elevation of surface tension of lung extracts, and a tendency to lung collapse similar to that found in hyaline membrane disease.

Against the aspiration theory is the failure to see a membrane in the first few hours of life. Intrauterine aspiration would be expected to line the airways with blood or squamous cells at the time of birth, and not several hours later. The endogenous origin of the membrane seems fairly well established on the basis of its high fibrin content. It is not inconceivable that aspirated fluid of altered pH could injure the distal airways and thus set the stage for later exudation and membrane formation (Benirschke et al., 1963; McAdams et al., 1973).

Against the background that aspiration of amniotic fluid or gastric contents could cause hyaline membrane disease, the suggestion was made that stomachs of all infants delivered by cesarean section should be aspirated at the time of delivery (Gellis et al., 1949; Freeman and Scott, 1954). This procedure, widely used since 1949, has not changed the incidence of hyaline membrane disease. If it is to be used for the purpose for which it was intended, it would be more reasonable to aspirate the gastric contents of all prematurely born infants than those delivered by cesarean section.

Others who consider aspiration to be important in the pathogenesis of the disease advocate positioning infants prone and slightly head down (Wright, 1961). There are no studies that show the efficacy of this position in prevention or therapy of the disease.

Asphyxia

The case for the role of asphyxia in the pathogenesis of the disease has been made most strongly by James (1959) and supported by the studies (previously cited) of Burns et al. (1961) and Miller (1962). On a statistical basis, there is little doubt that infants who subsequently die from hyaline membrane disease are more likely to be in difficulty in the delivery room than those who go on to survive. In the series of Rudolph et al. (1966) 70 per cent of the infants who had moderate to severe respiratory distress had an Apgar score of less than 6, indicative of respiratory depression at birth. Experimentally, asphyxia and prematurity together were associated with the disease in lambs. Immature animals developed the disease without asphyxia; mildly premature animals (130 to 136 days) developed the disease when the ewes were subjected to asphyxia; towards term, the disease occurred in only one of six animals after an asphyxial insult (Orzalesi et al., 1965). Now that techniques are available to measure fetal acidosis, it is possible to evaluate its role in the pathogenesis of respiratory distress more critically (Saling, 1964; Morris and Beard, 1965). It is certainly possible that prolonged fetal distress in the premature infant sets the stage for hyaline membrane disease.

Meanwhile, the therapeutic suggestion that arises from these observations on the relationship of asphyxia to the disease is to assist the onset of respiration by appropriate resuscitation in the delivery room.

Heart Failure

On the basis of clinical and pathologic findings, Lendrum (1955) argued that hyaline membrane disease might be a manifestation of heart failure. Shortly thereafter, the demonstration of fibrin in the membrane, presumably endogenous in origin, raised the possibility that increased capillary pressure, on the basis of left ventricular failure, could cause leakage of plasma proteins into the airspaces. The subsequent arguments in behalf of heart failure, reviewed by James (1959) and Smith (1960), consist essentially of the occasional demonstration of increased heart size, transient systolic murmurs thought to be ductal in origin, and catheterization evidence of large left-to-right shunts (Rudolph, 1961; Stahlman et al., 1972). Although the shunts in infants with respiratory distress were large, with pulmonary to systemic flow ratios of up to 3:7, there is no information about the size of the shunt in normal infants of comparable age and weight. Measurements of central venous pressure are lower in infants who succumb than in infants who recover (Bonham-Carter et al., 1956), but as James pointed out (1959), so too are pleural pressures, so that transmural venous pressure may be greater than normal. Further support for the role of heart failure came from the observations of Shanklin (1959) of cardiac malformations, chiefly atrial septal defect, in 34 of 132 cases of hyaline membrane disease. Shanklin's finding of associated cardiac malformations in some infants has not been duplicated with any statistical significance by others.

The outstanding argument against the primacy of heart failure in the pathogenesis of the disease is that many infants who die in the first days of life from lethal cardiac malformations and left ventricular failure do not have hyaline membrane disease. The pathology of pulmonary edema is distention of the alveoli with fluid, not atelectasis and membranes. Moreover, when one twin receives more than his share of the fetal placental circulation and the other is anemic, both may have hyaline membrane disease even though only one was in failure (Naeye, 1963).

Therapy based on this theory of pathogenesis has consisted of the use of digitalis. This drug has been widely used, but in a controlled study in which digoxin or a placebo were given to 196 premature infants, no benefit from digitalization was apparent. Deaths from hyaline membrane disease occurred in both groups (Martin, 1963).

Neither epinephrine nor norepinephrine has been widely used for circulatory support, despite the suggestion that they might be useful (Brown, 1959). Studies of plasma levels of epinephrine in infants with respiratory distress showed a fourfold increase over those of controls, while norepinephrine levels were about the same (Cheek et al., 1963). The significance of these findings is unclear, just as is the possible role of norepinephrine infusions in therapy.

Decreased Blood Volume

Perhaps the converse of the argument for heart failure is the suggestion that deprivation of the placental transfusion at birth, with consequent decreased blood volume, sets the stage for hyaline membrane disease (Bound et al., 1962). Possibly related to the concept of decreased blood volume is the suggestion of Moss et al. (1962) that delayed clamping of the umbilical cord will permit adequate perfusion of the pulmonary vascular bed, which could be impaired if the placental circulation were occluded before the lungs were inflated with air.

The background of Bound's hypothesis is as follows: (1) If the infant is delivered below the level of the placenta and the cord not clamped immediately, 30 to 100 ml. of blood will be transfused into the infant (Gunther, 1957; Secher and Karlberg, 1962). (2) Raised venous pressure appears to be beneficial in respiratory distress (Bonham-Carter et al., 1956). Moss theorized that if the cord is clamped prior to the initial aeration of the lungs when pulmonary vascular resistance is high systemic arterial pressure will rise and more blood will flow left to right through the ductus, perhaps with transudation into the air spaces (Moss et al., 1963).

More recently, extensive studies on the physiological consequences of the placental transfusion show that it can increase blood volume by more than 60 per cent. Blood volume then decreases over the next few hours to a level about 10 per cent greater at 72 hours than that of infants who did not receive the placental transfusion (Usher et al., 1963). Late clamping is associated with higher hematocrits, higher systemic and pulmonary artery blood pressures, higher right atrial and portal pressures, longer interval until the first breath, higher respiratory rates, and reduced lung compliance (Burnard and James, 1963; Arcilla et al., 1966; Oh et al., 1966, 1967). The longer the interval between onset of sustained respiration and cord clamping, the greater the size of the placental transfusion (Redmond et al., 1965). A possible note of caution arises from the observation of Danks and Stevens (1964) that a high hematocrit may contribute to respiratory distress.

The evidence in support of the efficacy of the placental transfusion is a comparison of deaths from hyaline membrane disease in one hospital during a two-and-a-half-year period in which the cord was usually clamped immediately after birth (7.3 deaths/100 live births of premature infants) with the experience in the same hospital over another two-year period in which the infant was held below the level of the labor bed and the cord clamped three to five minutes after delivery (2.5 deaths/100 live premature births). The infants were of comparable weight and hence presumably at comparable risk. In another study the incidence of clinical respiratory distress in infants in whom the cord was clamped before the second breath was compared with those in whom clamping was done after the second breath. Delayed clamping of the cord was associated with less clinical respiratory distress. The deaths in this group of 129 infants were too few to permit comparison of the incidence of hyaline membrane disease, since only two had the disease at autopsy (Moss et al., 1963).

Measurement of plasma volume with Evan's blue dye, which measures albumin space, showed no difference between premature infants with and without respiratory distress (Cassady, 1966).

The logical therapy suggested by this theory would be to hold the newborn infant below the level of the placenta and delay clamping the cord. It would also seem logical to give transfusions of fresh whole blood to infants sick with the disease in an attempt to combat clinical shock and provide an adequate circulating blood volume. The evidence in support of these hypotheses increases. Emmanouilides and Moss (1971) compared the incidence of respiratory distress in 147 infants under 2.5 kg. and 38 weeks' gestational age in whom the cord was clamped before the second breath or after it. Respiratory distress was evident in 40 per cent of the "early" clamped and in 11 per cent of the "late" clamped infants.

Pulmonary Hypoperfusion

A consequence of decreased blood volume, shock, or heart failure could be hypoperfusion of the pulmonary vascular bed. Asphyxia, as well, will tend to promote pulmonary vasoconstriction (Rudolph and Yuan, 1966). The possibility of pulmonary hypoperfusion at stages of hyaline membrane disease is supported by the demonstration of large right-to-left shunts (Strang, 1961; Prod'hom, 1965; Stahlman, 1966). Post-mortem, the lungs are difficult if not impossible to perfuse through the arteries (Lauweryns et al., 1961; Chu et al., 1965, 1967). The evidence for reduced perfusion of ventilated airspaces during the disease is clear; the primacy of hypoperfusion in the pathogenesis of the disease remains speculative.

Experimentally, a constrictive arteritis in the small arterioles of the lung was produced in premature lambs delivered of ewes previously stressed with promazine hydrochloride. The lambs subsequently developed many of the features of hyaline membrane disease (Stahlman et al., 1964). A search for vascular lesions in human lungs revealed no significant changes in the study of Kapteyn et al. (1963). Naeye (1966) found the small pulmonary arteries markedly constricted in infants with and without hyaline membrane disease who died on the first day of life.

Attempts to vasodilate the pulmonary vascular bed with acetylcholine or priscoline have not been uniformly successful, and the hazards of such therapy in the face of systemic shock are obvious. Oxygenation and the correction of acidosis will tend to promote pulmonary vasodilatation far more safely.

Disturbed Autonomic Regulation

The observation of low blood pressure, cool extremities, and edema suggests a disturbance in peripheral vasomotor tone. Moreover, the hypersecretion in the pulmonary epithelium may represent autonomic imbalance (Buckingham and Sommers, 1960). In small animals such as rabbits and guinea pigs, bilateral cervical vagotomy leads to pulmonary edema and occasionally to membrane formation (Farber, 1937; Miller et al., 1951). Thus, some degree of autonomic imbalance may be present; its etiology remains obscure.

A clinical trial with a beta-adrenergic drug, orciprenaline, was conducted by Helwig and Pullmann (1970). This compound, like isoproterenol, is said to elevate heart minute volume and blood volume in lung capillaries as well as to increase oxygen consumption. In infants of low birth weight with respiratory distress, 50 μg. of orciprenaline were injected intravenously. A deterioration in blood gases was found and was attributed to the increase in oxygen consumption. These authors, as well as Keuth et al. (1972), concluded that orciprenaline has no role in therapy of hyaline membrane disease. The use of such agents with blood volume expanders and careful monitoring of vascular pressures remains to be evaluated.

Enzyme Deficiencies

A depression in serum enzyme inhibitor concentrations in infants with respiratory distress was first noted by Evans et al. (1970). Subsequently, several groups of workers have demonstrated that a depression in concentrations of alpha₁-antitrypsin and alpha₂-macroglobulin occurred in cord blood of affected infants and bore some prognostic import. That is to say, if the concentrations increased in subsequent hours, survival was more likely than if they remained depressed (Mathis et al., 1973). Kotas et al. (1972) felt that a low level was predictive of potential fatality from respiratory distress syndrome and advocated its use to select those infants that should be transferred to a special care center. The measurement involves a spectrophotometric method and is inappropriate in hemolyzed specimens. It also requires approximately one hour to complete, so it cannot give the same rapid information that can be achieved with amniotic fluid using the Clements bubble stability test (Clements et al., 1972).

The reason for the depression in these proteins is not at all clear. They are in the globulin fraction and may contribute to the finding reported by Bland (1972) that total serum proteins are depressed below 4.6 gm. per cent in the cord blood of infants who subsequently have severe disease. Others have shown that the albumin concentrations do not differ between premature infants and those with respiratory distress; the possibility that the globulin fraction is different deserves further study. El-Bardeesy et al. (1972) studied a group of infants with hyaline membrane disease and other conditions. The depression in the serum inhibitory factors was more pronounced in hyaline membrane disease than in infants of comparable gestational age with other illnesses.

Cord bloods from infants who later develop respiratory distress have lower carbonic anhydrase concentrations than those of infants of similar gestational age who do not have respiratory distress (Kleinman et al., 1972). The overlap of values makes this measurement unreliable as a predictor of distress. The relevance of these measurements to the pathophysiology of hyaline membrane disease is unknown.

Enzyme and Other Protein Deficiencies

The demonstration that the membrane contained fibrin (Gitlin and Craig, 1956; van Breeman, 1961) and that there was a deficiency in plasminogen in premature infants led to the suggestion that the membrane resulted from the lack of the fibrinolytic enzymes. Lieberman postulated that the placenta, shown by him to have high levels of material capable of inhibiting the plasminogen activator, released this inhibitor into the fetal circulation. The inhibitor would prevent the dissolution of intra-alveolar fibrin; if life could be maintained during the critical hours after birth, the level of the inhibitor would decrease and recovery ensue (Lieberman, 1961). **In vitro** studies further show that fibrinogen can inhibit the activity of the surface-acting lipoprotein. If a capillary leak is a primary event, loss of the pulmonary surfactant could result (Taylor and Abrams, 1966).

The presence of fibrin in the membrane led several workers to suggest that fibrinolysins given by aerosol might be useful in therapy. Craig et al. (1958) showed that 600 units/ml. of fibrinolysin incubated three or more hours with tissue from lungs with hyaline membranes resulted in lysis of the membrane. A few preliminary reports suggest that some individuals who have used fibrinolysins are impressed by their efficacy (Villavicencio et al., 1960; Ebner, 1961; Ambrus et al., 1963); others are not (Combes et al., 1962; Gomez and Graven, 1964). In the most extensive study reported to date, combined therapy with urokinase-activated human plasmin given intravenously and by aerosol of the same substance resulted in survival of 72 per cent of the treated infants, whereas only 39 per cent of those given a placebo survived (Ambrus et al., 1966). Further studies with urokinase-activated plasmin are surely indicated.

TREATMENT

Oxygen Therapy

It follows from the clinical observations of cyanosis, and the laboratory demonstration of right-to-left shunts, that hypoxic infants would profit from increased concentrations of inspired oxygen (Warley and Gairdner, 1962). Nonetheless, the background of the use of oxygen in the treatment of hyaline membrane disease is complex. At one time, the use of oxygen was considered dangerous, since it has been shown that animals exposed for periods of several days to 100 per cent oxygen may develop a pulmonary lesion very similar to hyaline membrane disease (Bruns and Shields, 1954; De and Anderson, 1954; Berfenstam et al., 1958). These studies raised the question that perhaps even the oxygen in room air was toxic to the neonatal lung, just as it had been proved to be to the retinal vessels of small premature infants. (Ingalls, 1954). In fact, Sjöstedt and Rooth (1957) advocated administering 15 per cent oxygen as a routine prophylactic measure in infants, and noted no adverse effects, but no beneficial ones either.

The possibility that added oxygen may be a useful therapeutic aid was supported by the observations of Avery and Oppenheimer (1960) that deaths from the disease were greater during a four-year period in which no oxygen, or very little additional, was given to premature infants, compared with an earlier four-year period in which oxygen was used in higher concentrations. While these studies were retrospective and hence inconclusive, they failed to bear out the predictions that once retrolental fibroplasia was eliminated, hyaline membrane disease would also disappear.

Since dry gases are irritating to the airways, it is important that humidity be provided. Moreover, evaporative losses through the lungs at 30 to 40 per cent humidity average 8.6 gm./kg./day and may reach 12.3 gm./kg./day (Hooper et al., 1954), but insensible water losses are decreased in high humidity (O'Brien et al., 1954).

Hyperbaric oxygen has been used in the treatment of infants with hyaline membrane disease since it has been known that even 100 per cent oxygen at one atmosphere may not bring arterial oxygen tensions to levels compatible with life. In one study, eight infants with a deteriorating clinical condition were put in a chamber at two to three atmospheres for three to 20 hours. Arterial oxygen tensions were raised in all, but not sustained. Little change was observed in pH or carbon dioxide tensions, and all infants died (Cochran et al., 1965). In another study of six infants two to four atmospheres of oxygen at 40 to 100 per cent concentration failed to improve previous experience without hyperbaric therapy (Hutchison, 1962).

Assisted Ventilation

Respirators are indispensable in the treatment of severe hyaline membrane disease. The promise of encouraging case reports has been borne out in recent years (Benson et al., 1958; Colgan et al., 1960; Heese et al., 1963; Delivoria-Papadopoulos and Swyer, 1964; Thomas et al., 1965; Stahlman et al., 1965; Silverman et al., 1967). More extended experiences on both sides of the Atlantic were reviewed at a conference held in Paris in 1969 and were published in Biology of the Neonate, 16:1–196, 1970. Subsequently the introduction by Gregory et al. (1971) of continuous positive airway pressure, and by Chernick and Vidyasagar (1972) of continuous negative pressure, has added greatly to the efficiency of ventilatory assistance (see page 303).

Criteria for the use of continuous airway pressure include chiefly a low arterial oxygen tension that does not exceed 50 to 60 mm./kg. on 100 per cent inspired oxygen. If significant CO_2 retention has occurred (i.e., over 55 to 60 mm./kg.), artificial respiration in addition to continuous pressure is usually indicated (Stern et al., 1970; Daily and Smith, 1971; Outerbridge et al., 1972).

Complications of prolonged ventilatory assistance with 80 to 100 per cent oxygen have been reported. Infants so treated for more than 150 hours showed a chronic lung disorder, characterized by bronchiolar injury, hypertrophy of bronchiolar smooth muscle, increased numbers of macrophages, and perimucosal fibrosis. The condition was termed bronchopulmonary dysplasia. Radiographic changes of prominent lung markings and sometimes rounded areas of radio-

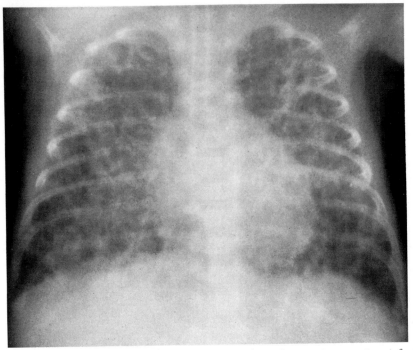

Figure 12–13. Diffuse, cyst-like areas of focal emphysema in premature infant who required long-term ventilatory assistance for respiratory failure. These findings are consistent with those seen in "bronchopulmonary dysplasia." (From Pusey, V. A., et al.: Canad. Med. Ass. J., *100:*451, 1969.)

lucency were noted (Fig. 12–13). Some of the infants died months later of respiratory insufficiency; some recovered. Whether the injury was related to the oxygen, mechanical injury from the respirator, or late effects of the disease, is not clear (Northway et al., 1967; Becker and Koppe, 1969).

More recent evidence lends weight to the possibility that most, if not all, of the lung injury in these late deaths relates to prolonged exposure to high concentrations of oxygen. The fact that oxygen can be toxic to the airways, and that the lesion is initially edema and late squamous metaplasia and fibrosis is now unequivocal. DeLemos et al. (1969) demonstrated the acute edematous response to oxygen in newborn lambs with or without artificial respiration, and Robinson et al. (1967) documented the chronic proliferative changes that oxygen induces in adult monkey lungs on prolonged exposure.

The human lung is also susceptible to oxygen toxicity as is now evident from a number of observations. Brewis (1969) reported on the severe lung changes in an adult epileptic treated with 90 per cent oxygen for 20 days; fortunately they reversed in time. Nash et al.

(1967) noted the similarity post-mortem in lungs of patients receiving high oxygen by artificial respiration, and the lesions produced expermentally from oxygen alone in animals. The evidence for pulmonary oxygen toxicity in humans was reviewed by Kafer (1971).

Unfortunately, we cannot establish safe limits of oxygen administration in the human, in part because of individual variability. Some infants have tolerated 100 per cent oxygen for over a week with no permanent adverse effects; others have shown significant lung lesions after only three to four days of pure oxygen. Clinical experience leads us to attest to the rarity of pulmonary oxygen toxicity in less than 60 per cent oxygen; if that concentration is sufficient to maintain arterial tensions at over 60 mm. Hg in the newborn infant, there seems little reason to exceed it.

Among the mechanical complications of artificial respiration are of course pneumotherax and pneumomediastinum. In addition, gas embolism may occur, as noted by Gregory and Tooley (1970). They suspected that gas was pushed into a pulmonary vein and subsequently distributed to both venous and arterial systems.

Prognosis

Since the evaluation of therapeutic measures depends on criteria for selection of infants to treat, it is important to weigh clinical and laboratory observations in an attempt to assign a prognosis.

The abnormalities in blood gases have been found most useful. Boston et al. (1966) described a low risk group as those infants who within 10 hours of birth had arterial oxygen tensions of over 100 mm. Hg when breathing 100 per cent oxygen, and a pH of greater than 7.20. The high risk group was more hypoxic and acidotic. Stahlman et al. (1967) introduced five variables in their system: oxygen tension while breathing 100 per cent oxygen, pH, birth weight, respiratory rate, and serum potassium level. By weighting these variables, they were able to assign a probability of survival. They stress, too, that the most meaningful single measurement from the aspect of prognosis is the arterial blood oxygen tension while breathing 100 per cent oxygen. Murdock et al. (1972) agreed that the most significant variable was P_aO_2, but advocate the use of a discriminant score that includes also birth weight (H^+), gestational age, P_ACO_2, blood pressure, serum phosphorus, respiratory frequency, and colonic temperature. Suitable weighting of each variable allows determination of the probability for survival.

Estimates of the number of infants who recover from hyaline membrane disease are not meaningful in the absence of systematic criteria for diagnosis. Probably the best general guide to efficacy of forms of management by those who do not have access to complex laboratory facilities is the overall mortality among low birth weight infants in groups designated by gestational age. Significant reductions in mortality are probably related to fewer deaths from hyaline membrane disease in those hospitals where it has been the leading cause of death among such infants. In parts of the world where infection is common, of course, overall death rates would not necessarily reflect mortality from hyaline membrane disease.

Follow-up of infants who have recovered from the disease shows that the majority have no further respiratory dysfunction. Increasingly, in recent years, reports of recurrent lower respiratory tract disease among survivors have raised the possibility that either the disease, or some feature of its therapy such as oxygen or respirators, may have left the lungs unusually susceptible to bronchiolitis. The infants reported by Outerbridge et al. (1972) differed from those described by Northway as bronchopulmonary dysplasia in that they were not all on respirators initially, nor was their problem a persistent one from the neonatal period. They had been discharged from the nursery as well, with normal chest roentgenograms. Lewis reported respiratory infection requiring hospitalization in 17.5 per cent of 63 survivors, and Shepard et al. (1968) described bronchiolitis and bronchopneumonia in 33 per cent of their nonventilated survivors and of 26 per cent of those who were on respirators.

Neurologic sequelae are found in surviving small premature infants, although they are not more frequent among survivors who recovered from respiratory distress than among other infants of similar birth weight (Robertson and Crichton, 1969; Outerbridge and Stern, 1973).

OTHER SUPPORTIVE MEASURES

Perhaps of central importance is the awareness of the metabolic cost of being chilled. Even the vigorous infant may show acidosis with cooling from the inability to meet the oxygen cost of added caloric expenditure (Gandy et al., 1964). The sick infant, in a cool environment, may require double his basal oxygen; in the presence of pulmonary disease, the increment in ventilation may not be possible (Scopes, 1966). Deaths in premature infants have been reduced when the incubator temperatures are kept at appropriate levels. Oxygen consumption is lowest when abdominal skin temperature is 36°C (Silverman et al., 1966).

The recognition of the disturbances in acid-base balance and the severity of the metabolic acidosis which may occur has led to wide use of intravenous alkali therapy. Usher (1963) showed a decrease in mortality, mostly in infants over 1.75 kg. when glucose and bicarbonate were infused from the first hours of life, or as soon as the diagnosis was made. He used a solution of 10 per cent glucose in water, to which was added sodium bicarbonate in concentrations of 5 to 15 mEq./100 ml. of solution depending on the pH of the infant's blood. The solution was infused at a rate of 65 ml./kg./body weight/day. Since then, wide experience with glucose and bicarbonate therapy has substantiated its effect in combatting the metabolic component of the acidosis. The route of administration may be through the umbilical artery, or a peripheral vein. The umbilical vein should not be used except in emergencies for short intervals, since inflammation of the vein and late cirrhosis of the liver have been noted.

The use of 10 per cent glucose is important to spare protein catabolism in stressed infants. As soon as active peristalsis can be demonstrated, and the infant voids well and has had a stool, cautious milk feedings by gavage seem appropriate. Forty-eight hours of starvation has been shown to be associated with significant nitrogen losses in premature infants, and as little as 40 cal./kg./day can lessen these losses (Auld et al., 1966). Severely ill infants may not tolerate oral feedings for some days. Intravenous alimentation with amino acid solutions and lipid preparations should be undertaken by the third day of life if oral feedings are not feasible (Heird et al., 1972).

THAM (tris-hydroxymethyl aminomethane) has been used by some in correcting the acidemia. The surprising finding of a rise in PO_2 after the use of THAM may have been the result of increased pulmonary perfusion with the correction of the acidosis (Gupta, 1965). No systematic comparisons of THAM and sodium bicarbonate have been done which would permit the endorsement of THAM at the present time. Its rapid distribution in the intracellular space is the theoretical reason for its superiority over sodium bicarbonate. Gupta et al. (1967) recommended a 0.3 M. solution with a pH of 8.8 at 37°C, at a rate of 1.0 ml./min. intravenously. They gave 1.0 ml./kg. for each 0.1 pH unit below 7.4. The Hammersmith group uses THAM only when the total sodium administered exceeds 15 mEq./kg. in the first 48 hours, or when the infant is on a ventilator, since they have observed apneic spells during or shortly after its administration (Davies et al., 1972).

Circulatory support, in the form of blood transfusions, seems appropriate when central venous pressure is low, or when relative anemia is present (hematocrit under 40 per cent). Again, systematic evaluation of this form of therapy is lacking.

PREVENTION

A controlled trial of prenatal administration of glucocorticoid to pregnant women has shown a significant reduction in respiratory distress in infants under 32 weeks' gestation whose mothers received the drug for more than 24 hours before birth (Liggins and Howie, 1972).[*] Toxemia was a contraindication for steroids. Further evaluation of this approach to prevention is surely indicated.

---

[*]Liggins, G. C., and Howie, R. N.: A controlled trial of antepartum glucocorticoid treatment for prevention of the respiratory distress syndrome in premature infants. Pediat., 50:515, 1972.

Chapter Thirteen

ASPIRATION SYNDROMES

One of the continuing controversies that face us in pediatric medicine concerns the problem of aspiration of fluid in utero or during delivery. Observations of fetal respiratory movements in utero do not establish that any significant fluid volume exchange occurs (pp. 27–28). However, some fluid continues to flow from the lungs of the exteriorized sheep fetus (Adams and Fujiwara, 1963), and an amount of fluid equal to about one-half of functional residual capacity appears to be present in the lung of the fetal goat at term (Avery and Cook, 1961). The question is, can the infant aspirate a volume of fluid so much in excess of that normally present as to interfere with ventilation of the lungs? The full answer to the question is not possible at this time. A partial answer is at hand from pathologic studies on a group of infants who aspirated particulate matter that was suspended in amniotic fluid, such as squamous cells and meconium. Such particles are readily apparent in the airways and alveoli at autopsy of some infants whose clinical course is characterized by labored breathing from birth and abundant crackling rales in the lung fields. Thus, aspirated particulate matter can be lethal to an infant. It remains to be demonstrated that clear amniotic fluid in the lungs is responsible for respiratory distress; conversely, it is established that squamous cells may be present in alveoli without causing serious respiratory difficulty. Camerer (1938) reviewed lung sections of 212 infants who died in the first week of life, and found squamous cells in 209 of them. Presumably the infants did not all have respiratory symptoms. Ahvenainen also found particulate material in lungs of all liveborn term infants and of nearly all premature infants under four days of age, even when the cause of death was not pulmonary in origin. Some squamous debris persisted as long as 14 days, but it was less prominent in the older infants (Ahvenainen, 1948) (Fig. 13–1).

234

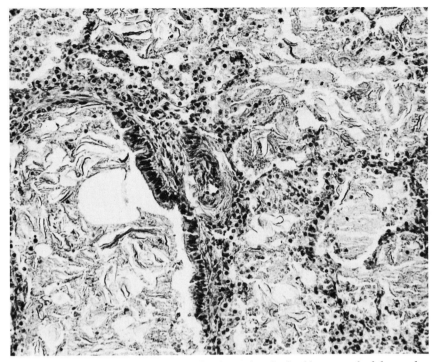

Figure 13–1. Lung of a 3.9-kg. infant born after the fetal heart rate had dropped to 80 beats/min. There was difficulty with the initiation of breathing and labored respiration throughout the six hours of life. Note the masses of squamous cells in the airspaces, which must have been aspirated in utero.

The possibility that fetal distress may predispose to aspiration is suggested by the finding that it is associated with gasping and aspiration in the experimental animal. Normally, a sphincter mechanism at the level of the arytenoid cartilages is closed, so that material injected into the nose or mouth of a fetal lamb is swallowed. Occasionally, the sphincter opens to allow lung liquid to be discharged into the pharynx. Section of the recurrent laryngeal nerves, or cord occlusion, results in relaxation of the sphincter (Adams et al., 1967).

Schaffer (1960) described "the massive aspiration syndrome" to delineate those infants in whom he felt that aspiration of amniotic fluid and its particulate matter was responsible for illness and sometimes death. He stated, "In our practice we make this diagnosis, we believe with justification, more frequently than that of any other disorder which produces dyspnea in the newborn infant." He studied 20 infants, eight of whom were postmature, eight at term, and four premature. Most of the infants had been delivered after asphyxial episodes in utero, which are known to incite gasping in some experimental animals. The illustrative cases he cites include three stillbirths in which alveoli distended with squamous cells were found. Of the six liveborn infants he cites, four were meconium stained, and the two who died had meconium in their lungs. The other two had minimal disease and recovered, so the etiology remains in doubt. Thus, there is unequivocal evidence of aspiration in association with stillbirths, and of death from aspirated meconium in the lungs. There is less evidence that aspiration of large amounts of uncontaminated amniotic fluid causes illness.

MECONIUM ASPIRATION

The incidence of the passage of meconium in utero is variously estimated as 10 to 20 per cent of all births (Desmond et al., 1957; Auld et al., 1961). Its presence is significantly associated with depression at birth (Auld et al., 1961). Thus it appears to be a sign of fetal distress, although not all infants who pass meconium in utero are in difficulty at birth.

Instillation of meconium labeled with tantalum into the tracheas of puppies before their first breath produced in the puppies findings similar to those found in infants. The meconium was cleared from the trachea and main bronchi within an hour, but peripheral migration occurred as well. This model seems suitable for study of the natural course of the disorder as well as evaluation of treatment (Gooding et al., 1971).

Clinical Findings. The infant who aspirates meconium is typically depressed at birth, and respirations may be irregular and gasping. If on prompt intubation a plug of meconium can be removed from the trachea, some benefit may result. More frequently, the inspissated meconium is in the distal airways so that suction at the trachea is of no avail. Respirations are labored, although the retractions are not always as obvious as those in the premature infant with hyaline membrane disease. Tachypnea is the rule, and rales may or may not be present. If the infant makes many forced inspirations, air trapping may occur distal to the partially obstructing meconium which then acts as a ball-valve mechanism. The chest appears to be enlarged.

Radiologic Signs. In contrast to the fine, reticulogranular pattern of hyaline membrane disease, radiographs of infants with meconium aspiration show coarse irregular pulmonary densities (Peterson and Pendleton, 1955) (Figs. 13–2 and 13–3). Gooding and Gregory (1971) have described patchy areas of diminished aeration or consolidation which usually cleared within 24 hours. There may be minimal associated pleural effusion. In this series of 30 infants with radiologic findings of meconium aspiration in the first hour after birth, hyperinflation of the lungs was surprisingly not a feature, but pneumomediastinum or pneumothorax was present in six. One of our patients who

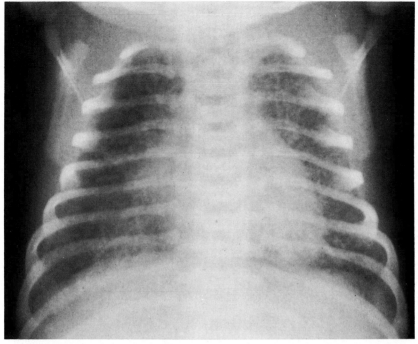

Figure 13–2. Chest film on the first day of life which shows diffuse, bilateral infiltrations from aspirated meconium.

had severe meconium aspiration developed cysts which resembled pneumatoceles (Fletcher et al., 1970) (Fig. 13–4A and B).

Course. Death may ensue a few minutes after birth if the aspirated meconium is abundant. More commonly the course is over some hours, but death, if it occurs, is likely within the first 24 hours. Infants who subsequently recover usually do so in a few days, but may have a very prolonged course of tachypnea for days or even weeks, with slow radiographic clearing.

Treatment. It is our policy to aspirate the stomachs of all infants who are meconium stained at the time of birth. The purpose of this procedure is to prevent further aspiration of meconium that may have been swallowed. If the infant makes gasping inspiratory efforts, indicative of upper airway obstruction, immediate inspection of the larynx with a laryngoscope and removal of any obstructing meconium by suction are essential. Positive-pressure resuscitation should be avoided until all meconium visible in the airway has been removed. Beyond these immediate measures, treatment is supportive. Oxygen is given in whatever concentration is required to keep the infant pink; full humidity and a neutral environmental temperature of 32 to 34°C are provided (Oliver and Karlberg, 1963). Antibiotics are indicated for two reasons: first, the differential diagnosis between bacterial pneu-

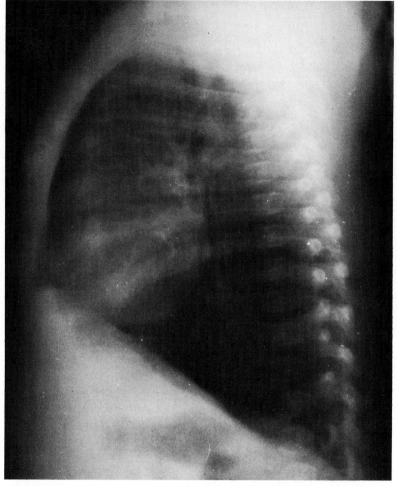

Figure 13-3. Lateral view of another infant with a significant degree of hyper-aeration after the aspiration of meconium.

monia and meconium aspiration is difficult; and second, intratracheal meconium has been shown to enhance the susceptibility to *E. coli* infection in rats (Bryan, 1967). The lungs at autopsy often show evidence of both aspiration and infection. The reaction in the lung may be considered as a chemical pneumonitis and the anti-inflammatory action of steroids may be helpful, although no controlled studies of their use in this condition have been reported.

PHARYNGEAL INCOORDINATION

It is not uncommon for a newborn infant to reject or regurgitate his first feeding of water. Less frequently, he takes it, but then chokes

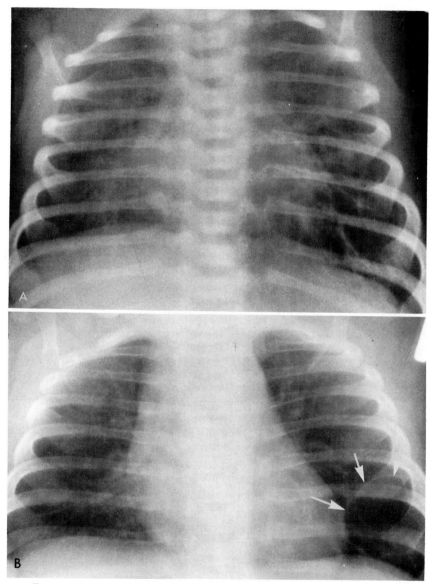

Figure 13–4. A, At 18 days, following severe meconium aspiration, residual pneumonitis is present bilaterally, and there are a number of cyst-like lucencies in the left lower lobe. *B*, By three months of age the pneumonitis has completely resolved. There is a single large thin-walled lucency remaining in the left lower lobe which resembles a pneumatocele. (From Fletcher, B. D., et al.: J. Canad. Assoc. Radiol. *21*:273, 1970.)

and frets for a few minutes. These events are the basis for the standing order in our nursery to withhold formula feedings until the infant has retained at least two feedings of water. The occasional infant who aspirates his feedings because of pharyngeal incoordination will presumably be in less difficulty if the substance aspirated is water rather than milk.

The reasons for temporary pharyngeal incoordination in the first days of life are unknown, but the frequency of the condition can be estimated from the findings of DeCarlo et al. (1952). One hundred normal newborn infants were given a swallow of an oily contrast medium at 12 to 24 hours of age. In 13 of them, the bolus divided at the larynx and a portion of it entered the trachea. This rarely happened after the second day of life, although in two infants it persisted for more than 144 hours. DeCarlo et al. noted that a barium swallow usually did not enter the trachea, whereas an oily contrast medium did. Although persistence of pharyngeal incoordination is rare, it is more common among infants with symptoms of choking or vomiting during feedings. Matsaniotis et al. (1971) found evidence of aspiration in 23 out of 44 infants from six days to six months of age with those symptoms. It was more common in the younger infants and tended to be self-limited. Three infants with chronic lung disease examined by Cumming and Reilly (1972) aspirated barium only after 3 to 4 ounces of feeding. In the absence of neurologic or structural abnormality, this suggested "fatigue" of the swallowing mechanism.

Occasionally, the inability to conduct liquids into the pharynx persists longer, and in the case of Morgan (1956) the infant who showed this phenomenon on fluoroscopy died on the sixth day of life with aspiration pneumonia. There were no visible anomalies of the pharynx at postmortem examination. Difficulty in swallowing from birth with repeated aspiration led to the death of an infant in South Africa. At autopsy, the pharyngeal cavity was dilated and there was hypertrophy of the pharyngeal constrictors. Histological sections of the esophagus showed an absence of ganglion cells in the upper third (Utian and Thomas, 1969).

We have observed this problem in a term infant delivered by elective cesarean section of a mildly diabetic mother. The infant turned blue after a feeding on the fourth day of life, and thereafter was tachypneic and had retractions. A chest film showed a pattern consistent with bilateral bronchopneumonia. On fluoroscopy, a swallow of contrast material was noted to puddle in the pyriform sinuses, then empty into the trachea as well as the esophagus (Fig. 13–5). No regurgitation was present. Thereafter the child had no more difficulty, and was discharged as recovered on the 12th day of life.

The late onset of symptoms in our patient is unusual in the light of DeCarlo's findings. The condition should be suspected whenever an infant chokes or coughs with feedings. Roentgenographic studies are essential to confirm the diagnosis and rule out an H-type tracheo-

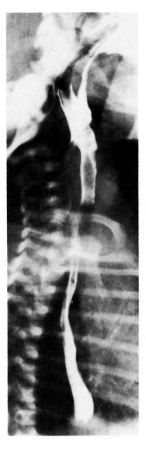

Figure 13–5. This infant had cyanotic spells during feedings. Note that the contrast material enters the trachea as well as the esophagus. The infant gradually improved and had no further symptoms after a week of age. (Frank, M. M., and Gatewood, O. B., Am. J. Dis. Child. *111*:178, 1966.)

esophageal fistula. The fatal outcome in Morgan's case suggests that formula should be given through a gastric tube, once the diagnosis is made. Occasionally, water may be offered by mouth as a test feeding to determine when the infant has acquired the normal degree of pharyngeal coordination. Apparently the process is self-limited in most infants. When it persists, the diagnosis of dysautonomia should be entertained (Neuhauser and Harris, 1962; Margulies et al., 1968).

Crichopharyngeal Achalasia

This very rare condition was described in an infant in 1972 by Blank and Silbiger. This condition differs from pharyngeal incoordination by the presence of good pharyngeal contraction, with persistence of a "cricopharyngeal bar" or ring-like compression of the esophagus in the region of the cricopharyngeal muscle at the entrance of the cervical esophagus. Their infant had some difficulty in swallowing and had choking, cyanotic spells with feeding. Subsequently recurrent febrile episodes with pulmonary infiltrates occurred. Improvement followed "vigorous dilatation."

Chapter Fourteen

PNEUMOTHORAX AND PNEUMOMEDIASTINUM

Spontaneous pneumothorax is more common in the newborn period than in any other time of childhood. Since it is one of the few treatable causes of respiratory difficulty in the early days of life, it is important to consider the predisposing factors, clinical findings, and indications for therapy.

INCIDENCE

The frequency of pneumothorax and pneumomediastinum in the newborn infant is apparent from the number of case reports and reviews in the literature. The first of these was by Ruge, who in 1878 reported a moderately asphyxiated infant who suddenly became cyanotic about 12 hours after a breech delivery. Subsequent writers have not always distinguished spontaneous pneumothorax from that associated with over-zealous artificial respiration. By 1957 Howie and Weed found 151 cases of both types in the English literature, and added nine more.

The detection of pneumothorax in newborn infants will depend on the degree of suspicion and availability of x-ray facilities. In 1903 Emerson reported 48 cases of pneumothorax from The Johns Hopkins Hospital, but none in newborn infants. By 1930, when Davis and Stevens reported on the value of routine radiographic examinations of newborn infants, they found six instances in 702 examinations. Solis-Cohen and Bruck (1934) found 11 pneumothoraces in chest roentgeno-

242

grams of 500 newborn infants. Without frequent radiographic studies, the presence of small pneumothoraces may be overlooked, as suggested by the incidence of only six in 8716 infants detected on physical examination by Harris and Steinberg (1954).

In contrast, routine radiography of 550 infants within two hours of birth showed pneumothorax and/or pneumomediastinum in 13, of which seven were asymptomatic. Pneumothorax occurred after routine vaginal delivery in 1.3 per cent, after cesarean section in 2 per cent, in 1 per cent of premature infants, and 6 per cent of intubated infants (Steele et al., 1971).

The report of Lubchenco (1959) emphasized the occurrence of pneumothorax in premature infants. Seventeen of the 27 infants she reported were of less than 2.5 kg. birth weight. The possibility of pneumothorax was suspected on the basis of respiratory distress, chiefly cyanosis and tachypnea, and unusual irritability or agitation relieved by administration of oxygen. There was an interesting inverse relationship between birth weight and age of onset: the more premature the infant, the later the onset. Others have noted the rarity of pneumothorax in premature infants except in association with hyaline membrane disease (Malan and Heese, 1966).

PATHOGENESIS OF PNEUMOTHORAX

Macklin (1939) demonstrated in the overdistended cat lung the mechanism of alveolar rupture and the dissection of air along vascular sheaths to the lung root. He observed rupture of mediastinal walls, and air entry into the pleural space as well as the mediastinum. The rarity of rupture of an alveolus in a normal lung depends on the inability of the diaphragm or chest wall to expand much beyond total lung capacity. The pressure that can be applied to the lung at large volume is no more than about 30 cm. H_2O, or too little to rupture it. In the presence of atelectasis, however, the diaphragm has sufficient mechanical advantage to apply a much longer stroke, hence much larger pressures across aerated alveoli, with the possibility of rupture and dissection of air along vascular sheaths.

In eight of a series of 15 infants reported by Chernick and Avery (1963), the probability of aspiration of blood, meconium, or squamous debris was evident. The association of meconium and mucus aspiration was also apparent in the series of Emery (1956), Malan and Heese (1966), and Chasler (1964). A partial obstruction of a bronchiole or small bronchus may result in a ball-valve mechanism. A sudden maximal inspiratory effort might fully distend an airspace distal to the obstruction, and the next forced expiration fail to empty it. In time, a forcible inspiratory effort, such as accompanies a cry, could result in rupture of such an airspace.

A unique aspect to the first breath of the newborn infant poses a mechanical problem of such moment that perhaps the pertinent question would be why every infant does not have a spontaneous pneumothorax with his first breath. Introduction of air into the airless lung requires the application of high pressures to overcome the viscosity of fluid in the airway and the forces of surface tension, and to stretch the lung parenchyma (Avery, 1962). Karlberg has shown that the normal newborn infant applies transient pressures of 40 to 80, and sometimes even 100 cm. H_2O with the first breath (1957). The normal lung inflates promptly, with ventilatory units opening serially, but almost all units are nearly open after the first few breaths. If for any reason portions of the lung do not inflate promptly, those units already open "see" all of the pressure applied to those not yet open. Thus, the newborn infant, with his first few breaths, may rupture a few alveoli, and more rarely, has a symptomatic pneumothorax.

Pneumothoraces which are frequently large, bilateral, and associated with pneumomediastinum may occur in infants with hypoplastic lungs associated with Potter's syndrome, cystic renal dysplasia and obstructive urologic malformations (Stern et al., 1972). The urologic abnormalities may not be immediately detectable (Renert et al., 1972) and the presence of unexplained extrapulmonary air in the immediate newborn period should suggest the presence of underlying renal malformations even in the absence of the typical Potter's facies (Fig. 14–1).

Pneumothorax is also a problem in association with congenital diaphragmatic hernia and pulmonary hypoplasia. While ipsilateral pneumothorax is commonly present postoperatively, a contralateral pneumothorax either before or after operative correction of the hernia suggests a bad prognosis (Fliegel and Kaufmann, 1972).

A rare cause of unilateral pneumothorax in the newborn is spontaneous rupture of the esophagus with esophagopleural fistula (Tolstedt and Tudor, 1968). Hydropneumothorax was recognized in the case of Harell et al. (1970). The site of perforation can be determined by an esophagogram. The cause is unknown.

DIAGNOSIS AND THERAPY

The early recognition of the presence of pneumothorax will be enhanced if chest films on all infants with respiratory distress are required. The diagnosis of isolated pneumomediastinum is sometimes more difficult than that of pneumothorax. The physical findings on percussion and auscultation are hard to elicit and often not "typical," but a shift of the apical cardiac impulse is one of the most reliable signs.

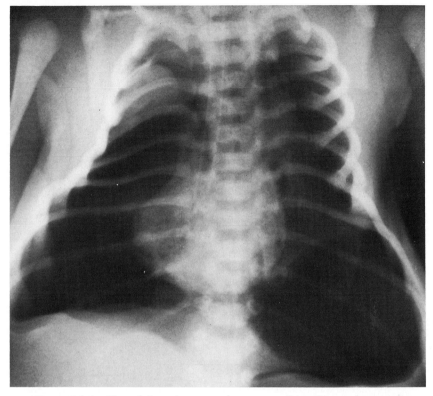

Figure 14–1. Huge bilateral pneumothoraces resulting from pulmonary hypoplasia associated with severe bilateral renal dysplasia in a three-hour-old infant. (From Stern, L., et al.: Amer. J. Roentgen. *116*:785, 1972.)

Tachypnea is a nearly uniform finding; grunting and retractions may be present. A prominent chest bulge on the same side as a unilateral pneumothorax, or a central sternal bulging are important signs and sufficiently pathognomonic to make the presumptive diagnosis if chest films are not available. Unusual irritability and restlessness occur frequently. Once it is suspected that a pneumothorax is present, the infant should be on special observation with pulse and respirations recorded at least every 15 minutes. Any sudden change in vital signs should alert the physician to the possibility of air under tension, and needle aspiration should be done if there is deterioration in the clinical status. A number 18 needle, a three-way stop-cock, and a syringe should be available. If repeated aspirations are required, they should be carried out by the physician until such time as a catheter and water-seal section are available for continuous drainage at −10 to −15 cm. H_2O.

If the infant is cyanotic and there is difficulty in establishing continuous suction, administration of 100 per cent oxygen by mask may prove lifesaving. The inspired oxygen will facilitate nitrogen washout

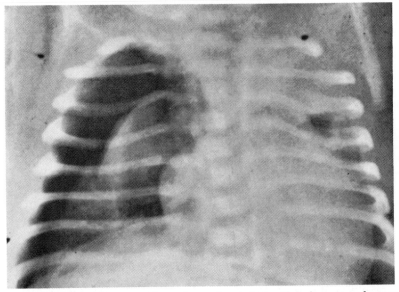

Figure 14–2.   Film at two days of age of an infant with tachypnea and cyanosis from a tension pneumothorax on the right. The mediastinum is shifted to the left.

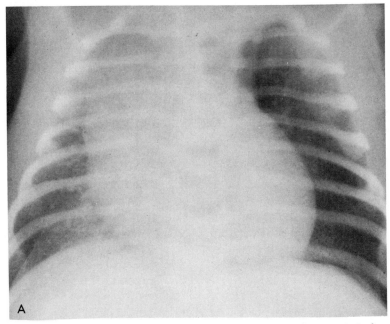

Figure 14–3.   One-day-old infant with severe respiratory distress. A, Left pneumothorax suspected on AP radiograph because of overexpanded, hyperlucent left hemithorax.   *(Illustration continued on opposite page.)*

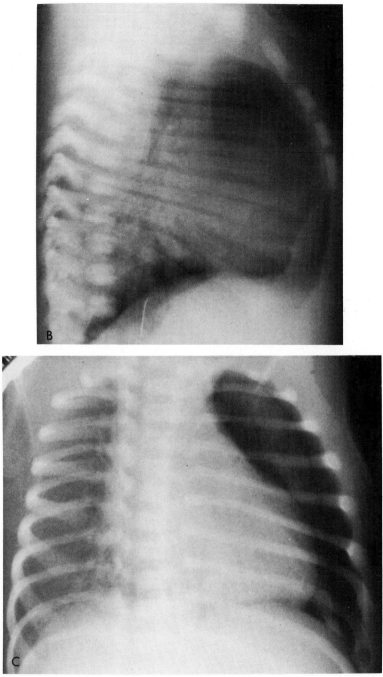

Figure 14–3 Continued. B, On horizontal beam lateral projection, an ill-defined collection of air is seen in the retrosternal area and also under a lung posteriorly. *C,* The right lateral decubitus view shows a well-defined large pneumothorax. (From Tchou, C.-S. et al.: J. Canad. Assoc. Radiol. 23:85, 1972.)

of the blood and tissues, and thus establish a difference in the gas tensions between the loculated gases in the chest and those in the blood. Oxygen tensions in the venous blood and tissues will not rise very high because of its utilization and the shape of the hemoglobin dissociation curve. Chernick and Avery (1963) demonstrated in rabbits that the removal of loculated gas in the chest was about six times as fast with oxygen breathing as with air breathing.

The precautions of having a needle, a syringe, and a stopcock by the bedside, and making frequent observations, seem justified for all infants with pneumothorax despite the knowledge that only a few will require aspiration. For all infants it seems reasonable to prevent vigorous crying if possible. Early and frequent small feedings may be useful in this regard. Restricting the numbers of observers carrying out physical examinations may prevent the one hard cry which produces the tension phenomenon.

Radiologic Diagnosis

A tension pneumothorax is usually easily recognizable in infants: a large amount of air is frequently seen in the pleural space and the mediastinum is displaced to the contralateral side (Fig. 14–2). However, a surprisingly large amount of intrapleural air may not be apparent, and these pneumothoraces may be overlooked in recumbent infants if only anteroposterior or lateral views are obtained with a vertical beam. MacEwan et al. (1971) suggested a horizontal beam lateral film of the recumbent infant. Since air rises to the uppermost region, it can often be demonstrated in the retrosternal region of the supine baby. A lateral decubitus view will demonstrate a pneumothorax not evident on the other views (Fig. 14–3).

In isolated pneumomediastinum, air is seen adjacent to the borders of the heart on anteroposterior projection (Han et al., 1963; Morrow et al., 1967). The mediastinal air can elevate the thymus away from the pericardium, resulting in a crescentic configuration resembling a spinnaker sail (Moseley, 1960). The mediastinal air is frequently more easily visualized on the lateral view, as in Figure 14–4. Occasionally apparent dextroversion of the heart results from pneumomediastinum (Franken, 1970). In contrast to older children, air rarely dissects into the soft tissues of the neck when pneumomediastinum occurs in the newborn infant (Fig. 14–5).

OTHER MANIFESTATIONS OF
ALVEOLAR AIR EXTRAVASATION

Interstitial Emphysema

Pulmonary interstitial emphysema occurs when air from a ruptured alveolus extravasates into the perivascular spaces (Macklin,

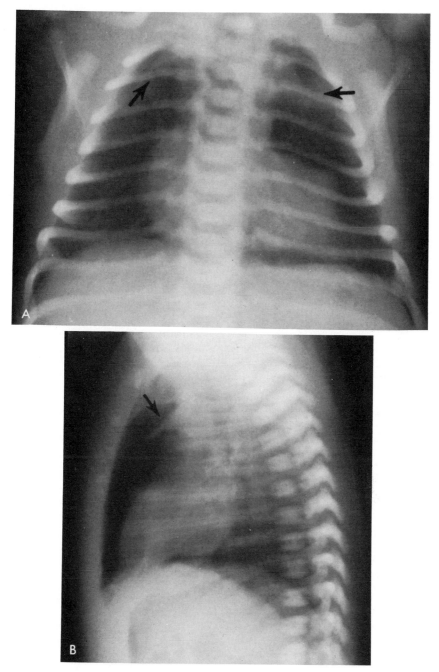

Figure 14–4. A, On the AP view, the pneumomediastinum is very poorly defined. The thymic lobes however, are elevated (arrows) indicating air in the mediastinum. B, In the same patient, the horizontal beam lateral view clearly shows a collection of air in the mediastinum anterior to the heart. The displacement of the thymus (arrow) away from the anterior border of the heart is well demonstrated.

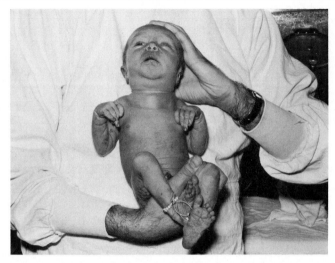

Figure 14–5. Rarely air dissects along the mediastinal structures into the subcutaneous tissues. The prominence of this infant's neck is from subcutaneous emphysema in association with a small pneumomediastinum. Both resolved in 48 hours without treatment.

1939). The presence of air in the interstitium can compromise pulmonary vascular circulation and ventilation of the lungs. Although it is difficult to identify in otherwise normal lungs, interstitial emphysema causes a roentgenologically characteristic fine "bubbly" pattern when it occurs in infants with hyaline membrane disease (Fletcher et al., 1970; Campbell, 1970) (Fig. 14–6). This appearance which is associated with increased volume of the lungs occurs rapidly either spontaneously or when respiration is mechanically assisted and is associated with sudden clinical deterioration. If it is bilateral and unassociated with pneumothorax or pneumomediastinum, death rapidly ensues. We have seen emphysema localized to one lung or lobe in which the prognosis was favorable.

Pneumopericardium

This rare occurrence in the newborn infant may happen spontaneously, probably due to rupture of air through the pericardial reflections of the great vessels. Resorption of air using high oxygen concentrations has been successful therapy (Gershanik, 1971). Needle aspiration, however, may be necessary to prevent fatal tamponade (Grosfeld et al., 1970). On chest radiographs, the pneumopericardium completely surrounds the heart, unlike pneumomediastinum which does not extend under the inferior margin of the cardiac silhouette (Fig. 14–7).

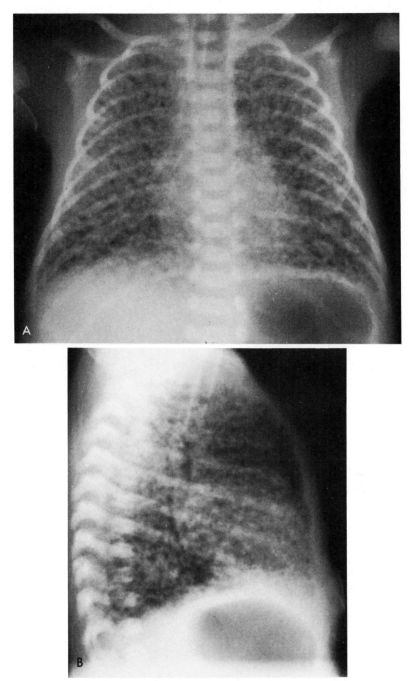

Figure 14–6. Bilateral pulmonary interstitial emphysema in small premature infant, managed with positive-pressure respirator for hyaline membrane disease. Radiologic changes seen on AP (*A*) and lateral (*B*) views accompanied dramatic deterioration of the patient's condition. Note the voluminous lungs with a diffuse "bubbly" pattern of lucent air-containing spaces, contrasting with densities due to atelectasis.

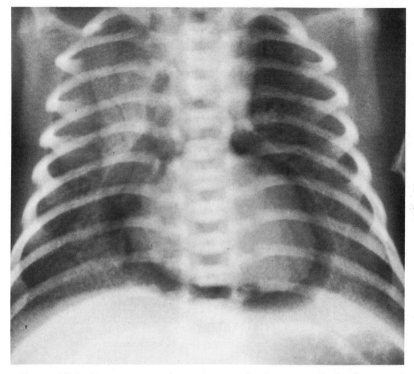

Figure 14–7. Pneumopericardium. Air completely surrounds the heart and is limited by the pericardial sac.

Extrathoracic Air

If abdominal distention is also present, pneumoperitoneum should be suspected. Apparently air under pressure can dissect along vascular sheaths and ultimately rupture into the peritoneal cavity (Aranda et al., 1972). Lee and Kuhn (1971) described an infant who developed pneumatosis intestinalis, preceded by pneumomediastinum. Clinically, this could not be differentiated from necrotizing enterocolitis. Sudden fatal extravasation of air into the circulatory system (pulmonary gas embolism) can occur and is apparently due to rupture of pulmonary veins in conjunction with high alveolar pressures (Gregory and Tooley, 1970).

Chapter Fifteen

PULMONARY
HEMORRHAGE

One of the challenges to an attempt to understand the causes of respiratory difficulty in newborn infants is the problem of pulmonary hemorrhage. Whereas our ignorance as to the pathogenesis of many infections, hyaline membrane disease, and the disposition of fluid in the lungs at birth is all too obvious, at least there are a number of studies to consider. As for pulmonary hemorrhage, about all that is possible is to cite its incidence and symptoms, and speculate on its etiology.

INCIDENCE

Pulmonary hemorrhage is a common post-mortem finding in still-births and early neonatal deaths. In a review of histologic material from 758 liveborn infants who survived less than two weeks, massive pulmonary hemorrhage, defined as involvement of all areas in two or more lobes, with and without other lesions, was present in 17.8 per cent (Esterly and Oppenheimer, 1966). The incidence of the finding was 3.8 per 1000 live births in the Johns Hopkins series representing a population with about an 11 per cent incidence of babies under 2.5 kg. Pulmonary hemorrhage was less common in the British Perinatal Study, 0.7 per 1000 live births in a population with 6.7 per cent of infants born under 2.5 kg. (Butler and Bonham, 1963). In all studies, the lesion has been noted most frequently in infants of low birth weight, with a predisposition for those of small size for their gestational age.

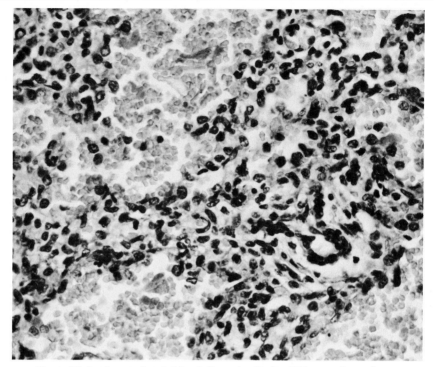

Figure 15–1.   Lung of an 1.1-kg. infant who died at 37 hours of age after respiratory distress. Bloody material was suctioned from the oropharynx. Note the extensive intra-alveolar hemorrhage and intrabronchial hemorrhage. × 400.

PATHOLOGY

The hemorrhage may be predominantly alveolar, interstitial, or mixed. Interstitial hemorrhage occurs most frequently in infants who die in the first day of life; alveolar hemorrhage is more common in those who die later (Fig. 15–1). The lesion can coexist with other pulmonary lesions such as hyaline membrane disease, aspiration, and pneumonia, and may be associated with hemorrhage in other organs. When present in term infants, other major problems such as congenital heart disease, or a history of thoracotomy, or severe asphyxia are usually evident.

CLINICAL FINDINGS

The onset of respiratory distress in infants who have pulmonary hemorrhage at autopsy is usually within the first hours of life. Retractions, cyanosis, and tachypnea are common; and it is not possible to

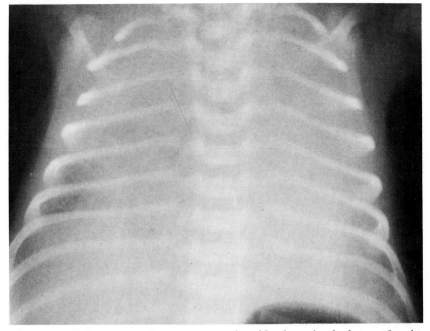

Figure 15-2. A 34-week gestation, one-day-old infant who died soon after this radiograph was obtained. Autopsy showed massive pulmonary hemorrhage.

distinguish the infants from those with hyaline membrane disease. Bleeding from the upper airway occurs in nearly half the infants and is the most nearly pathognomonic finding. The radiographic findings are not specific. Occasionally a reticulogranular appearance dominates the lung fields; sometimes coarse nodular densities are found; and rarely a homogeneous opacification of a whole lung field is present (Rowe and Avery, 1966). (See Fig. 15-2.)

PATHOGENESIS

Factors which could predispose to pulmonary hemorrhage, on the basis of a statistical association, include prenatal and perinatal asphyxia from any cause, and breech presentation.

The association of the pulmonary hemorrhage with infection was noted by Landing (1957), Ahvenainen and Call (1952), and Ahvenainen (1956). *Staph. albus, Alcaligenes faecalis, E. Coli, para-colon,* and *Proteus* were isolated from lungs at autopsy. Ahvenainen and Call (1952) also produced hemorrhagic pneumonia in kittens by the intratracheal injection of *E. coli* alone and with gastric contents. No relationship between infection and hemorrhage was found in the Hopkins series. However, only careful routine bacteriological and viral studies can answer the question.

The possibility that the central nervous system plays a role in pulmonary hemorrhage is suggested by the association of kernicterus and hemorrhage. In Ahvenainen and Call's series, four of 10 patients with kernicterus had combined alveolar and septal hemorrhages; the other six had alveolar hemorrhage alone. They did not cite the total number of kernicteric infants without pulmonary hemorrhage. Silverman (1961) could not find an association between the two conditions in his patients. Only speculation is possible with regard to the meaning of this association, if it exists. If kernicterus in some way interferes with central vagal connections, it is possible that the lesion is on the basis of vascular congestion similar to that which occurs after vagotomy. Evidence of increased intracranial pressure and anoxic brain injury is frequently present in infants who die with pulmonary hemorrhage (McAdams, 1967).

Pulmonary hemorrhage may occur in infants with congenital malformations of the heart in which there is an increase in pulmonary blood flow, such as a widely patent ductus arteriosus or ventricular septal defect. Perhaps the phrase hemorrhagic pulmonary edema would be more suitable under such circumstances. Adamson et al. (1969) analyzed the bloody fluid in the upper respiratory tract of two infants who died with massive pulmonary hemorrhage, and noted hematocrits of 4 and 7 per cent, suggesting that the fluid was a filtrate from pulmonary capillaries. Subsequently, Cole et al. (1972) provided convincing arguments that acute left ventricular failure, usually related to asphyxia, increased filtration of liquid from pulmonary capillaries to alveoli.

A bleeding diathesis such as hemorrhagic disease of the newborn may be associated with pulmonary hemorrhage, although bleeding from the gastrointestinal tract is more common. Ahvenainen and Call (1952) were unable to produce more than petechial hemorrhages in rats given large doses of anticoagulants in combination with ANTU (alpha-naphthylthiourea) which produces pulmonary edema.

In England, infants who are delivered at home in poorly heated houses and thus exposed to cold may arrive at the hospital with body temperatures lower than 90°F. Of 14 such infants reported by Mann and Elliott (1957), eight died; five of these eight had massive pulmonary hemorrhages, which with one exception were not associated with evidence of infection. The symptoms of lethargy, pitting edema, and sclerema with red extremities occur in the first week or two of life. It is not clear from the published cases whether other predisposing conditions such as infection, hernicterus, or a hemorrhage diathesis could have been present, nor are there adequate experimental studies of the effects of cold on pulmonary vessels in newborn animals.

The many similarities between pulmonary hemorrhage and hyaline membrane disease suggested that they could at times have a common pathogenesis (Rowe and Avery, 1966). The association of the two lesions has been noted for many years. Blystad et al. (1951) noted hemorrhage in 45 per cent of infants with hyaline membranes; in 21 per cent of the infants studied by Rowe and Avery membranes were present. In the case of twins, one may have hemorrhage, the other membranes. Injury to the terminal airways, either from lack of the pulmonary surfactant or from its alteration, could lead to transudation not only of fibrin but of whole blood as well.

Aspiration of maternal blood can be a cause of alveolar hemorrhage, as proven by finding sickle cells in the alveoli of an infant, but not in his vascular bed (Ceballos, 1968).

TREATMENT

There is no proven treatment of pulmonary hemorrhage. Since the infants appear to be in shock, and may have clotting defects, we elect to give small transfusions of fresh blood immediately. We find a donor who is blood Group O, Rh negative, withdraw 10 ml. of blood into a heparinized syringe, and give it to the infant over about a five-minute period. If the infant survives for a while, we treat with antibiotics and repeat the transfusions on indication of a low hematocrit level or clinical shock. A warm environment and sufficient oxygen to maintain good color appear to be useful supportive measures. We have no evidence that these measures are helpful, but feel they are reasonable at this time.

Chapter Sixteen

PULMONARY EDEMA

The classic findings in pulmonary edema of cyanosis, tachypnea, fine bubbly rales, and occasionally froth at the mouth may occur in the first days of life just as they do at other ages. Left ventricular failure in the newborn period may be associated with tachypnea before rales are audible, and sometimes no murmur can be heard.

CAUSES IN THE NEWBORN

Keith (1956), in his review of causes of congestive heart failure, cites aortic atresia as the most common example in the first week of life. Twenty per cent of his series of 1580 patients with congenital heart disease were in failure in the first week of life. Of these, 44 per cent had aortic atresia, 10 per cent coarctation of the aorta, 10 per cent patent ductus arteriosus, 8 per cent pulmonary stenosis or atresia, and 8 per cent Ebstein's disease. An important and frequently overlooked cause of congestive heart failure in the newborn period accompanied by dyspnea and cyanosis is the infradiaphragmatic type of total anomalous pulmonary venous return (Johnson et al., 1958). This may present with the radiologic picture of acute pulmonary interstitial edema (Heitzman and Ziter, 1966).

Heart failure may also be secondary to paroxysmal tachycardias, myocarditis, and arteriovenous aneurysms and fistulas. Increasingly in recent years heart failure has been reported as the presenting symptom of intracerebral aneurysms (Holden et al., 1972). The diagnosis may be suspected in the absence of other causes of failure and is usually confirmed by the presence of a cerebral bruit; occasionally no bruit is audible. Cerebral angiography is confirmatory. Resection may be required. At least one infant is reported to have recovered with medical management of the heart failure (Sunderland et al., 1971). Arterial-venous shunting in giant hepatic hemangioma may lead to death from cardiac failure (Berdon and Baker, 1969).

When the circulation is overloaded, as in hydrops fetalis or in the placental transfusion syndrome in which one twin receives more than his share of the fetal blood supply, the infant may be in failure (Naeye, 1963).

In severe asphyxia, cardiac enlargement is evident on roentgenographic studies (Burnard and James, 1961), and left atrial pressures are elevated. If the infant receives a placental transfusion after stripping of the umbilical cord, and is asphyxiated as well, further cardiac dilatation occurs and atrial pressures are elevated up to 10 mm. Hg (Burnard and James, 1963). However, in the absence of other cardiac or pulmonary lesions, the group of infants with cardiac dilatation and modest elevations of atrial pressures associated with asphyxia at birth were "healthy be accepted standards." Obstruction of the upper airways can cause pulmonary edema in the newborn as well as in older children (Jeresaty et al., 1969).

CLINICAL SIGNS

One of the earliest signs of congestive failure in infancy is tachypnea, sometimes up to 150/min. Tachycardia is usually present, and not infrequently the heart rate and the respiratory rate are the same. The liver may enlarge with amazing rapidity and decrease in size after digitalization just as fast. The enlarged liver feels firm; when it pulsates obstruction or insufficiency of the tricuspid valve is suggested. Venous engorgement is evident, but peripheral edema is not often present; when apparent, it is a late finding and a poor prognostic sign. Aside from tachypnea, the pulmonary findings are fine bubbling rales and harsh breath sounds. Retractions may be present. The cardiac signs include enlargement, which is difficult to ascertain clinically but may be evident on the chest film, tachycardia and a gallop rhythm, and occasionally murmurs that depend on the nature of the lesion. Murmurs tend to be less audible at high rates, so their absence by no means rules out shunts or valvular defects.

The problem of distinguishing the tachypnea of heart failure from that of pulmonary disease by clinical means poses some difficulties. The old adage that a good cry will reverse the cyanosis of pulmonary disease and aggravate that of heart disease has not been helpful in our experience. When it is recalled that right-to-left shunts occur in hyaline membrane disease just as they do in some forms of congenital heart disease, it is evident that a good cry will not necessarily make an infant with hyaline membrane less cyanotic; often it makes him more cyanotic. Cyanosis may lessen or deepen with crying in either cardiac or pulmonary disease. The most useful generalization would seem to be that intense cyanosis in the absence of marked retractions is more likely to be on a cardiac basis than to represent a lung disorder. A chest film is most useful, since an abnormal cardiac contour, such as the narrow base of the heart with transposition of the great vessels, marked cardiomegaly, or prominent pulmonary vessels, will point to heart disease. Electrocardiographic changes may likewise indicate heart disease.

RADIOGRAPHIC FEATURES

Pulmonary edema may involve the interstitium or airspaces of the lung. Although interstitial edema precedes airspace involvement, a combination of the two patterns is frequently present. The former (Fig. 16–1A) is characterized by loss of definition of the hila and pulmonary vascular markings and thickening of the interlobular septa. Right-sided predominance is not uncommon. There may be minimal pleural effusion. When the edema fluid enters the airspaces, the lungs acquire a more homogeneous density in which an air bronchogram can be seen (Fraser and Paré, 1970) (Fig. 16–1B).

TREATMENT

The fulminating nature and grave prognosis of congestive failure in infancy make immediate treatment imperative. Oxygen, the upright position and warmth and humidity are all indicated. Digitalis should be given. Keith (1955) recommends digoxin, 0.07 mg./kg. in four divided doses given intramuscularly for the first 24 hours. The daily maintenance dose after full digitalization is about one-fourth to one-fifth the total digitalizing dose given in two divided doses per day. Markowitz (in Schaffer, 1971) states his preference for a lower total digitalizing dose of 0.05 mg./kg., since this is often effective and is associated with less toxicity. The individual variability of tolerance to digitalis preparations, particularly in premature infants, makes frequent electrocardiograms necessary (Levine and Blumenthal, 1962). Sapin et al. (1956) believe that S-T segment and T wave changes are not signs of serious toxicity, but that conduction defects and arrhythmias are indications to withhold further digitalis until they revert to normal.

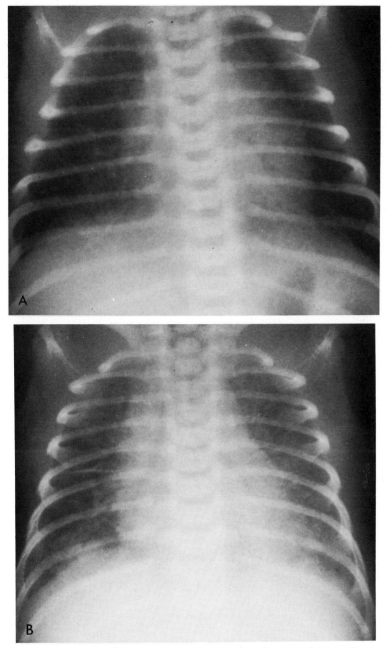

Figure 16–1. A, Pulmonary edema associated with severe birth asphyxia. The edema is mainly interstitial. The pulmonary vascular markings are ill-defined, and there is a small pleural effusion in the right costophrenic angle. The heart is not enlarged. *B,* The severe edema in this patient involves the airspaces particularly in the lower lobes where homogeneous densities are present. There is also a faint "air bronchogram" in the right lower lobe. Note thickening of the minor fissure, due to pleural effusion.

In acute distress, morphine in a dose of 0.2 mg./kg. is indicated.

Diuretics may be necessary if the response to digitalis is inadequate.

Oral feedings should be withheld during the acute phase of congestive failure because of the risk of vomiting and aspiration. Intravenous fluids can be given in amounts calculated to provide maintenance needs, although the infants usually respond to digitalization and rarely need intravenous fluids. When the infant can tolerate oral feedings, low-sodium formulas are useful. Frequent small feedings help reduce fatigue. Occasionally, infants who receive a restricted sodium intake and mercurial diuretics become depleted in sodium so that determinations of the serum sodium levels are indicated.

Finally, respirators should be considered for support of an infant in whom pharmacologic measures have been ineffective. Positive end-expiratory pressure may prove useful in the management of pulmonary edema in infants just as it has in adults.

Chapter Seventeen

MISCELLANEOUS CONDITIONS

CHYLOTHORAX

This unusual condition in the newborn infant is as puzzling as it is rare. The onset of symptoms is usually in the first days of life, but may be at several months of age. Approximately one-half of the infants are symptomatic within 24 hours of birth. Tachypnea, retractions, and cyanosis occur as they do with many pulmonary disorders in the newborn period. When the disorder is unilateral, the diagnosis is suggested by a shift of the mediastinum to the side away from the effusion, and dullness to percussion with decreased breath sounds on the side of the effusion. Radiologically, fluid is seen in the pleural space; a large volume of fluid may depress the ipsilateral diaphragmatic dome and displace the mediastinum to the opposite side. A thoracentesis in the first days of life will reveal clear fluid; after the infant is on oral feedings, the fluid becomes opalescent, with a protein content usually of 2 to 4 per cent, and visible fat globules (Randolph and Gross, 1957; Perry et al., 1963).

Chylothorax has been reported in males twice as commonly as in females, more commonly on the right side, and bilaterally at least once (Forbes, 1944; Yancy and Spock, 1967). The amount of fluid present may be very slight, and it may disappear after a single thoracentesis. More commonly, in the reported cases at least, its reappearance has required repeated thoracenteses. Boles and Izant (1960) removed a total of 1955 ml. during 27 thoracenteses in one infant over a

263

period of 30 days. Wessel's patient (1944) required 12 aspirations in which a total of 1278 ml. was removed over a 14-day period. As much as 200 ml. was aspirated on one occasion. The infant recovered spontaneously.

Some of these infants have succumbed to their disease. No obstructive lesions have been found to account for the leakage of chyle. The thoracic duct was not identified in Forbes's patient despite a careful search. At least three patients have come to operation after the failure of multiple thoracenteses to prevent accumulation of chyle in the pleural space. Randolph and Gross (1957) reported one patient in whom no leaks were identified; the surgeons roughened the pleural surface and the patient recovered after operation. They reported another in whom several leaks were noted in the mediastinal pleura. These were ligated, as was the thoracic duct, and recovery ensued. The patient of McKendry et al. (1957) showed a generalized weeping of serous fluid from the entire pleural surface. These authors also reported one patient with generalized lymphedema, including chylothorax and chylous ascites, in whom it was thought that peripheral lymphatic vessels failed to communicate with the main channels. In the case of Gates et al. (1972), radionuclide lymphangiography showed leakage of the thoracic duct into the left pleural space.

The majority of infants have recovered after single or multiple thoracenteses. Although there may be recurrences some weeks after initial response, as in one of Randolph and Gross's patients (1957), usually there are none, nor are there associated problems. Chernick and Reed (1970) point out that recurrent effusions may require insertion of a chest tube. Continuous drainage of chyle can lead to protein depletion and inanition. Feeding a medium-chain tryglyceride formula to lessen chyle formation would seem appropriate.

The etiology of chylothorax is unknown, but trauma to the lymphatic ducts during delivery, and congenital weakness of the duct wall, have been considered. The early onset of symptoms in most cases is consistent with either possibility. However, the protected position of the thoracic duct, and the absence of a history of obstetrical trauma, make injury unlikely in most cases. The evidence for a congenital anomaly of the duct system is inferential. Randolph and Gross suggested the possibility of a failure of fusion of the primordial duct structures, with formation of true congenital fistulas, and thought the multiple sites of leakage in their patient to be consistent with this hypothesis. Whatever the etiology, it is clear that other lymphatic vessels in the body are not affected in most of these infants. The failure to demonstrate obstructive lesions in the thoracic duct, the absence of known trauma in many cases, and the localization of the lesion in the chest, as well as the probability of spontaneous recovery, are factors that must be considered in any hypothesis about the pathogenesis of chylothorax.

A FORM OF PULMONARY INSUFFICIENCY IN PREMATURE INFANTS: WILSON-MIKITY SYNDROME, ? PULMONARY DYSMATURITY

In 1960 Wilson and Mikity described a respiratory disease in premature infants characterized by a unique roentgenographic picture of multiple cyst-like foci of hyperaeration that alternated with a coarse thickening of the interstitial supporting structures. Since then other infants with similar roentgenograms and clinical courses have been reported, so that the syndrome appears to be a clinical entity, although a rare one (Butterfield et al., 1963; Baghdassarian et al., 1963; von Hottinger et al., 1963). In the past, many infants with this condition probably were thought to have had congenital cystic disease of the lung. It seems worthwhile to distinguish infants with the features described by Wilson and Mikity from that group, however, since some infants recover completely.

Clinical Features.   Nearly all infants reported have been premature by weight, the smallest being 0.86 kg. While maternal hemorrhage has been present in nearly half the cases, no unusual obstetrical problems were present in the others, except the premature onset of labor. Males and females alike have been affected, but no familial tendency has been noted.

The onset of symptoms was at birth or as late as 35 days thereafter. The chief feature was the infant's dependence on oxygen to overcome cyanosis. The respiratory rates were normal or slightly elevated, with occasional periodic breathing. Rales were sometimes present, and retractions noted, although they were not of the severity associated with respiratory distress from many other causes. Wheezing has been heard in two of the patients, but not constantly.

The functional derangement, in the few infants in which it has been studied, consists of an intrapulmonary shunt with arterial hypoxemia, decreased lung compliance, and increased expiratory flow resistance (Swyer et al., 1965; Bucci et al., 1966). Significant elevation of pulmonary artery pressure may occur late in the disease. Persistent patency of the ductus arteriosus has also been described (Grossman et al., 1972).

Death has occurred in nearly half the reported cases; one infant died 12 hours after birth, the other infants at two or four months of age. The remainder have gradually improved, and chest roentgenogram and physical examination have been normal at six months to one year of age.

Roentgenographic Features.   These patients are distinguished by the similarity and characteristic appearance of the roentgenographic picture. The changes are diffuse and bilateral, with coarse thickening of the interstitial supporting structures which alternates in

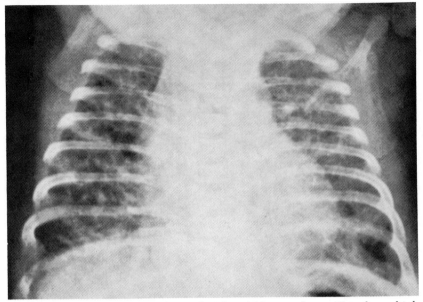

Figure 17–1.   Film of an infant with Wilson-Mikity syndrome. Note the multiple cyst-like foci throughout both lungs. In some infants these have resolved after several months. (From Baghdassarian et al.: Am. J. Roent. 89:1020, 1963.)

a lacy fashion with minute to 10 mm. cyst-like foci of hyperaeration. As the disease progresses, the cystic foci at the bases coalesce, and eventually the lower lobes are overexpanded with flattening of the diaphragms. Residual strands persist in the upper lobes for months to years. The last abnormality to disappear is the overexpansion, and eventually, completely normal chest films are found in the survivors. The cardiovascular structures are normal throughout the course of the disease as is the peripheral pulmonary vasculature. Angiographic studies may reveal prominence of the pulmonary artery and tapering of the peripheral arteries. Spontaneous rib fractures have occurred in a few patients with the Wilson-Mikity syndrome (Mikity et al., 1967) (Fig. 17–1).

Laboratory Examinations.   There are no consistent hematological changes. Routine bacteriologic cultures have failed to reveal a pathogenic organism. Viral studies by Wilson and Mikity were negative, but Butterfield et al. (1963) found type 19 ECHO virus in the lung of one infant who succumbed. Corresponding serologic changes were not demonstrated in the mother or infant, however. Skin tests for tuberculosis and histoplasmosis have been negative, and the concentration of chloride in the sweat was normal.

Pathology.   The lungs at autopsy were voluminous and aerated, and readily distensible. On inflation, the interlobar markings appeared to be retracted and the lobules themselves overdistended (Fig.

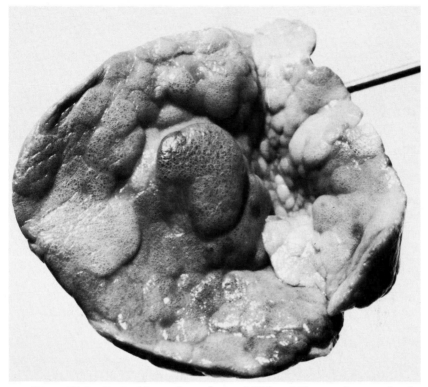

Figure 17–2. Excised lung of an infant with Wilson-Mikity syndrome inflated to 30 cm. H₂O pressure. The distal airspaces are overdistended, and restricting septa give this diaphragmatic surface of the lung a hobnail appearance. (From Baghdassarian et al.: Am. J. Roent. 89:1020, 1963.)

17–2). The histological features were septal thickening in places, variation in size and outline of terminal airspaces, and an apparent decrease in alveolar divisions. A mononuclear response was present in some areas, as was focal lobular hemorrhage. Capillaries may be reduced in many alveolar septa, although normal in others (Swyer et al., 1965).

Etiology. The etiology is obscure. The features that have been consistent and require explanation are (1) occurrence in premature infants, (2) possibility of complete recovery, (3) prolonged course in most infants, (4) absence of fever, white count changes, and bacteria, (5) hyperaeration of lobules of the lung on roentgenogram, and (6) persistent cyanosis.

The concept of retarded and uneven postnatal development of lung alveoli was suggested by Mithal and Emery (1961) and is consistent with the finding of lack of distensibility of some areas of lung and of overdistention of others. Baghdassarian et al. suggested the term "dysmaturity" to imply unequal maturation of parts of the lung parenchyma, chiefly a failure of alveolar proliferation. The concept of dysmaturity allows for the possibility of ultimate normal architecture in time as new lung growth occurs.

Treatment.   No specific therapy is known, but added oxygen to overcome cyanosis has been associated with survival of some of these infants. Cortisone has not been effective.

TRANSIENT TACHYPNEA OF THE NEWBORN

First described as a syndrome in 1966 on the basis of eight infants with very similar signs and clinical course, the pathogenesis is unknown and the diagnosis is one of exclusion of other known causes of respiratory distress (Avery et al., 1966). "Transient respiratory distress of the newborn" (Swischuk, 1970) and "Wet-lung disease" (Wesenberg et al., 1971) have been offered as alternative names for this syndrome; a number of these babies, however, had birth asphyxia.

The infants are usually born at term, with no specific antenatal events in common. In the first hours of life, they exhibit elevated respiratory rates, up to 120/min., in the absence of significant retractions or rales. They may be minimally cyanotic, but alveolar ventilation is normal as measured by blood pH and Pco_2. No cardiovascular abnormalities have been found. Sundell et al. (1971) reported 36 infants with similarities to those described by Avery et al. They used the name type II respiratory distress to designate their infants, most of whom were born prematurely, although late in gestation. Mild depression at birth was common in the series described by Sundell. Prompt increase in oxygenation on administration of oxygen distinguished these infants from those with hyaline membrane disease. A benign course was emphasized by both groups reporting on this disorder.

The chest radiographs show prominent, ill-defined vascular markings, edematous interlobar septa, and pleural effusions in the costophrenic angles and interlobar fissures, typical of interstitial edema (Kuhn et al., 1969). On occasion, alveolar edema may be present. The lungs tend to be slightly hyperaerated. Clearing of the lungs is usually evident the next day, although complete clearing may require three to seven days (Fig. 17–3).

One suggested mechanism for the tachypnea is a delay in resorption of fetal lung liquid. The prominent perihilar streaking may represent engorgement of the periarterial lymphatics, which have been shown to participate in clearance of alveolar liquid with the initiation of air breathing. Fletcher et al. (1970) tested the possibility that delayed clearance of lung liquid could account for the findings by sequential chest films in newborn lambs. When lung water content was elevated, and radiographic abnormalities were present, the respiratory rates were increased.

Sequential films in asymptomatic newborn infants sometimes show vascular engorgement in the first two hours of life. Northway et al. (1971) and Steele and Copeland (1972) pointed out that the vascular engorgement was not always associated with tachypnea.

The process is self-limited, and infants followed as long as one year had no recurrence of tachypnea or other evidence of pulmonary dysfunction.

Persistent Liquid-filled Lung

Animal experiments involving fetal tracheal ligation established the fetal lung as a secretory organ in which liquid could accumulate. (Jost and Policard, 1948; Lanman et al., 1971). It is hardly surprising, then, that bronchial occlusion in utero can promote liquid accumulation in the affected lobe. Griscom et al. (1969) reported two infants in whom bronchial obstruction was present with a space-occupying radiopaque mass noted on roentgenogram. At operation liquid-filled lung distal to the obstruction was noted. With removal of the obstruction, aeration occurred in one; in the other, normal lung was resected.

Respiratory Distress from Pulmonary Vascular Disorders

Both pulmonary arterial and veno-occlusive disease have been described in the lungs of infants. Wagenvoort et al. (1971) added the 12th patient to the literature with intimal thickening of the pulmonary veins in association with a chronic interstitial pneumonia and subacute myocarditis. Their infant was symptomatic from birth, with cyanosis and cough. The chest film showed a reticular pattern, but the heart was normal size. On cardiac catheterization pulmonary artery pressure was 110/45, and left atrial pressure was 3. Wedge pressure was 15. The infant died at eight weeks of age. The only hint as to pathogenesis was a respiratory infection in the mother during the last weeks of pregnancy.

A less severe and perhaps more common problem was described by Siassi et al. in a group of five full-term infants who presented with cyanosis and tachypnea at birth, persisting for five to seven days. On cardiac catheterization pulmonary artery pressures were elevated with the mean between 48 and 68 mm. Hg. Four of them had right-to-left ductal shunts. One infant died at three days of age, and on histological examination of the lung, thickening of the media or the arterioles was noted. No inflammation was noted. The authors considered intrauterine hypoxia or hypervolemia as perhaps etiologic in the persistent pulmonary hypertension.

Progressive and fatal pulmonary hypertension in two infants born at term who died in the third month of life was described by Burnell et al. (1972). No associated cardiac or respiratory disease was present.

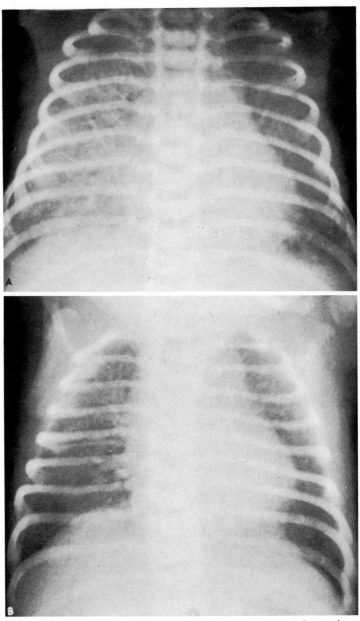

Figure 17–3. Sequential radiographs of the chest of a term infant with tachypnea in the first days of life. *A*, Four hours of age, with diffuse haziness of lung fields and prominent vascular markings. *B*, Twenty-four hours of age, showing some clearing but persistent interstitial edema.

(Illustration continued on opposite page).

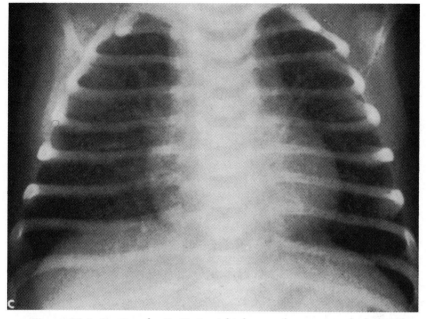

Figure 17-3 Continued. C, Forty-eight hours of age, normal chest. These changes are thought to represent delay in the clearance of lung fluid after birth.

Mean pulmonary artery pressures persisted at fetal levels of 66 mm. Hg in one infant and 42 mm. Hg in the other. Pressures fell to normal on breathing oxygen in one infant, but not in the other. At autopsy the pulmonary vessels showed an abnormal pattern of branching with thickening of the walls of the preacinar arteries. Intimal thickening was described in some vessels.

MUSCULAR WEAKNESS

Impaired ventilation of the lungs may be the result of weakness of the muscles of respiration from a variety of causes. It would be rare to have isolated weakness of only the muscles of respiration, except with diaphragmatic paralysis (discussed on pages 162–164). More commonly there is generalized muscle weakness, so that hypoventilation could be anticipated in some flaccid infants. Among the illnesses likely to impair muscle strength in the newborn period are myasthenia gravis, the amyotonia congenita syndrome, and congenital poliomyelitis. Perhaps the first condition to consider is myasthenia gravis since it is amenable to drug therapy.

Myasthenia Gravis

Myasthenia in the newborn may be of a transient variety in the infant of a myasthenic mother, or persistent if the infant is born of a normal mother, according to Teng and Osserman (1956), who reviewed 217 cases that were reported in the literature and seen by them since the first reported case by Strickroot et al. (1942). In a single case reported by Greer and Schotland (1960), an infant of a normal mother had symptoms for only six days.

Symptoms. In congenital myasthenia gravis, in which the mothers are normal, fetal activity is often decreased. The infant's cry is characteristically weak and swallowing difficult in both congenital and transient forms of the disease. Ptosis and even ophthalmoplegia may be present in the newborn period. The infants of myasthenic mothers are usually symptomatic at birth, but may not be symptomatic until two or three days of age. This is the more severe form and has been lethal. The life-threatening dangers are aspiration from poor swallowing, and hypoventilation (Kibrick, 1954).

Treatment. An intramuscular or subcutaneous injection of 0.1 to 0.2 mg. of neostigmine methylsulfate or 1.0 mg. of edrophonium chloride should result in an improvement in muscle strength within 10 to 15 minutes, and may thus be used as a diagnostic test. If therapy is required for a few days in the transient form of the disease, it should be noted that recovery may occur so suddenly that there is a danger of overdose of neostigmine.

Poliomyelitis

The fetus can be infected with the viruses of poliomyelitis, or the disease can be acquired in the neonatal period (Schaeffer et al., 1954). Bates (1955) reported an infant normal at birth, febrile by 40 hours of age, and without reflexes the next day. The pathologic findings are similar to those in older individuals, although often severe and widespread. Encephalomyelitic signs are frequent, with irritability, vomiting, and diarrhea. Localized groups of muscles may be involved, as well as the muscles of respiration. The diagnosis should be suspected in the presence of maternal poliomyelitis or during an epidemic.

Amyotonia Congenita (Werdnig-Hoffmann Disease)

Fetal movements are often weak or absent in this rare familial disease. The infant may be areflexic and limp at birth, although sensation and sphincter tone are normal. Occasionally, the onset of symptoms is rather sudden in the early days of life. In a severe case, the only movements the infant may make are side-to-side turning of the head and slight digital movement. Since the intercostal muscles are paralyzed before the diaphragm is involved, marked retractions are present. Fibrillations of the tongue and poor sucking eventually occur.

The diagnosis can be made on the basis of the family history, or in sporadic cases with a muscle biopsy. There is atrophy of the muscle secondary to degeneration of the motor neurons in the spinal cord (Clark in Nelson, 1969).

Other Causes of Muscle Weakness in the Newborn

Muscular dystrophy, primarily of the diaphragmatic musculature, was described in two siblings by Lewis and Besant (1962). The infants were irritable, and nursed poorly by the second week of life; thereafter they showed progressive respiratory difficulty until death at six and nine weeks of age, respectively. The diaphragmatic musculature showed degenerative changes consistent with muscular dystrophy. In one infant, the pectoral muscle was also involved, although other muscles were normal.

The differential diagnosis of persistent muscle weakness at birth should include atonic diplegia, cerebral lipoidosis, cerebral von Gierke's disease, kernicterus, spinal cord injury or tumor, polymyositis, chronic infection, and benign congenital hypotonia, in addition to myasthenia gravis, poliomyelitis, and Werdnig-Hoffmann disease. For a discussion of differential diagnosis, see Clark in Nelson (1969).

Chapter Eighteen

PERSISTENT PULMONARY DYSFUNCTION IN PREMATURE INFANTS

It is increasingly apparent that there is a group of low birth weight infants who demonstrate significant abnormalities of pulmonary function, sometimes associated with symptoms and radiographic changes for many weeks. The infants were first thoroughly studied by Burnard et al. (1965) who chose to consider them part of a spectrum of disease in which the Wilson-Mikity syndrome is an extreme example. Since the radiographic features may be very different from those described by Wilson and Mikity (1960), it seems useful to preserve the eponym for the infants who fulfill the radiographic criteria, and consider the changes described by Burnard in a separate category.

INFANTS AT RISK

The observations of persistent abnormalities of pulmonary function are mostly in those infants below 1.5 kg. birth weight and less than 34 weeks' gestational age, studied in the first few months of life.

SYMPTOMS AND SIGNS

The infants with pulmonary dysfunction may have slightly higher respiratory rates, but frequently do not direct attention to themselves.

274

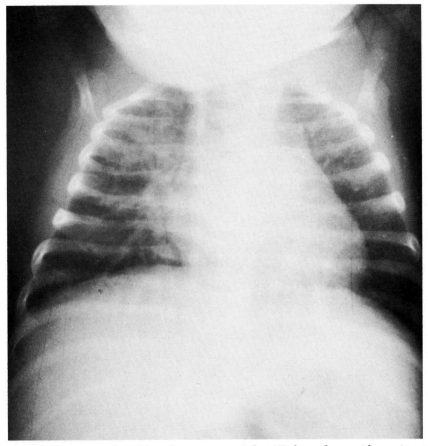

Figure 18–1. Chest film of a premature infant 58 days of age with persistent pulmonary dysfunction similar to that described by Burnard. The chest film was normal at four months of age.

Burnard found radiographic changes in about one-third of a group of infants under 1.8 kg. selected at random. He described a fine pattern of branching—interlaced markings which tapered from hilum to periphery. Ill-defined opacities were noted in many lung fields (Fig. 18–1). The findings usually became evident at one to two months of age, and persisted for some months thereafter.

PATHOPHYSIOLOGY

Infants who had been normal had moderate elevations in Pco_2 by two weeks of age. The arterial Pco_2 rose from 35 mm. Hg to 40 to 65 mm Hg, with an arterial-end-tidal gradient of as high as 10 mm Hg.

The oxygen tension of temporal artery blood of low birth weight infants may be in the range of 70 mm. Hg and in some infants as low as 40 mm. Hg for some months, according to the findings of Thibeault et al. (1966).

Lung volume and compliance fell by approximately 25 per cent between the first and second weeks in some infants studied serially. The ratio of compliance to lung volume did not change, which suggested the fall in compliance reflected the loss of volume. Resistance to airflow was elevated for several months in some infants, but not in all.

Some of the abnormalities seen on the radiographs may relate to the phenomenon of gas-trapping, documented by Krauss and Auld (1971) in a series of infants under 1750 gm. birth weight. Little functional impairment was found in Krauss and Auld's patients, since the trapped gas (as measured plethysmographically) was apparently minimally ventilated and perfused. It should be noted, in addition, that the trapped gas was most evident in the first week of life, whereas the abnormalities seen by Burnard occurred later.

COURSE

The outcome is on the whole favorable. Although long-term follow-up of low birth weight infants with respect to lung function has not been done, the patients studied by Burnard et al. (1965) improved over a period of months. The frequency of the abnormalities in lung function in a low birth weight group of infants, and their apparent recovery, suggest the changes are related in some manner to immaturity. Burnard suggested the predominantly diaphragmatic breathing of the small infant could subject the lungs to regional pressure differences in expiration, and the very compliant airways could collapse with subsequent uneven distribution of ventilation.

These infants will be seen in increasing numbers as those of very low birth weight survive long enough to develop the pulmonary dysfunction. The clinical significance of the changes described is not clear at this time; nor is any active treatment known or indicated beyond supportive measures.

Chapter Nineteen

NONPULMONARY
CAUSES OF BREATHING
IRREGULARITIES

The observation of rapid breathing or hyper- or hypoventilation calls attention first to the respiratory system, and in the majority of instances a pulmonary basis for the abnormal respiration can be found. The lungs may be involved secondary to heart disease and pulmonary edema (pp. 258–262), but here again there are usually changes in the lungs which are detectable on auscultation or on a chest film. Infants occasionally have marked changes in the depth and rate of ventilation in the presence of normal findings on examination of the chest. In our experience the most common extracardiopulmonary causes of abnormal respiration are the effects of drugs, central nervous system disease, and metabolic acidosis.

DRUGS THAT AFFECT RESPIRATION OF THE INFANT

Most medications given to the mother cross the placenta and affect the fetus, although the concentrations in the fetal circulation vary widely. A few agents such as isoniazid are in higher concentration in the fetus than the mother; others such as epinephrine enter the fetal circulation in very small amounts (Baker, 1960). Surely the last word has not been written about the complicated interactions of drugs ingested by the mother on fetal development and function. With the numbers of new agents appearing each year, it can be anticipated that

277

mothers will receive analgesics and anesthetics long before their effect on the infant-in-utero is known, and the pediatrician responsible for the care of the newborn infant is well advised to be on the alert for clinical syndromes that might relate to maternal medications. It is not always easy to sort out the effects of the drugs from the effects of the maternal condition for which the drugs were given. For example, if a mother has preeclampsia, the disease itself may affect the infant adversely; on the other hand, the narcotics or antihypertensive agents she receives may likewise depress the infant.

Almost all sedative or anesthetic agents cross the placenta. Thus the drugs widely used in the management of labor and delivery can be expected to depress the infant. Clinical experience teaches that most such agents used in moderate doses do not interfere seriously with the initiation of respiration, although the unresponsive infant in the nursery with ether on his breath testifies that maternal anesthesia can put the baby to sleep. While ether anesthesia in particular does tend to lower the Apgar score (Auld et al., 1961), there is as yet no evidence that the infants are jeopardized by being sleepy (Smith and Barker, 1942). However, long-term follow-up studies of children to evaluate the role of maternal medications have not been done.

Given a history of excessive maternal medication in the absence of maternal illness, it seems justifiable to attribute depression of the infant to the medications. Characteristically, depressed infants initiate spontaneous respiration, although the cry is feeble and the respirations are shallow. Labored breathing should not be attributed to medication. The infants gradually wake up and appear to be more vigorous, hence specific therapy is rarely indicated. The morphine antagonist N-allylnormorphine may be given in the umbilical vein in a dose of 0.2 mg./kg. body weight if the depression of the infant is caused by morphine or related compounds. Analeptic agents such as nikethamide and vanillic acid diethylamide are of potential value in the profoundly depressed infant. Barrie (1963) has shown that both drugs may be absorbed from the buccal mucosa, and recommends that 0.5 ml. of a 25 per cent solution of nikethamide or 0.5 ml. of a 25 per cent solution of vanillic acid diethylamide be placed on the tongue. Intramuscular use of these or other agents is not likely to be effective, since there is a delay of at least 15 minutes in absorption of them. Intravenous administration carries more risk of convulsions than does buccal absorption (Barrie, 1963).

Stimulation of ventilation of the infant from maternal medication must be very rare, but can occur with salicylates. The infant reported by Earle (1961) was born at term to a mother who had ingested 15 to 18 gm. of aspirin with suicidal intent 27 hours before the child was born. The baby was hyperpneic with a respiratory rate of 110/min., and had some retractions but no cyanosis. A chest film was negative. The infant, whose salicylate level was 35 mg. per cent, recovered after an exchange transfusion.

Another drug-induced respiratory disturbance in the newborn infant is the "stuffy-nose syndrome" from reserpine given to the mother. Mothers who receive reserpine within 15 minutes to 50 hours before delivery may give birth to infants with nasal discharge, cyanosis, and retractions. Two of the 12 infants reported by Budnick et al. (1955) died from occlusion of the upper airway. Antihistamines and nasal decongestants have not been impressive in treatment. The use of an oral airway is indicated for the period of one to five days over which symptoms persist. The disturbance is self-limited.

METABOLIC ACIDOSIS

A renal disorder should be considered in a newborn infant whose heart and lungs are normal, but who appears to be hyperpneic. A number of renal anomalies can occur which may be severe enough to interfere with the excretion of fixed acids. The accompanying acidosis stimulates ventilation, and the infant blows off carbon dioxide in an attempt to compensate for the acidosis. Usually renal anomalies of such severity in the newborn period are associated with oliguria and an elevated urea nitrogen level in the blood. A decrease in the carbon dioxide combining power or pH of the blood would be present, with a reduction in the partial pressure of carbon dioxide, if the hyperpnea were secondary to a metabolic derangement.

After the first few days of life, diarrhea and dehydration may be present with acidosis and hyperpnea. Transient diabetes mellitus may occur in the first days of life, but here again the dehydration is more striking than the hyperpnea (Keidan, 1955).

CENTRAL NERVOUS SYSTEM IRRITATION

Gross cerebral hemorrhage and increased intracranial pressure are likely to be associated with respiratory depression. In fact, the sudden appearance of apneic spells in an infant who has been doing well is the chief sign of a sudden intracranial hemorrhage. Grossly irregular respirations, sometimes accompanied by twitching of the arms and legs or a myoclonic jerk, may occur with brain damage. At any other time of life we would call such movements convulsions, but in premature infants, at least, we confess our inability to distinguish "jitteriness" that is within the range of normal from that which is associated with central nervous system pathology.

Central nervous system injury may also cause hyperventilation, which can resemble respiratory distress from pulmonary disease. Usually retractions and rales are absent, and cyanosis less likely when the tachypnea is from central neural stimulation. If a chest film is clear, and blood pH normal or mildly alkalotic, and other neurologic symptoms present, a central nervous system etiology for the respiratory distress would be likely. However, respiratory stimulation is far less common than respiratory depression in association with brain injury in the newborn infant.

The diagnosis of intracranial hemorrhage during life is difficult. It can be suspected in premature infants, or after a traumatic delivery. There are usually no localizing signs that serve to distinguish hemorrhage from the cerebral edema of asphyxia. The spinal fluid may contain red blood cells from a traumatic tap. Even with a technically satisfactory puncture, a few red blood cells and some xanthochromia may be present in an infant who is neurologically normal; thus their presence need not imply significant central nervous system hemorrhage. Moreover, intracerebral hemorrhage may be present when the spinal fluid is normal. A lumbar puncture is nonetheless indicated in any infant whose depression and irregular respirations may be due to a central nervous system lesion, because it is the only way to rule out meningitis.

PART III

Artificial
Respiration

Chapter Twenty

RESUSCITATION
AT BIRTH

The apneic newborn infant is frequently a candidate for artificial respiration. It is hardly surprising that almost every conceivable technique to stimulate respiration has been employed at one time or another and that success has been frequent enough with most methods so that each has its advocates (Cook et al., 1956). The success of many methods has depended more on the certainty that the majority of infants will breathe in time without any stimulation than it has on the efficacy of the method. Nonetheless there are infants in whom effective artificial respiration prevents severe asphyxia and may be life-saving. The numbers of articles, books, and films devoted to this subject through the years testify to the demand for information about safe and effective methods of assisting the onset of breathing. The evidence that death or severe disability relates to the delayed onset of breathing is less clear-cut; and even more difficult to document is the question whether cerebral damage was responsible for the failure to breathe, or the failure to breathe responsible for the cerebral damage.

Deaths around the time of birth continue to occur in large numbers. In 1955, for example, 86,124 deaths of infants before or during birth were reported in this country, and 77,351 of these were deaths of liveborn infants in the neonatal period. A comparison of perinatal deaths in 1942 (50.0 per 1000 births) with those in 1955 (35.6 per 1000 births) would point to improvement. It is evident on closer analysis, however, that the improvement has been most marked in the survival

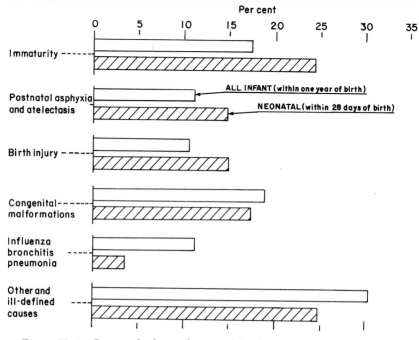

Figure 20–1. Causes of infant and neonatal deaths (percentages of total infant and total neonatal deaths). (Canada Yearbook, 1970-1971. Dominion Bureau of Statistics, Ottawa, Canada.)

of infants over three days and under 27 days of age. Fetal deaths and neonatal deaths in the first three days of life have decreased somewhat; fetal deaths have decreased from 25 per 1000 births in 1942 to 16.8 per 1000 births in 1955, but deaths in the first three days of life have decreased only 17.7 to 14.7 per 1000 births (Eliot, 1958). There is no way to be certain from such national statistics how many of these early neonatal deaths might have been prevented by adequate resuscitation. When they are indexed for statistical purposes, postnatal asphyxia and atelectasis (which includes hyaline membrane disease) are grouped together. This group, however, accounts for 4.1 deaths per 1000 live births (from the Canada Yearbook, 1970–1971).

An estimate of the number of deaths from asphyxia at birth is available from the Perinatal Mortality Survey in England in March, 1958. There were 104 infants listed as liveborn, but in whom respiration was never established, out of a total of 17,000 infants registered in the study (Butler, 1963). From these data, it would appear that one in 1700 infants will die an asphyxial death after birth; how many would be saved by appropriate artificial respiration cannot be known.

INFANTS AT SPECIAL RISK OF ASPHYXIA

While apnea at birth cannot always be anticipated, certain conditions are associated with birth asphyxia so frequently as to suggest the possible need for resuscitation of the infant (Table 20–1).

EXPERIMENTAL AND CLINICAL EVIDENCE OF THE EFFECTS OF ASPHYXIA ON THE BRAIN

The suggestion that abnormal factors in the perinatal period may be the cause of neurologic deficit in later years was first stressed in detail in the writings of Little (1861). His studies were retrospective,

Table 20–1. Conditions Sometimes Associated
with Asphyxia at Birth

I. Mechanical factors
   A. Cephalopelvic disproportion, shoulder dystocia (Fenton and Steer, 1962)
   B. Malposition of the infant
   C. Abnormal uterine contractions
   D. Prolapse of the umbilical cord or cord entanglements
   E. Multiple pregnancy
   F. Difficult forceps delivery
II. Maternal hemorrhage
   A. Abruptio placentae
   B. Placenta praevia
   C. Other antepartum hemorrhage
III. Other maternal conditions
   A. Maternal age over 35 years
   B. Grand multiparity
   C. Toxemia of pregnancy
   D. Diabetes
   E. Cardiorespiratory disease
   F. Intrauterine infection
   G. Postmaturity
   H. Prolonged labor
IV. Iatrogenic factors
   A. Excessive maternal analgesia
   B. Excessive maternal anesthesia (Auld et al., 1961)
   C. Antihypertensive agents
   D. Maternal hyperventilation (Moya et al., 1965)
V. Fetal factors
   A. Erythroblastosis fetalis
   B. Passage of meconium (Desmond et al., 1957)
   C. Pneumonia
   D. Sepsis
   E. Malformations
   F. Fetal tachycardia (> 160/min.) and bradycardia (< 100/min.)
      (Brady and James, 1963)

for the most part, but he did elicit a history of difficulties around the time of birth, especially asphyxia, in 46 of 47 children with generalized spasticity.

Banker (1962) has stressed the vulnerability of the brain of the premature and term newborn infant to lack of oxygen. Her detailed clinical and pathologic studies on a series of 51 infants who died in the first month of life, 74 per cent of whom were premature, showed a correlation between hypoxic episodes and the presence of periventricular leukomalacia. Without exception, the infants in this series suffered severe hypoxic spells before the terminal episode. All of them also had some pulmonary pathology. While the external configuration of their brains was normal, there were changes in the periventricular zones characterized by necrosis, astrocytic degeneration, microglial proliferation, and later, astrocytic and macrophage proliferation. When the lesions were more than 24 hours old, vascular proliferation was evident, followed by scarring and ependymal loss. More subtle changes in the gray matter were characterized by neuronal loss and astrocytosis. Hemorrhages were present in only five instances, and usually in the distribution of the vena terminalis.

Banker noted further that the only experimental lesions that resembled the ones she found so frequently in the infants studied were those produced by exposure to low concentrations of oxygen and to potassium cyanide, but even these lesions differed in distribution from the ones seen in the human infants. She suggested that the pathology in infants was related to the stage of vascularization of the brain. Changes were found in the border zones between the portions of the brain vascularized by the anterior, middle, and posterior cerebral arteries. In the newborn infant the vessels in these areas are thin-walled and do not appear to be fully developed. Perhaps in the event of shock or temporary hypoxia, flow to the periventricular white matter is inadequate. Ischemic damage to the brain may also occur in the subcortical white matter, especially in the parietal area at the zones of vascularization between the internal and external vascular systems.

Yates (1959) described lesions in the base of the brain from traumatic injury to the vertebral arteries. He found evidence of distortional trauma to the cervical spine in 27 of 60 infants examined at autopsy; in 24 infants there were hemorrhages into the adventitial coat of one or both vertebral arteries which narrowed the lumen.

Attempts to document the sequelae of asphyxia in the living human infant have been only partially revealing, although a number of prospective studies that relate the condition of the infant at birth to future mental development have been reported. Graham et al. (1957) showed a decreased mental capacity in childhood in those who as infants had had difficult deliveries. The group of 156 children studied as newborns and also at ages seven to nine years by Schachter and Apgar (1959) showed some decrement in IQ and performance on the Bender-

Gestalt Test, Sorting Test, and Critical Flicker Frequency Test, when perinatal complications had been present. In this carefully studied group of patients, there was no correlation between umbilical vein or heel blood oxygen contents and subsequent mental performance. Moreover, while the infants with perinatal distress scored less well than their more vigorous counterparts, the differences were not marked; the children who were distressed as infants averaged only 4.87 points lower in IQ, and no differences were recorded in a number of special tests. The perinatal complications that did correlate with poorer function were fetal distress, prematurity, and the need for prolonged resuscitation (more than five minutes) or "essential resuscitation," defined as oxygen under pressure for delayed crying time of more than two minutes, inadequate breathing for more than two minutes, poor general condition, or excessive maternal medication. The inclusion of prematurity as a perinatal complication in this study weights the "complicated" group with infants whose mental defect may be on a basis other than asphyxia.

In a review of 2432 obstetric charts, Usdin and Weil (1952) compared infants who were apneic for three or more minutes with ones who breathed promptly. They excluded premature infants, those with neurologic findings at birth or subsequently, those born by cesarean section, and those in whom hemorrhage or trauma could have occurred. Of 90 apneic infants and 90 controls, about one-half were available for follow-up at ages 13 to 14 years. These authors found no differences in the IQ of the infants in their two groups. However, the broad categories of exclusion may well have eliminated infants in whom anoxia caused neurologic lesions. On the other hand, Pasamanick and Lilienfeld (1955) reviewed the obstetrical records of 1107 retarded children and their matched controls and found that there were more complications of pregnancy, prematurity, and abnormal neonatal occurrences, such as asphyxia and convulsions, in the group of retarded children than there were in the control group.

More marked differences in follow-up neurologic status of distressed and vigorous infants were found by Prechtl and Dijkstra (1959), who studied infants at age 48 hours and ages two to four years. Of those who had been abnormal at 48 hours, 68 per cent were abnormal at two to four years, whereas only 8 per cent of the normal group were later impaired. The relationship of the abnormalities to asphyxia is not clear, however, since the initial evaluation was at 48 hours of age.

While studies on humans may be inconclusive, animal studies leave little doubt that asphyxia at birth can impair neurologic performance. Perhaps the most significant of such studies are those of Windle (1963), since they were performed on monkeys in which it was possible to time the duration of anoxia. Windle induced asphyxia by performing cesarean sections near term and removing the fetus with membranes intact. Asphyxia was timed from the moment of placental separation and continued for intervals up to 20 minutes.

The severity of the damage was roughly proportional to the duration of the asphyxia. Very little clinical disturbance was noted in less than 10 minutes of asphyxia, although discrete lesions in the thalamus and inferior colliculus were present at autopsy. Monkeys asphyxiated for 15 or 16 minutes, then successfully resuscitated, showed bizarre behavioral disturbances, would not swallow, and occasionally went into status epilepticus. If the animals survived, they had marked neurologic impairment that resembled cerebral palsy.

The neuropathology in the monkeys consisted of bilateral diencephalic and brainstem lesions, and sometimes neocortical and cerebellar damage. Cerebral hemorrhage was not seen. Windle suggests that hemorrhages in the human may be traumatic; since the head of the monkey is so small, less trauma might be anticipated. Alternately, he suggests that hemorrhages may represent a terminal agonal artifact. The reasons for the differences in lesions between asphyxiated monkeys and asphyxiated human infants remain to be determined. The fact of neurologic damage to the newborn monkey from about 15 minutes of asphyxia at birth is clearly established.

TOLERANCE OF THE NEWBORN TO ANOXIA

The observation of the survival of newborn animals for longer than adult animals in an oxygen-free environment dates from Robert Boyle in 1670. Mott (1961), in a review of the ability of young animals to withstand oxygen lack, pointed out that from mid-gestation to the early neonatal period, the younger the animal the longer the survival in total anoxia. She also noted that in general the animals which are more immature at birth, such as rats, puppies, and rabbits, survive longer than the animals more mature at birth, such as guinea pigs, sheep, and monkeys.

The metabolic pathways that make possible anaerobic metabolism are not yet fully understood. Chief among them, however, is glycolysis. The work of Himwich et al. (1942) demonstrates the central importance of glycolysis. Inhibition of glycolysis by iodoacetate or fluoride decreased the ability of newborn rats to withstand 100 per cent N_2 from a survival time of 50 minutes to three and 16 minutes, respectively.

Later, Stafford and Weatherall (1960) showed that the ability of the newborn rat to survive anoxia was closely correlated with the cardiac glycogen stores. Studies in kittens, guinea pigs, and rabbits also point to the close association between the ability to survive anoxia and the content of glycogen in heart muscle (Mott, 1961). While the association does not prove cause and effect, it does lead to the interpretation that carbohydrate stores are important at birth, and that prolonged or repeated bouts of hypoxia may deplete them in utero or at birth.

Other sources of energy in fetal tissues must be available to account for the tolerance to hypoxia, since glycolysis is relatively inefficient and does not alone explain the long survival in anoxia. (Villee, 1958). However, evidence for other metabolic pathways of significance has not been produced.

The consequence of anaerobic metabolism is an increase in blood lactate levels. Although lactate can cross the placenta in either direction, in severely depressed infants umbilical vein concentrations exceed those in maternal arteries. Blood lactate levels rise even more in the moments after birth, reaching a maximum level at 10 minutes of age (Daniel et al., 1966).

Body temperature is another factor apparently related to the duration of survival in an oxygen-free environment. Bert (1870) first noted that the survival of newborn kittens was prolonged if they were drowned in cold water, as compared to their survival in warm water drowning. More recently, Miller and Behrle (1958) demonstrated the prolongation of survival of guinea pigs, puppies, and rabbits in a cool environment. Presumably, the fall in metabolic rate associated with cooling to less than 30°C. permits longer survival in the absence of oxygen. Some evidence for that view is that the cardiac glycogen of hypothermic asphyxiated guinea pigs was not reduced as much as that of normothermic asphyxiated animals (Miller et al., 1964). Hypothermia is, unfortunately, less effective in prolonging gasps in monkeys previously asphyxiated (Daniel et al., 1966). Although Westin et al. (1959) advocate hypothermia in the treatment of asphyxiated infants, the lack of controlled observations in infants and the greater benefit, in monkeys, from sustained artificial respiration than hypothermia, force the conclusion that hypothermia is not indicated in resuscitation of the human infant.

Some experimental studies suggest that barbiturate-produced narcosis may enhance resistance to asphyxia perhaps by a suppression of metabolism. The oxygen uptake of narcotized newborn guinea pigs was reduced in both normothermic and hypothermic states, and survival in a nitrogen atmosphere prolonged (Miller and Miller, 1962). Although the reasons for the favorable effects of barbiturates are not clear, it is of interest that those drugs depress central medullary discharges and block catecholamine production.

Thus we have to face a kind of paradox. Pathologists and other students of the relationship of asphyxia to subsequent neurologic function have shown unequivocally that the premature infant is more frequently afflicted with ischemic necrosis of the brain from apneic episodes than is the term infant. On the other hand, the immature animal can survive an acute hypoxic episode longer than the term animal, perhaps because of greater stores of carbohydrate in the myocardium. These findings are not necessarily contradictory, because studies of brains of immature animals after acute lethal anoxia are not comparable to those reported in infants in whom the hypoxic episodes have been more prolonged and less intense. Moreover, perhaps the hypoxic insult that is lethal to the term infant may not be lethal to the premature infant, so that the morbidity in terms of brain damage is more evident in the surviving prematures. We cannot know in a given infant the extent of intrauterine hypoxia. We can be sure that it may be damaging at any age, so that little comfort is provided by the knowledge that the newborn infant has some special adaptive mechanisms to withstand anoxia.

EVALUATION OF THE INFANT AT BIRTH

Since 1953, when Apgar introduced her method of evaluation of the infant in the first minutes of life, many investigators and clinics have used her system, with the consensus that it improves the quality of observations and helps in retrospective evaluation of the severity of asphyxia.

The method of scoring is shown in Table 20-2.

Thus a score of 10 — two points for each of the five signs — indicates the best possible condition (Apgar et al., 1958).

The simplicity of the score itself, aided perhaps by the epigram proposed by Butterfield and Covey (1962), has been important in its wide acceptance.

A = appearance
P = pulse
G = grimace
A = activity
R = respiration

The equal weight given to signs of unequal importance has been noted (Apgar et al., 1958; Auld et al., 1961), but the tendency of many of the signs to be decreased or absent in the presence of asphyxia, and of most to be present in vigorous infants, means that the populations of distressed and normal infants are usually well separated.

Table 20-2.   Apgar Evaluation Method

Sign	0	1	2
Heart rate	Absent	< 100/min.	> 100/min.
Respiratory effort	Absent	Weak cry Hypoventilation	Good strong cry
Muscle tone	Limp	Some flexion of extremities	Well flexed
Reflex irritability (response of skin stimulation to feet)	No response	Some motion	Cry
Color	Blue; pale	Body pink, extremities blue	Completely pink

Apgar and James (1962) reviewed their experience with the scoring system in 32,962 infants born over an eight-year period at Sloane Hospital for Women in New York. It is clear from their large experience that infants who score less than 3 at age one minute are at much greater risk of dying than those who score over 7 one minute after birth. The lower the score, the more profound the acidosis that accompanies asphyxia (James et al., 1958). Apgar and her group have used the score to judge the need for resuscitation; when the infant is profoundly depressed, artificial inflation of the lungs is undertaken at once (Apgar and James, 1962). Auld et al. (1961), in a smaller study at the Boston Lying-In Hospital, used the Apgar score to evaluate the effect of maternal conditions on the status of the infant at birth, as well as the need for resuscitation. They thought it was of little help in evaluating the necessity for resuscitative procedures, since infants with marked depression often improved promptly without artificial respiration. While these authors agreed that the risk of death was greater in low-score infants, they noted the many exceptions to the prognostic value of the score and felt that the score had little predictive value for a given infant. There is no question, however, that careful evaluation of every infant at birth is essential before criteria for resuscitation can be established or evaluated, and the Apgar scoring system is the most widely used approach.

CRITERIA FOR RESUSCITATION

If there were a way of knowing the duration of intrauterine hypoxia, the tolerances of a given infant to hypoxia, and the cause of the apnea at birth in each infant, precise criteria for resuscitation could be outlined. The clinical situation does not make this ideal world possible. Signs of maternal illness or fetal distress may suggest chronic hypoxia, but these signs may be absent at the birth of infants just as distressed. In the absence of precise criteria, the physician responsible for the infant must make this judgment on the basis of the clinical situation.

Perhaps the most sensitive indicator of severe hypoxia is the heart rate. If it is less than 100 beats/min. and becomes even slower in time, prompt resuscitation is indicated. As long as it is over 100 beats/min., the chance of the spontaneous onset of respiration is excellent. The indications for resuscitation and the measures we advocate are shown in Table 20–3. These steps are put forth as a modus operandi that seems reasonable and workable, but many variations are equally reasonable.

An excellent review of criteria and management of artificial respiration in infants was published by Gregory (1972).

Table 20-3.   Indications for Resuscitation

Indication	Treatment
Fetal heart beat present just before delivery, absent at birth	Immediate intubation and external cardiac massage
Profound depression; heart beat < 100 and falling; no respiratory effort, or strenuous respiratory efforts and no air entry into lungs (obstruction)	Immediate intubation and mouth-to-tube respiration
Moderate depression; heart rate > 100	Mask oxygen with intermittent positive pressure to 35 cm. H_2O
Mild depression; heart rate > 100; occasional gasp	Mask oxygen only

All infants receive gentle suction of secretions in oropharynx and gentle manual stimulation of skin.

Drugs: morphine antagonists if mother received morphine or morphine derivatives.

TECHNIQUES OF RESUSCITATION

General Care

As noted in Table 20-3, all infants should receive gentle suction of secretions in the oropharynx with a bulb syringe or a catheter. Removal of fluid from the upper airway is helped by positioning the infant slightly head down, with the head turned to either side. The habit of suspending an infant by his heels to aid in removal of secretions or for the purpose of obtaining a measure of length seems unnecessary and perhaps dangerous, since cerebral venous pressure would increase with risk of hemorrhage during such a maneuver. No strong evidence of harm is available; on the other hand, there is no evidence that the maneuver is necessary.

The next steps in resuscitation depend on the condition of the infant. For the infant without a heart beat, but in whom one had been heard just before delivery, external cardiac massage and intubation with active inflation of the lungs should be started immediately.

External Cardiac Massage

There are some well-documented instances of infants, born with no audible heart beat, resuscitated with intubation and cardiac massage, and normal in all respects months to years later (Sutherland and Epple, 1961; Moya et al., 1962; Mathews et al., 1963). If the fetal heart was present just before delivery, and is absent at birth, immediate intubation of the trachea and mouth-to-tube resuscitation with oxygen-enriched air are indicated. While these procedures are under way, compression of the middle portion of the sternum will massage the heart as it rests on the vertebral column (Thaler and Stobie, 1963). External cardiac massage should be stopped when the lungs are inflated, and resumed on expiration, at a rate of 100 to 120 times/min. Mouth-to-tube respirations should be 30 to 40 times/min. ordinarily, or perhaps fewer when cardiac massage is under way (Fig. 20-2).

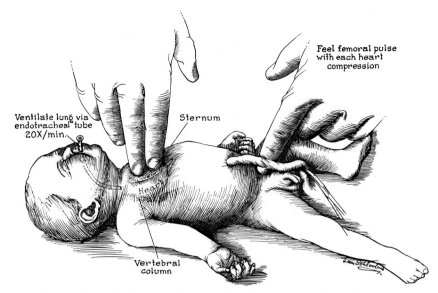

Figure 20–2. Technique of external cardiac massage. (From Mathews et al.: J.A.M.A. *183*:964, 1963.)

Intubation

1. Place infant on his back, head down slightly, with a towel under the shoulders.
2. Hold the infant laryngoscope in one hand and enter one side of the infant's mouth. When the glottis is in view, shift the laryngoscope to midline, tilt the blade up to raise the epiglottis, and expose the trachea.
3. Apply suction to the upper trachea with a soft rubber catheter.
4. Introduce a suitable endotracheal tube (one that slides in easily and does not injure the tracheal mucosa). Advance the tube along one side of the laryngoscope up to the flange.
5. Gently withdraw the laryngoscope.
6. Insert a tube that will deliver oxygen to your mouth, and blow the oxygen-enriched air from your mouth through the endotracheal tube. Observe the movements of the infant's chest and use a stethoscope to verify the position of the tube. Your cheek muscles are sufficient to propel air into the infant's lungs (Fig. 20–3).

Intermittent Positive Pressure by Mask

Resuscitation equipment should be available in the delivery rooms and the nurseries. The equipment we use is shown in Figure 20–4.

Numerous devices are available or can be readily assembled to permit the intermittent application of pressure by means of a mask

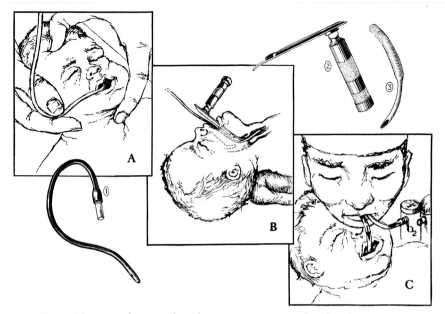

Figure 20–3. Technique of intubation. *A,* Suction with soft catheter (1); *B,* position of laryngoscope (2); and *C,* mouth-to-tube insufflation through endotracheal tube (3).

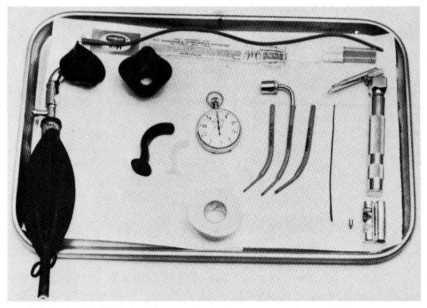

Figure 20–4. Useful equipment in delivery rooms and nurseries.

that covers the infant's nose and mouth. While there is no agreement on the optimal pressures or duration of time of their application, experience with such devices suggests that pressures of 35 cm. H_2O for intervals of one to two seconds are safe, may be required, and are sometimes effective (Hustead and Avery, 1961).

Correction of Acidosis

Since the asphyxiated infant has a lactic acidemia and metabolic acidosis, which may be profound, use of alkali and glucose seems reasonable. Support for these measures came from studies on newborn monkeys, asphyxiated after delivery. Those given 0.5 molar solution of tris-hydroxymethyl aminomethane (THAM) in 3.5 per 100 ml. glucose adjusted to pH 8.85 in a dose of 12 ml./kg. over two to four minutes had fewer sequelae than those not given glucose and alkali (Dawes et al., 1964; Adamsons et al., 1964).

Although no studies are available on the results of rapid correction of pH in asphyxiated infants, infusion of 5 to 10 ml. of a solution of 25 mEq./100 ml. of sodium bicarbonate in 10 per cent glucose by push is reasonable. In infants with continuing respiratory depression, measurement of blood pH, PCO_2 and HCO_3 would indicate the need for subsequent intravenous therapy.

Persistent hyponatremia, with hypertonic urine and normal renal function was reported by Feldman et al. (1970) in three infants on the days following an asphyxial episode at delivery. All three recovered by a week of age. The excretion of hypertonic urine in the face of hypotonic plasma implies continuing, hence inappropriate ADH secretion in these infants. The authors speculate that an insult to the central nervous system served as the stimulus to ADH secretion.

Drugs

The use of drugs as analeptics in the delivery room is not to be recommended. We do inject a morphine antagonist, N-allylnormorphine, or levallorphan, 0.2 mg./kg. intravenously, if it is clear that the depression of the infant is due to excessive amounts of morphine or related compounds given to the mother. Barrie (1963) has recommended nikethamide, 0.5 ml. of a 25 per cent solution, or vanillic acid diethylamide, 0.5 ml. of a 5 per cent solution, placed on the tongue. We have not had any experience with these agents given by that route. Intramuscular caffeine sodium benozoate, epinephrine, or nikethamide will not be absorbed for at least 15 minutes, hence have little role in resuscitation. The intravenous use of these agents is hazardous. (See page 278.)

Hyperbaric Oxygenation

The use of hyperbaric chambers in delivery rooms to facilitate oxygenation of the apneic infant was shown to be effective by Hutchison et al. (1963). Their studies did not show that hyperbaric oxygenation was more effective than intubation and artificial inflation of the lungs with air or oxygen. Controlled trials of resuscitation of asphyxiated young rabbits with hyperbaric oxygenation or positive pressure breathing with air and with oxygen failed to support hyperbaric oxygenation. Indeed it was significantly less effective than positive pressure breathing with air or oxygen (Campbell et al., 1966).

Two physiologic problems militate against hyperbaric oxygenation of the infant with primary apnea: first, the fluid in the fetal lung does not permit the diffusion of significant volumes of oxygen into the blood, and second, the elimination of carbon dioxide is an essential part of resuscitation.

Chapter Twenty-One

USE OF RESPIRATORS

The past decade has been characterized by an increasing use of respirators in the care of infants in the first days of life. Apneic spells in infants in the nursery may be transient, and infants who have them need not receive more than the occasional tactile stimulus, suction, or oxygen delivered by mask. But other infants, particularly those profoundly depressed by excessive maternal analgesia or anesthesia, may require several hours of assisted breathing before they are capable of adequate spontaneous respiration. Still others have such severe respiratory illness that they seem to tire themselves, and succumb from hypoventilation. It is these latter two groups of infants who may profit from appropriate artificial respiration. There are many reasons why there has only recently been widespread success in the maintenance of assisted respiration in such infants. First, the patients vary greatly in size and hence in appropriate volumes for tidal respiration. Second, smaller infants require respirators designed with a minimum of dead space and low resistance valves. Third, distensibility of the lungs is not the same in all infants and is particularly impaired in those with hyaline membrane disease. Fourth, pressures that may be required to move an appropriate volume of air may need to be so high and sustained as to impede the circulation of blood through the pulmonary vascular bed. Fifth, the problems of the constant application of a mask to a small face, or a sealed collar to a soft neck, or prolonged use of endotracheal tubes or tracheostomies have discouraged some who have hoped to maintain ventilation in infants over a period of days. None of these problems need be insurmountable; however, their complexity is sufficiently great that it seems worthwhile to analyze them to the best of our ability as a first step in establishing the requirements for suitable respirators.

PRINCIPLES OF ARTIFICIAL RESPIRATION

To achieve adequate ventilation, it is necessary to distend both lungs and thorax over an appropriate volume range. The volume-pressure characteristics of the lungs and thorax of infants and adults are illustrated in Figure 21–1. Normal breathing takes place over a portion of the volume-pressure curve of lungs and thorax where the most

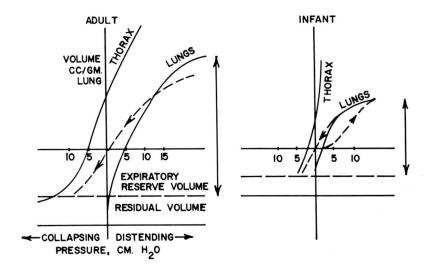

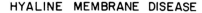

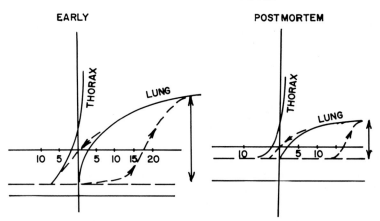

Figure 21–1. Relaxation pressure-volume curves. The ordinates are all volumes, the abscissas are pressures. Note that the thorax of the infant distends more for a given change in pressure than that of the adult, when compared on the basis of lung weight. In hyaline membrane disease, the residual volume is reduced, and larger changes in pressure are required to achieve a given volume than in the normal infant. Thus the compliance of the lung ($\Delta V/\Delta P$) is reduced in hyaline membrane disease.

volume is achieved for the smallest applied pressure. Note that to move air from the expiratory reserve volumes would require a much higher pressure than that needed to move an equal volume of air into the inspiratory reserve volume such as occurs in normal breathing. This property of the lungs and chest wall explains the failure to ventilate apneic individuals adequately by application of pressure on the back of the chest when they are prone. Thus, the first principle of artificial respiration is to move air in and out of the inspiratory reserve volume.

There are at least six methods of accomplishing effective artificial respiration in adults (Whittenberger, 1955).

Method	*Comment*
1. Intermittent positive pressure applied at the nose or mouth or through an endotracheal tube	Most widely used method in infants
2. Intermittent "negative" pressure applied to the body by a tank respirator or chest cuirass	Tank respirator is effective in infants
3. Changes in gas density without thoracic movement	Probably effective but has not been properly evaluated in infants
4. Electrical stimulation of the phrenic nerve	Effective but difficult
5. Manual methods with an active inspiratory maneuver such as arm-lift followed by back pressure	Ineffective in infants
6. Diaphragmatic shift with position such as occurs with rocking	Ineffective in infants

Mechanics of Movement of Air

For air to flow from one region to another, there must be a pressure difference between the two regions. In normal breathing, the descent of the diaphragm and contraction of the intercostal and spinal muscles enlarge the thorax so that the pressure in the airways is less than atmospheric pressure during inspiration. During inspiration, the pressure in the lung may be 754 mm. Hg, when atmospheric pressure is 760 mm. Hg. At end-inspiration, when no air is moving, the pressure in the alveoli is atmospheric pressure. The pressure in the pleural "space," or rather, that pressure which can be measured by the insertion of a needle between the parietal and visceral pleura, is less than atmospheric not only during inspiration but at end-inspiration as well. The difference in pressure between the pleural space and the alveoli at end-expiration results from the elasticity of the lung, which, when stretched, exerts a force in the direction of decreasing size; and from the elasticity of the thorax, which in the range of quiet breathing exerts a force in the direction of increasing size. Expiration is accomplished by the decrease in thoracic size which raises the pressure of air in the lung above atmospheric pressure. In adults, expiration is usually passive, since the potential energy created by contraction of the inspiratory muscles is "stored" in the elastic structure of the lung. In infants, expiration often has an "active" component so that end-expiratory pressures may be positive. Elasticity is the property of restoration to the original shape after that shape has been distorted by an external force; it represents the tendency of the lungs to recoil after being stretched by the action of the thoracic muscles, including the diaphragm.

Since movement of air depends on a difference in pressure between two regions, movement will be the same regardless of whether the pressure is raised at one point or lowered at another. From the point of view of distention of the lung, the effect of positive pressure at the mouth is identical with the effect of negative pressure around the chest. The only circumstance in which the effects on intrathoracic structures of the two methods could be different is in the event of an air-containing space that is temporarily not in communication with the airway. Its volume would increase with negative pressure around the chest and would decrease with positive pressure applied at the mouth. This single exception is so unusual, however, that the general rule stands that the effects on the airways and alveoli are identical to the two types of applied pressures.

Circulatory Effects

The effects of positive- and negative-pressure breathing on the heart and peripheral circulation are not so obvious. Since the heart and great vessels are in the thorax, they are surrounded by the same pressures as those which surround the lung. In fact, the evidence that mediastinal structures are at pleural pressure is secure in that a pressure-sensing device in the esophagus has been used to measure pleural pressure. Simultaneous pleural and esophageal pressure recordings are very similar (Mead and Gaensler, 1959; Daly and Bondurant, 1963). In normal respiration, the decrease in pressure around the heart facilitates its filling with blood from the systemic veins. However, since the pressures normally required to ventilate the lung are so small, they have very little effect on the cardiovascular dynamics. The effects of moderate positive pressure in the airway on the circulation (although similar to those of negative pressure around the body) are different from those in normal breathing in adults; they were summarized as follows by Maloney and Whittenberger (1957):

1. Cardiac output remains the same or decreases slightly
2. Venous pressure rises
3. Peripheral vascular resistance increases
4. Arterial pressure rises
5. Blood is displaced from the thorax to the peripheral venous bed
6. Blood volume falls slightly

Positive-pressure breathing can be deleterious in the event of shock, barbiturate poisoning, or anything that interferes with peripheral circulatory adjustments. Circulatory support with transfusions, however, can maintain cardiac output in such individuals as long as artificial respiration is indicated. In the newborn infant with peripheral vascular instability, and in the distressed infant in shock, circulatory embarrassment may be lethal when positive-pressure breathing is instituted.

The effects of tank respirators on the circulation are identical with the circulatory effects of positive-pressure respiration. The reason for this is that both thoracic structures and peripheral vascular bed are surrounded by the same pressures, which are subatmospheric with tanks, atmospheric with positive-pressure breathing. (The proportion of the circulation which goes to the head is such a small part of the total that it can be ignored.) When the body is in a tank respirator, there is no augmentation of venous return such as occurs with normal inspiration, since the peripheral vessels are surrounded by the same subatmospheric pressure as the intrathoracic vessels.

The circulatory effects of negative-pressure breathing with a chest cuirass are probably identical with those of normal respiration, although adequate information is not available. This method would thus appear to be ideal in the event of systemic hypotension which limits the usefulness of either positive-pressure or tank-type respiration. Its limitation is in the ability to make a tight seal around the neck and lower rib cage, particularly in small infants. Recently an ingenious solution to this problem was proposed by Bancalari et al. (1973). They used commercially available plastic iris diaphragms on either end of a 22 × 22 × 8.5 cm. plastic box to achieve a seal around the neck and pelvic area of an infant. The box was equipped with an aneroid manometer and attached to wall suction or a vacuum pump to achieve negative pressure around the thorax. This device permits application of continuous negative pressure, but could be modified to cycle as well.

The adverse circulatory effects of positive-pressure breathing can be reduced if the time of applied pressure is short and the mean mask pressure is kept low. Cournand et al. (1948) showed that if expiration occupied at least 50 per cent of the respiratory cycle, and if expiratory mask pressures during expiration were close to atmospheric pressure, there were no significant adverse circulatory effects. With mean mask pressures of 7 to 10 mm. Hg, cardiac output fell about 15 per cent in normal adults. Werkö (1947) showed that when the mean mask pressure exceeded 5 mm. Hg, the decrease in cardiac output was roughly proportional to mean mask pressure. Cournand et al. (1948) summarized the desirable characteristics of intermittent positive-pressure breathing as follows: (1) a gradual increase in pressure during inspiration, (2) a rapid drop in pressure after cycling occurs, (3) mean mask pressure during expiratory period as near atmospheric pressure as possible, (4) expiratory time equal to or more than inspiratory time.

Changes in Gas Density without Thoracic Movement

This method, introduced by Thunberg (1926), consists of rhythmic changes in barometric pressure in a chamber that surrounds the entire patient. The pressures used are sufficient to change the density of gases in the chest so that tidal molecular displacements occur without motion of the chest. The success of the method depends on the presence of some gas in the chest at end-expiration. If in a normal adult the functional residual capacity is 3 liters, and a tidal volume 500 ml., then a change in pressure of one-sixth of an atmosphere would cause a change in volume of one-sixth of 3 liters, or 500 ml. Thus if the chamber "cycled" from 700 to about 820 mm. Hg, adequate gas exchange could occur. Approximately the same pressures would successfully ventilate an infant who had a functional residual capacity of 80 ml. and required a tidal volume of 12 to 15 ml. If, on the other hand, the functional residual capacity were greatly reduced, as it is in hyaline membrane disease, greater changes in pressure would probably be required. The physiological limitation to this method is the effect on gases in other parts of the body such as the intestine and middle ear, where changes in volume would also occur with the risk of discomfort and possible rupture of the tympanic membrane. The mechanical limitation is the necessity for the suitable chamber that could produce changes in pressure at the normal respiratory frequencies. Barach's modification of Thunberg's barospirator consists of a double chamber in which the pressure around the body is 5 to 6 cm. H_2O less at the start of the positive cycle, and 4 to 5 cm. H_2O higher at the start of the negative cycle than pressures around the head. This lag in pressures adjusts for airway-resistive pressures so that ventilation is accomplished with no chest movement. The method has been used successfully in adults (Barach, 1940) but awaits evaluation in infants.

Phrenic Stimulation

External electrical stimulation of the phrenic nerve has proved to be feasible in the management of some patients with bulbar poliomyelitis. Studies on animals and patients have shown that aeration of the lung on the unstimulated side also occurs (Sarnoff et al., 1950). Some success with this method of maintaining respiration in asphyxiated infants has been reported in a few studies; however, the degree of skill needed to apply the electrode effectively to the skin, and the hazard of damage to the nerve with implantation of the electrode, have limited the usefulness of this method (Cross and Roberts, 1951; Day and Sanford, 1955). In infants, insignificant aeration of the unstimulated side was noted. Day and Sanford concluded that the results were more encouraging in stimulating the apneic newborn than in the maintenance of respiration after birth; however, their experience of 11 deaths in 25 apneic infants resuscitated by phrenic stimulation led them to conclude that the procedure was not developed sufficiently for general usage.

Methods that Increase Lung Volume

Continuous positive airway pressure (CPAP), positive end-expiratory pressure (PEEP), and continuous negative pressure on the chest wall (CNP) all serve to increase lung volume at end-expiration, hence to reduce the lung's tendency to collapse when the surfactant is deficient. These adjuncts to assisted ventilation, used with or without cyclic ventilation, have been shown to increase greatly the oxygenation of the infant and to decrease mortality from hyaline membrane disease (Gregory et al., 1971; Chernick and Vidyasagar, 1972).

Previous attempts to increase lung volume in hyaline membrane disease include the hook on the sternum, advocated by Townsend and Squire (1956). The first systematic study of the use of positive pressure to achieve prevention of atelectasis was reported by Gregory et al. in 1971. They showed marked increases in oxygenation with little reduction in carbon dioxide, suggesting that an improvement in the relationship of ventilation to perfusion and reduction of the intrapulmonary shunt are the main consequences of positive airway pressure. Pressures up to 12 mm. Hg were delivered through an endotracheal tube and were lowered as determined by serial measurements of arterial oxygen tension. As the infant improved, a reduction in inspired oxygen and a lowering of airway pressure were accomplished. As little as 2 mm. Hg airway pressure favorably effects oxygenation. Applied pressures are deleterious to cardiac output when the lung is normal; in hyaline membrane disease, presumably, the high surface forces in the airspaces limit the amount of pressure transmitted to the vessels.

Increase in lung volume can also be achieved by application of continuous negative chest wall pressure. Chernick and Vidyasagar (1972) reported an average elevation of arterial oxygen tension of 40 mm. Hg on the same inspired concentration in 23 infants after application of negative chest wall pressure. Initially they used 10 cm. H_2O pressure, and on occasion 15 cm. H_2O without adverse circulatory effects. They first lowered the inspired oxygen concentration to 40 per cent; then they raised the pressure applied to the chest wall in 3 to 5 cm. H_2O increments. An advantage to the negative pressure approach is the avoidance of an endotracheal tube or mask. Maintaining the ability of the infant to grunt is an advantage noted by Harrison et al. (1968). A small modification of the Air-Shields negative pressure respirator may be required if pressures above 10 cm. H_2O are desired. (Vidyasagar and Chernick, 1971; Chernick, 1973; Bancalari et al., 1973).

Other Ineffective Methods of Artificial Respiration in Infants

The last two methods listed on page 299 and noted as ineffective are nonetheless worthy of comment because of the persistence of some workers in their application.

Back Pressure. Back pressure combined with air lifting has been extensively evaluated in adults and has been conclusively demonstrated to be less effective than pressure applied at the mouth (Safar et al., 1958). Moreover, back pressure never has been feasible for the maintenance of respiration since it requires rather complicated sequential acts by a trained operator, and in adults, at least, is tiring to the operator. No systematic studies of this approach have been made in infants, other effective methods being available, and such studies scarcely seem indicated.

The Rocking Principle. This principle, which depends on the force of gravity to move the abdominal viscera and hence the diaphragm, is effective in ventilating adults but ineffective in infants. A 600 ml. inspiration occurs at a foot-down tilt of 30 degrees from horizontal in a normal adult 6 feet tall (Colville et al., 1956). The simplicity of rocking an infant on the arm tempts one to apply the method in the hope that proportionate diaphragmatic displacement will occur (Eve and Forsyth, 1958; Miller and Davies, 1946; Millen et al., 1955). However, studies on the shift in end-expiratory position in normal newborn infants with changes in body position show no consistent movements (Avery and O'Doherty, 1962). Normal infants with aerated lungs would be more likely to show a shift — if any were to occur — than apneic infants with abnormal lungs. The reasons for the lack of effect in rocking of infants were proposed by Colville et al. (1956); the degree of movement of abdominal viscera, hence the force applied against the diaphragm, is a function of abdominal length. Pressures required to ventilate infants are the same as those required to ventilate adults, but infants' shorter abdomens afford less pressure of viscera upon the diaphragm. Also, the rib cage being more compliant in infants than in adults makes any small diaphragmatic displacement less effective in moving air.

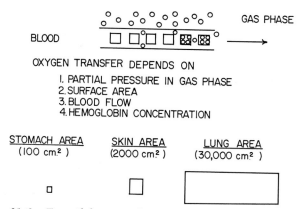

OXYGEN TRANSFER DEPENDS ON

1. PARTIAL PRESSURE IN GAS PHASE
2. SURFACE AREA
3. BLOOD FLOW
4. HEMOGLOBIN CONCENTRATION

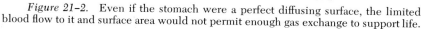

Figure 21-2. Even if the stomach were a perfect diffusing surface, the limited blood flow to it and surface area would not permit enough gas exchange to support life.

Gastric Oxygen. Little theoretical reason and no convincing experimental evidence are available to support the idea of oxygenating an apneic infant by insufflation of the gastrointestinal tract with oxygen. Figure 21–2 illustrates the theoretical limitations to the use of the stomach as an oxygenating surface. The small surface area and limited perfusion of the stomach and intestine mean that even if the gut wall imposed no barrier to the diffusion of gas, little effect could be expected when venous blood from the stomach mixed with venous blood from other tissues. Moreover, a few measurements in infants in whom reflux into the trachea was ruled out clearly showed the lack of effect of gastric oxygen on arterial saturation (James et al., 1959, 1963). This approach to resuscitation, in common with methods that utilize oxygenation through the skin, fails to achieve adequate oxygenation and likewise omits consideration of the removal of carbon dioxide. Effective resuscitation must not only oxygenate the infant but eliminate carbon dioxide as well.

USE OF MASKS AND ENDOTRACHEAL TUBES

Since positive-pressure breathing is feasible and numerous respirators are available for use on infants, the problem of how to apply pressure to the upper airway becomes a practical one.

Masks may be used with respirators if suitable precautions are observed. First, the mask should be of low dead space and should fit tightly over the infant's nose and mouth. Helmrath et al. (1970) described their success with masks in infants with hyaline membrane disease. They used a face mask* held in place with a disposable

---

*Puritan Compressed Gas Corp., Kansas City, Mo.

diaper and anesthesia straps. An orogastric tube was inserted to lessen gastric distention. Some success with intermittent mask and bag therapy was also reported by Gruber and Klaus (1970).

The importance of added dead space in any type of artificial respiration is apparent, since a single breath must fill that space as well as the oropharynx, trachea, bronchi, and the portions of the lung in which gas exchange takes place. Thus, in a sense, a part of each breath is wasted in terms of the ultimate purpose of respiration, which is to exchange oxygen and carbon dioxide. To enlarge that portion of a tidal volume which does not undergo gas exchange is to require deeper breaths for the same alveolar ventilation. When alveolar ventilation is inadequate, carbon dioxide tension in the blood rises, oxygen tension falls, and the chemoreceptors are stimulated to increase ventilation. In the apneic individual with accumulated carbon dioxide and severe hypoxia, the chemoreceptors may no longer respond, and a vicious circle becomes apparent. If artificial respiration is undertaken with added dead space, deeper breaths must be given which require higher pressures, and the deleterious effects on the circulation, mentioned earlier, may follow.

Endotracheal tubes are the mainstay of resuscitation in the delivery room and are also used with respirators in the maintenance of respiration thereafter. They should be firm but flexible, tapered, snugly but not tightly fitting, and approximately 12 cm. in length to avoid passage beyond the carina with danger of occlusion of one bronchus. Some tubes are abruptly narrowed to prevent insertion too far. While such narrowing is in that sense an advantage, it also results in some decrease in airway diameter. The wall of the tube should be thin, but rigid enough to prevent collapse.

Nasotracheal intubation has been advocated for infants who require assisted ventilation. A Portex tube of uniform bore, at least one size smaller than the infant would have for anesthesia, is used to allow for some edema. The tube, moistened with water, is introduced along the floor of the nose, and guided into the glottis under direct vision with a laryngoscope. A rule of thumb, proposed by Sinclair, for the distance for insertion (from nares to mid-trachea) is 21 per cent of the baby's crown-heel length. The tube should be fixed rigidly to the skin. Humidification of the inspired air is important to prevent occlusion of the tube by dried secretions. Hourly suctioning with strict sterile technique is essential (Smith, 1966).

The time over which it is safe to leave an endotracheal tube in place is not established. If the first intubation is atraumatic, and the tube does not fit too tightly, 72 hours of continuous intubation are possible without significant laryngeal edema. Nasotracheal tubes have been used instead of tracheostomies for weeks in some infants, although complications have been reported particularly when the larynx is inflamed, as in croup (McDonald and Stocks, 1965; Downes et al., 1966).

In a series of 172 infants who died after intubation and artificial respiration, Joshi et al. (1972) found mild lesions in the larynx or trachea of 63 per cent, and relatively severe inflammatory lesions in 16 per cent. The lesions were most commonly seen in the vocal cords and were related to the duration of intubation and presence of infection. Occasionally hoarseness has been noted in the survivors of prolonged intubation.

Recently, with increased use of continuous negative pressure, intubation has been required less frequently (Chernick and Vidyasagar, 1972). Application of continuous positive airway pressure by face mask (Rhodes and Hall, 1973) or by a molded nasal piece (Kattwinkel et al., 1973) has been reported and is now widely used. Tracheostomy has been done (Weseman, 1960) but is rarely indicated.

TYPES OF RESPIRATORS

Positive-pressure Breathing

All respirators that employ a mask applied to the airway or endotracheal tube depend on a device to restrict flow to the lung. The restriction may be by a needle valve or other resistance in the line through which the gas flows, or by limitation of the volume of the source of gas (Radford in Whittenberger, 1962).

Respirators designed to ventilate an infant with positive-pressure breathing are of two principal types: the first has a cycling mechanism that depends on a pressure-sensitive element; the second is designed to deliver a fixed volume of gas, usually with a pressure limitation.

The advantage of the first or pressure-cycled type is that no knowledge of an appropriate volume is required. The gas flow and pressures depend on air interaction of the respirator and the patient's lungs and thorax. On the other hand, upper limits of the pressures which are safe in all circumstances are not known. High pressure applied briefly is less hazardous than high pressure applied for a longer time, since there is a pressure drop initially from flow-resistive forces (Day et al., 1952). However, too brief application of pressure will not allow time for inflation of the lung. Moderate pressures applied for over half the respiratory cycle may not allow time for circulatory compensations to occur (Cournand et al., 1948). Low pressures may be inadequate to move sufficient air. The problem is compounded by lack of knowledge of the state of the lungs that require ventilation. Lungs of infants with hyaline membrane disease may have a greatly reduced compliance so that high pressures are needed to distend them (Karlberg et al., 1954). Lungs of a narcotized infant may be quite normal so that pressure changes of only 4 to 6 cm. H_2O are required. It would thus appear that respirators that depend on pressure settings would have to be provided with devices to adjust the pressure, and the operator must determine the suitable pressures for each infant.

The second type of respirator, which is piston driven to deliver a known volume, as well as pressure limited, would appear to be an advance over pressure-limited devices without volume adjustments. If the endotracheal tube were snug so that no leaks could occur, the average tidal volume of an infant could be delivered at his usual frequency. Infants of about 1.5 kg. require 6 to 10 ml. tidal volumes; infants of 3 kg. require 15 to 20 ml. tidal volumes. As in any situation that requires the use of respirators, an occasional "deep breath" is helpful in overcoming atelectasis which tends to occur with fixed tidal volumes (Mead and Collier, 1959; Ferris and Pollard, 1960). The potential danger of a volume-limited respirator is that it will be used in infants in whom some portions of the lung are completely obstructed. All of the volume would then go to the lung in communication with the airway, which could be overstretched, and rupture. Some pressure limitation is desirable in such a respirator. Again it is hard to know what the pressure should be. Excised lungs of infants usually tolerance 35 cm. H_2O pressure without rupture (Gribetz et al., 1959). There is no indication that the rupture pressures of lungs of premature infants differ from those of adults' lungs. We have sustained 50 cm. H_2O pressure across excised lungs of infants without leakage, although interstitial dissection of air was not ruled out. As noted earlier, higher pressures could be tolerated for brief periods.

Some respirators have been devised so that the infant can cycle them on demand (Donald, 1954). With each respiratory effort the infact receives an "assist" from the respirator. While this refinement has advantages in some infants, most who require artificial respiration do not fight the respirator but rather let it take over. Muscle relaxants have been used in infants who tend to fight the respirator, but their role has not been evaluated in a large series.

Tank-type Respirators

The small size of the infant makes it seem feasible to construct some simple tank-type respirator to apply artificial respiration. These devices operate by changing the pressure around the body, with the head outside, and do not restrict flow to the patient. The chief advantage of such respirators would be that they could be used without intubation of the infant. The problems have been with regard to the fit of a cuff around the neck. Loose-fitting cuffs can be used if the pressure changes are made sufficiently large; however, such leakage results in movement of air over the body, and subsequent cooling. Many of these problems were overcome by the Isolette respirator, (Air Shields, Hatboro, Pa.) which operates on the tank principle, but keeps the infant's head in another portion of the incubator. Cooling is prevented by an infant servo heating unit (Stern et al., 1970).

Chapter Twenty-Two

CLINICAL SUMMARY

The multiple causes of respiratory distress in the first days of life, discussed in the previous sections, may leave one feeling that the differential diagnosis must be extensive and diagnostic procedures may need to be exhaustive. In practice, it is a fairly straightforward matter to sort out the difficulties in the majority of infants. Occasionally we remain perplexed when an infant shows isolated tachypnea for a few days and then recovers, or retracts for some hours and then mysteriously ceases to do so, or has apneic spells for no obvious reason. Far more commonly, we can arrive at a likely diagnosis with a minimum of disturbance to the baby.

Table 22–1 lists events in the mother's history which predispose the infant to certain conditions, as well as findings in the infant which should suggest certain diagnoses. While any such attempt to relate cause and effect is oversimplified, it is useful to see how helpful a few clues might be in predicting the likelihood of a specific type of respiratory distress. Note that all the information required to entertain the likely diagnoses in the right-hand column comes from knowledge of the maternal history and inspection and palpation of the infant.

The most useful single diagnostic aid in distinguishing the causes of respiratory distress is a chest film. Indeed, it is so essential that it would be obvious neglect to care for infants in an institution where chest films were not available 24 hours a day. The most skilled physician can overlook a pneumothorax or even diaphragmatic hernia on physical examination. Knowledge of their presence will mean the initiation of treatment that can be lifesaving.

While history, physicial examination, and chest film are the sine qua non of differential diagnosis of respiratory distress, other procedures are sometimes indicated. Good bacteriologic facilities are

Table 22–1. Clues to Diagnosis of Types of Respiratory Distress

Information from Maternal History	*Most Likely Condition in Infant*
Prematurity	Hyaline membrane disease
Diabetes	Hyaline membrane disease
Hemorrhage in the days before premature delivery	Hyaline membrane disease
Infection	Pneumonia
Premature rupture of membranes	Pneumonia
Prolonged labor	Pneumonia
Meconium-stained amniotic fluid	Meconium aspiration
Hydramnios	Tracheoesophageal fistula
Excessive medications	Central nervous system depression
Reserpine	Stuffy nose
Traumatic or breech delivery	Central nervous system hemorrhage
	Phrenic nerve paralysis
Fetal tachycardia or bradycardia	Asphyxia
Prolapsed cord or cord entanglements	Asphyxia
Postmaturity	Aspiration

Signs in the Baby	*Most Likely Associated Condition*
Single umbilical artery	Congenital anomalies
Other congenital anomalies	Associated cardiopulmonary anomalies
Scaphoid abdomen	Diaphragmatic hernia
Erb's palsy	Phrenic nerve palsy
Cannot breathe with mouth closed	Choanal atresia
	Stuffy nose
Gasping with little air exchange	Upper airway obstruction
Overdistention of lungs	Aspiration, lobar emphysema, or pneumothorax
Shift of apical pulse	Pneumothorax
	Chylothorax
	Hypoplastic lung
Fever, or rise in temperature in a constant temperature environment	Pneumonia
Shrill cry, hypertonia, or flaccidity	Central nervous system disorder
Atonia	Trauma, myasthenia, poliomyelitis, amyotonia
Frothy blood from larynx	Pulmonary hemorrhage
Head extended in the absence of neurologic findings	Laryngeal obstruction or vascular rings
Choking after feedings	Tracheoesophageal fistula or pharyngeal incoordination

needed for an intelligent approach to the treatment of infection. Stains of gastric aspirate and frozen sections of the umbilical cord may reveal microscopic signs of inflammation. The pH, P_{CO_2}, and bicarbonate levels in the arterial or arterialized capillary blood are the most important biochemical determinations. The oxygen tension in the arterial blood is of great interest, and now that it can be measured in most hospitals, it will doubtless enhance the rational use of oxygen in the treatment of conditions associated with cyanosis. The hematocrit value is helpful in the evaluation of the significance of cyanosis. Measurement of arterial and central venous pressures in very sick infants is a useful guide for appropriate circulatory support. A white blood cell count and urinalysis occasionally contribute information of use, and a lumbar puncture at times reveals the central nervous system basis of respiratory disturbances, just as an electrocardiogram may reveal the cardiovascular basis of labored breathing.

In summary, it is not the intent of this concluding section to list all the procedures that might be useful, but rather to stress that respiratory distress in the newborn period may result from many causes. The most likely condition can be suspected by history and inspection and palpation of the infant. The chest film is an indispensable aid. If the diagnosis continues to be elusive, the readily available laboratory procedures widely used on most pediatric services will make it possible to establish a diagnosis in the majority of instances. The challenge for the future is to find more effective forms of therapy for the many life-threatening respiratory problems of the newborn infant.

REFERENCES

Abbas, T. M., and Tovey, J. E.: Proteins of the liquor amnii. Brit. Med. J. 1:476, 1960.

Abel, S., and Windle, W. F.: Relation of the volume of pulmonary circulation to respiration at birth. Anat. Rec. 75:451, 1939.

Abler, C.: Neonatal varicella. Amer. J. Dis. Child. 107:492, 1964.

Ablow, R. C., and Markarian, M.: The advantages of an intensive care nursery radiographic room. Radiology 104:119, 1972.

Ablow, R. C., and Orzalesi, M. M.: Localized roentgenographic pattern of hyaline membrane disease. Evidence that the upper lobes of human lung mature earlier than the lower lobes. Amer. J. Roentgen. Rad. Ther. Nucl. Med. 112:23, 1971.

Ablow, R. C., Greenspan, R. H., and Gluck, L.: Advantages of the direct magnification technique in the newborn chest. Radiology 92:745, 1969.

Ablow, R. C., and Effman, E. L.: Hepatic calcifications associated with umbilical vein catheterization in the newborn infant. Amer. J. Roentgen. 114:380, 1972.

Aborelius, M., Jr., Gustafsson, T., Kjellman, B., Lundstrom, N. R., and Mortensson, W.: Xe^{133} radiospirometry for evaluation of congenital malformations of pulmonary arteries. Pediatrics 47:529, 1971.

Adams, F. H., and Lind, J.: Physiologic studies on the cardiovascular status of normal newborn infants (with special reference to the ductus arteriosus). Pediatrics 19:431, 1957.

Adams, F. H., and Fujiwara, T.: Surfactant in fetal lamb tracheal fluid. J. Pediat. 63:537, 1963.

Adams, F. H., Fujiwara, T., and Rowshan, G.: The nature and origin of the fluid in the fetal lamb lung. J. Pediat. 63:881, 1963.

Adams, F. H., Desilets, D. T., and Towers, B.: Control of flow of fetal lung liquid at the laryngeal outlet. Resp. Physiol. 2:302, 1967.

Adams, J. M.: Primary virus pneumonitis with cytoplasmic inclusion bodies: Study of epidemic involving thirty-two infants with nine deaths. J. A. M. A. 116:925, 1941.

Adams, J. M.: Congenital pneumonitis in newborn infants. Am. J. Dis. Child. 75:544, 1948.

Adamson, T. M., Boyd, R. D. H., Normand, I. C. S., Reynolds, E. O. R., and Shaw, J. L.: Hemorrhagic pulmonary oedema in the newborn. Lancet 1:494, 1969.

Adamson, T. M., Hawker, J. M., Reynolds, E. O. R., and Shaw, J. L.: Hypoxemia during recovery from severe hyaline membrane disease. Pediatrics 44:168, 1969.

Adamsons, K., Jr., Behrman, R., Dawes, G. S., James, L. S., and Koford, C.: Resuscitation by positive-pressure ventilation and tris-hydroxymethylaminomethane of rhesus monkeys asphyxiated at birth. J. Pediat. 65:807, 1964.

Addison, W. H. F., and How, H. W.: On the prenatal and neonatal lung. Am. J. Anat. 15:199, 1913.

Agostoni, E., Taglietti, A., Agostoni, F., and Setnikar, I.: Mechanical aspects of the first breath. J. Appl. Physiol. 13:344, 1958.

Agostoni, E.: Volume-pressure relationships of the thorax and lung in the newborn. J. Appl. Physiol. 14:909, 1959.

Aherne, W., and Dawkins, M. J. R.: The removal of fluid from the pulmonary airways

312

after birth in the rabbit, and the effect on this of prematurity and pre-natal hypoxia. Biol. Neonat. 7:214, 1964.

Ahlfeld, F.: Über bisher noch nicht beschriebene intrauterine Bewegungen des Kindes. Deutsch. Ges. Gynäk. 2:203, 1888.

Ahvenainen, E. K.: On changes in dilatation and signs of aspiration of foetal and neonatal lungs. Acta Paediat. (Suppl. 3) 35:1948.

Ahvenainen, E. K., and Call, J. D.: Pulmonary hemorrhage in infants. A descriptive study. Amer. J. Path. 28:1, 1952.

Ahvenainen, E. K., and Call, J. D.: Pulmonary hemorrhage. Experimental studies. Amer. J. Path. 28:193, 1952.

Ahvenainen, E. K.: Massive pulmonary hemorrhage in newborn. Ann. Paediat. Fenn. 2:44, 1956.

Alescio, T., and Cassini, A.: Induction in vitro of trahceal buds by pulmonary mesenchyme grafted on tracheal epithelium. J. Exptl. Zool. 150:83, 1962.

Alexander, W. J., and Dunbar, J. S.: Unusual bone changes in thymic alymphoplasia. Ann. Radiol. 11:389, 1967.

Allen, A. C., and Usher, R.: Renal acid excretion in infants with the respiratory distress syndrome. Pediat. Res. 5:345, 1971.

Allen, R. J., Towsley, H. A., and Wilson, J. L.: Neurogenic stridor in infancy. Am. J. Dis. Child. 87:179, 1954.

Allen, R. P., Taylor, R. L., and Reiquam, C. W.: Congenital lobar emphysema with dilated septal lymphatics. Radiology 86:929, 1966.

Altstatt, L. B., Dennis, L. H., Sundell, H., Malan, A., Harrison, V., Hedvall, G., Eichelberger, J., Fogel, B., and Stahlman, M.: Disseminated intravascular coagulation and hyaline membrane disease. Biol. Neonate 19:227, 1971.

Alzamora-Castro, V., Battilana, G., Abugattas, R., and Sialer, S.: Patent ductus arteriosus and high altitudes. Am. J. Cardiol. 5:761, 1960.

Ambrus, C. M., Weintraub, D. H., Dunphy, D., Dowd, J. E., Pickren, J. W., Niswander, K. R., and Ambrus, J. L.: Studies on hyaline membrane disease. I. The fibrinolysin system in pathogenesis and therapy. Pediatrics 32:10, 1963.

Ambrus, C. M., Weintraub, D. H., and Ambrus, J. L.: Studies on hyaline membrane disease. III. Therapeutic trial of urokinase-activated human plasmin. Pediatrics 38:231, 1966.

Anderson, G. S., Green, C. A., Neligan, G. A., Newell, D. J., and Russel, J. K.: Congenital bacterial pneumonia. Lancet 11:585, 1962.

Angus, G. E., and Thurlbeck, W. M.: Number of alveoli in the human lung. J. Appl. Physiol. 32:483, 1972.

Anselmino, K. J., and Hoffman, F.: Die ursachen des icterus neonatorum. Arch. Gynak. 143:477, 1930.

Apgar, V.: A proposal for a new method of evaluation of the newborn infant. Anesth. Analg. (Paris) 32:260, 1953.

Apgar, V., Holaday, D. A., James, L. S., Weisbrot, I. M., and Berrien, C.: Evaluation of the newborn infant—Second report. J. A. M. A. 168:1985, 1958.

Apgar, V., and James, L. S.: Further observations on the newborn scoring system. Am. J. Dis. Child. 104:419, 1962.

Aranda, J. V., Stern, L., and Dunbar, J. S.: Pneumothorax with pneumoperitoneum in a newborn infant. Amer. J. Dis. Child. 123:163, 1972.

Arcilla, R. A., Oh, W., Lind, J., and Blankenship, W.: Portal and atrial pressures in the newborn period. Acta Paed. 55:615, 1966.

Arcilla, R. A., Oh, W., Lind, J., and Gessner, I. H.: Pulmonary arterial pressures of newborn infants born with early and late clamping of the cord. Acta Paediat. Scand. 55:305, 1966.

Ardran, G. M., and Kemp, F. H.: The nasal and cervical airway in sleep in the neonatal period. Amer. J. Roentgen. 108:537, 1970.

Ardran, G. M., and Kemp, F. H.: The mechanism of changes in form of the cervical airway in infancy. Med. Radiol. Photog. 44:26, 1968.

Arrechon, W., and Reid, L.: Hypoplasia of lung with congenital diaphragmatic hernia. Brit. Med. J. 1:230, 1963.

Arthurton, M. W.: Stridor in a paediatric department. Proc. Roy. Soc. Med. 63:712, 1970.

Auld, P. A. M., Rudolph, A. J., Avery, M. E., Cherry, R. B., Drorbaugh, J. E., Kay, J. L., and Smith, C. A.: Responsiveness and resuscitation of the newborn. The use of the Apgar score. Am. J. Dis. Child. 101:713, 1961.

Auld, P. A. M., Nelson, N. M., Cherry, R. B., Rudolph, A. J., and Smith, C. A.: Measurement of thoracic gas volume in the newborn infant. J. Clin. Invest. 42:476, 1963.

Auld, P. A. M., Bhangananda, P., and Mehta, S.: The influence of an early caloric intake with i-v glucose on catabolism of premature infants. Pediatrics 37:592, 1966.

Auld, P. A. M.: Delayed closure of the ductus arteriosus. J. Pediat. 69:61, 1966.

Avery, M. E., and Mead, J.: Surface properties in relation to atelectasis and hyaline membrane disease. Am. J. Dis. Child. 97:517, 1959.

Avery, M. E., Frank, N. R., and Gribetz, I.: The inflationary force produced by pulmonary vascular distention in excised lungs. The possible relation of this force to that needed to inflate the lungs at birth. J. Clin. Invest. 38:456, 1959.

Avery, M. E., and Oppenheimer, E. H.: Recent increase in mortality from hyaline membrane disease. J. Pediat. 57:553, 1960.

Avery, M. E.: In Fomon, S. J., (ed.): Normal and abnormal respiration in children. Report 37th Ross Conf. on Pediatric Research. Columbus, Ohio, 1961.

Avery, M. E., and Cook, C. D.: Volume-pressure relationships of lungs and thorax in fetal, newborn, and adult goats. J. Appl. Physiol. 16:1034, 1961.

Avery, M. E.: The alveolar lining layer. Pediatrics 30:324, 1962.

Avery, M. E., and O'Doherty, N.: Effects of body-tilting on the resting end-expiratory position of normal infants. Pediatrics 29:255, 1962.

Avery, M. E., Chernick, V., Dutton, R. E., and Permutt, S.: Ventilatory response to inspired carbon dioxide in infants and adults. J. Appl. Physiol. 18:895, 1963.

Avery, M. E.: Prevention of hyaline membrane disease (commentary). Pediatrics 50: 513, 1972.

Avery, M. E., Chernick, V., and Young, M.: Fetal respiratory movements in response to rapid changes of CO_2 in the carotid artery. J. Appl. Physiol. 20:225, 1965.

Avery, M. E., and Said, S.: Surface phenomena in lungs in health and disease. Medicine 44:503, 1965.

Avery, M. E., Gatewood, O. B., and Brumley, G.: Transient tachypnea of the newborn. Am. J. Dis. Child. 111:380, 1966.

Baden, M., Bauer, C., Colle, E., Klein, G., Taeusch, H. W., Jr., and Stern, L.: A controlled trial of glucocorticoids in the treatment of respiratory distress syndrome. Pediatrics 50:526, 1972.

Baden, M., Papageorgiou, A., Joshi, V. V., and Stern, L.: Upper airway obstruction in a newborn secondary to hemangiopericytoma. C.M.A. Journal. 107:1202; 1972.

Baghdassarian, O., Avery, M. E., and Neuhauser, E. B. D.: A form of pulmonary insufficiency in premature infants? Pulmonary dysmaturity. Amer. J. Roentgen. 89:1020, 1963.

Baker, D. C., Jr.: Congenital disorders of the larynx. New York State. J. Med. 54:2458, 1954.

Baker, D. H., Berdon, W. E., and James, L. S.: Proper localization of umbilical arterial and venous catheters by lateral roentgenograms. Pediatrics 43:34, 1969.

Baker, J. B. E.: The effects of drugs on the foetus. Pharmacol. Rev. 12:37, 1960.

Balis, J. U., and Conen, P. E.: The role of alveolar inclusion bodies in the developing lung. Lab. Invest. 13:1215, 1964.

Balis, J. U., Delivoria, M., and Conen, P. E.: Maturation of postnatal human lung and the idiopathic respiratory distress syndrome. Lab. Invest. 15:530, 1966.

Ballard, P. L., and Ballard, R. A.: Glucocorticoid receptors and the role of glucocorticoids in fetal lung. Proc. Nat. Acad. Sci., USA 69:2668, 1972.

Bancalari, E., Gerhardt, T., and Monkus, E.: Simple device for producing continuous negative pressure in infants with IRDS. Pediat. 52:167, 1973.

Bancalari, E., Garcia, O. L. and Jesse, M. J.: Effects of continuous negative pressure on lung mechanics in idiopathic respiratory distress syndrome. Pediat. 51:485, 1973.

Banker, B. Q.: Periventricular leukomalacia of infancy. A.M.A. Arch. Neurol. 7:32, 1962.

Barach, A. L.: Immobilization of lungs through pressure. Am. Rev. Tuberc. 42:586, 1940.

Barclay, A. E., Franklin, K. J., and Prichard, M. M. L.: The foetal circulation and cardiovascular system, and the changes that they undergo at birth. Blackwell Sci. Pub., Oxford, 1944.

Barcroft, J., and Karvonen, M. J.: The action of carbon dioxide and cyanide on foetal respiratory movements; the development of chemoreflex function in sheep. J. Physiol. 107:153, 1948.

Barrett, C. T., Heymann, M. A., and Rudolph, A. M.: Alpha and beta adrenergic receptor activity in fetal sheep. Amer. J. Obstet. Gynec. 112:114, 1972.

Barrie, H.: Placental transfusion and hyaline membrane disease. Lancet *11*:92, 1962.
Barrie, H.: Resuscitation of the newborn. Lancet *1*:650, 1963.
Bárta, K., Dvořáček, Č., and Kadlec, A.: Komplement-Bindungs-Reaktion bei Pneumocysten-Pneumonien. Schweiz. Ztschr. allg. Path. *18*:22, 1955.
Barter, R. A., and Maddison, T. G.: The nature of the neonatal pulmonary hyaline membrane. Arch. Dis. Child. *35*:460, 1960.
Barter, R. A.: Pulmonary hyaline membrane. Arch. Dis. Child. *37*:314, 1962.
Barton, E. G., and Campbell, W. G., Jr.: Further observations on the ultrastructure of pneumocystis. Arch. Path. *83*:527, 1967.
Bates, T.: Poliomyelitis in pregnancy, fetus, and newborn. Am. J. Dis. Child. *90*:189, 1955.
Battaglia, F. C., Prystowsky, H., Smisson, C., Helleghers, A., and Bruns, P.: Fetal blood studies XVI on the change in total osmotic pressure and sodium and potassium concentrations of amniotic fluid during the course of human gestation. Surg. Gynec. Obstet. *105*:509, 1959.
Bauer, C. R., Elie, K., Spence, L., and Stern, L.: Hong Kong influenza in a neonatal unit. J. A. M. A. *223*:1233, 1973.
Baugh, C. D., and O'Donoghue, R. F.: Teratoma of the tonsil causing respiratory obstruction in the newborn. Arch. Dis. Child. *30*:396, 1955.
Baum, G. L., Racz, I., Bubis, J. J., Molho, M., and Shapiro, B. L.: Cystic disease of the lung. Am. J. Med. *40*:578, 1966.
Bauman, W. A.: The respiratory distress syndrome and its significance in premature infants. Pediatrics *24*:194, 1959.
Bazaz, G. R., Manfredi, O. L., Howard, R. G., and Claps, A. A.: Pneumocystis carinii pneumonia in three full-term siblings. J. Pediat. *76*:767, 1970.
Beard, R. W., and Morris, E. D.: Foetal and maternal acid-base balance during normal labour. J. Obstet. Gynaec. Brit. Common. *72*:496, 1965.
Beaudoing, A., Valois, J., and Lagier, A.: Le goitre néonatal secondaire à l'absorption d'iodure de potassium par la mère. Pediatrie *19*:121, 1964.
Becker, M. J., and Koppe, J. G.: Pulmonary structural changes in neonatal hyaline membrane disease treated with high pressure artificial respiration. Thorax *24*:689, 1969.
Behrle, F. C., Gibson, D. M., and Miller, H. C.: Role of hyaline membranes, blood, exudate, edema fluid and amniotic sac contents in preventing expansion of the lungs of newborn infants. Pediatrics *7*:782, 1951.
Behrman, R. E., Lees, M. H., Peterson, E. N., deLannoy, C. W., and Seeds, A. E.: Distribution of the circulation in the normal and asphyxiated fetal primate. Amer. J. Obstet. Gynec. *108*:956, 1970.
Beinfield, H. H.: Ways and means to reduce infant mortality due to suffocation, importance of choanal atresia. J. A. M. A. *170*:647, 1959.
Belanger, R., LaFlèche, L. R., and Picard, J. L.: Congenital cystic adenomatoid malformation of the lung. Thorax *19*:1, 1964.
Benesch, R., and Benesch, R. E.: The effect of organic phosphates from the human erythrocyte on the allosteric properties of hemoglobin. Biochem. Biophys. Res. Comm. *26*:162, 1967.
Benirschke, K., and Clifford, S. H.: Intrauterine bacterial infection of the newborn infant: Frozen sections of the cord as an aid to early detection. J. Pediat. *54*:11, 1959.
Benirschke, K.: Routes and types of infection in the fetus and the newborn. Am. J. Dis. Child. *99*:714, 1960.
Benirschke, K., Samuels, A. J., and Moore, E.: Enhanced proteolytic activity at pH 2 in lungs of infants dying from hyaline membrane disease. Proc. Soc. Exp. Biol. Med. *112*:697, 1963.
Benitez, R. E.: Degenerative changes in liver associated with aspiration of vernix and hyaline membrane formation in lungs in intrauterine anoxia. Arch. Path. (Chicago) *54*:378, 1952.
Bensch, K., Schaefer, K., and Avery, M. E.: Granular pneumonocytes; electron microscopic evidence of their exocrine function. Science *145*:1318, 1964.
Benson, F., Celander, O., Haglund, G., Nilsson, L., Paulsen, L., and Renck, L.: Positive-pressure respirator treatment of severe pulmonary insufficiency in the newborn infant. Acta Anaesth. Scand. *2*:37, 1958.
Berdon, W. E., and Baker, D. H.: Radiology of the newborn. Pediat. Clin. N. Amer. *13*:1017, 1966.

Berdon, W. E., and Baker, D. H.: Giant hepatic hemangioma with cardiac failure in the newborn infant. Value of high-dosage intravenous urography and umbilical angiography. Radiology 92:1523, 1969.

Berdon, W. E., Baker, D. H., and James, L.: The ductus bump. A transient physiologic mass in chest roentgenograms of newborn infants. Amer. J. Roentgen. 95:91, 1965.

Berdon, W. E., Baker, D. H., and Amoury, R.: The role of pulmonary hypoplasia in the prognosis of newborn infants with diaphragmatic hernia and eventration. Amer. J. Roentgen. 103:413, 1968.

Berezin, A.: Histochemical study of hyaline membrane of newborn infants and of that produced in guinea pigs. Biol. Neonat. 14:90, 1969.

Berfenstam, R., Edlund, T., and Zettergren, L.: The hyaline membrane disease. A review of earlier clinical experimental findings and some studies on pathogenesis of hyaline membranes in O_2-intoxicated rabbits. Acta Paediat. 47:82, 1958.

Berger, A., Altman, M., and Winter, S. T.: Neonatal asphyxia caused by teratoma of pharynx. Am. J. Dis. Child. 109:584, 1965.

Berger, M., Ferguson, C., and Hendry, J.: Paralysis of the left diaphragm, left vocal cord and aneurysm of the ductus arteriosus in a 7-week-old infant. J. Pediat. 56:800, 1960.

Berggren, S. M.: The oxygen deficit of arterial blood caused by non-ventilating parts of the lung. Acta Physiol. Scand. 4, suppl. 11, 1942.

Berglund, G., and Karlberg, P.: Determination of the functional residual capacity in newborn infants. Acta Paediat. 45:541, 1956.

Berkovich, S., and Taranko, L.: Acute respiratory illness in the premature nursery associated with respiratory syncytial virus infections. Pediatrics 34:753, 1964.

Bernard, C.: De la matière glycogène considérée comme condition de développement de certains tissues chez le foetus avant l'apparition de la fonction glycogénique du foie. J. Physiol. (Paris) 2:326, 1859.

Bernstein, J., and Wang, J.: The pathology of neonatal pneumonia. Am. J. Dis. Child. 101:350, 1961.

Bert, P.: Leçons sur la physiologie comparée de la respiration. (Trente et unième leçon.) Baillière, Paris, 1870.

Bertalanffy, F. D., and LeBlond, C. P.: The continuous renewal of the two types of alveolar cells in the lung of the rat. Anat. Rec. 115:515, 1953.

Bertalanffy, F. D., and LeBlond, C. P.: Structure of respiratory tissue. Lancet II:1365, 1955.

Bhagwanani, S. G., Fahmy, D., and Turnbull, A. C.: Prediction of neonatal respiratory distress by estimation of amniotic-fluid lecithin. Lancet I:159, 1972.

Binet, J. P., Nezelof, C., and Fredet, J.: Five cases of lobar tension emphysema in infancy; importance of bronchial malformation and value of postoperative steroid therapy. Dis. Chest 41:126, 1962.

Bingham, J. A. W.: Two cases of unilateral paralysis of the diaphragm in the newborn treated surgically. Thorax 9:248, 1954.

Biscoe, T. J., and Purves, M. J.: Types of nervous activity which may be recorded from the carotid sinus nerve in the sheep foetus. J. Physiol. 202:1, 1969.

Bishop, H. C., and Koop, C. E.: Acquired eventration of the diaphragm in infancy. Pediatrics 22:1088, 1958.

Black, M. M., and Speer, F. D.: Structure of lymph nodes in hyaline membrane disease. Am. J. Clin. Path. 33:303, 1960.

Blackburn, W. R., Travers, H., Kelley, J. S., and Rhoades, R. A.: Biochemical studies of fetal rat lung after in utero decapitation (abstract). Fed. Proc. 31:238, 1972.

Blanc, W. A.: Amniotic and neonatal infection: Rapid cytologic diagnosis. Gynaecologia 136:101, 1953.

Blanc, W. A.: Amniotic infection syndrome. Pathogenesis, morphology and significance in circumnatal mortality. Clin. Obstet. Gynec. 2:705, 1959.

Blanc, W. A.: Pathways of fetal and early neonatal infection. J. Pediat. 59:473, 1961.

Bland, R. D.: Cord-blood total protein level as a screening aid for the idiopathic respiratory distress syndrome. New Eng. J. Med. 287:9, 1972.

Blattner, R. J.: Unilateral paralysis of the diaphragm without involvement of the brachial plexus. J. Pediat. 20:223, 1942.

Blumberg, J. B., Stevenson, J. K., Lemire, R. J., and Boyden, E. A.: Laryngotracheoesophageal cleft, the embryologic implications: Review of the literature. Surgery 57:559, 1965.

Blumenthal, B. I., Capitanio, M. A., Queloz, J. M., and Kirkpatrick, J. A.: Intrathoracic mesenchymoma. Observations in two infants. Radiology 104:107, 1972.

Blumenthal, S., and Ravitch, M. M.: Seminar on aortic vascular rings and other anomalies of the aortic arch. Pediatrics 20:896, 1957.

Blystad, W., Landing, B. H., and Smith, C. A.: Pulmonary hyaline membranes in newborn infants. Pediatrics 8:5, 1951.

Blystad, W.: Blood gas determinations on premature infants. III. Investigations on premature infants with recurrent attacks of apnea. Acta Paediat. 45:211, 1956.

Boeckman, C. R., Krill, C. E., Jr.: Bacterial and fungal infections complicating parenteral alimentation in infants and children. J. Pediat. Surg. 5:117, 1970.

Boles, E. T., and Izant, R. J., Jr.: Spontaneous chylothorax in the neonatal period. Amer. J. Surg., 99:870, 1960.

Bonar, B. E., Blumenfeld, C. M., and Fenning, C.: Studies of fetal respiratory movements. Am. J. Dis. Child. 55:1, 1938.

Bonham-Carter, R. E., Bound, J. P., and Smellie, J. M.: Mean venous pressures in the first hours of life. Lancet 11:1320, 1956.

Bookstein, J. J., and Voegeli, E.: A critical analysis of magnification radiography: laboratory investigation. Radiology 98:23, 1971.

Born, G. V. R., Dawes, G. S., Mott, J., and Rennick, B. R.: The constriction of the ductus arteriosus caused by oxygen and by asphyxia in newborn lambs. J. Physiol. 132:304, 1956.

Bosma, J. F., and Lind, J.: Roentgenologic observations of motions of the upper airway associated with establishment of respiration in the newborn infant. Acta Paediat. (Suppl. 123) 49:18, 1960.

Boss, J. H., and Craig, J. M.: Reparative phenomena in lungs of neonates with hyaline membranes. Pediatrics 29:890, 1962.

Boston, R. W., Humphreys, P. W., Reynold, E. O. R., and Strang, L. B.: Lymph-flow and clearance of liquid from the lungs of the foetal lamb. Lancet II:473, 1965.

Boston, R. W., Geller, F., and Smith, C. A.: Arterial blood gas tensions and acid-base balance in the management of the respiratory distress syndrome. J. Pediat. 68:74, 1966.

Bound, J. P., Harvey, P. W., and Bagshaw, H. B.: Prevention of the pulmonary syndrome of the newborn. Lancet I:1200, 1962.

Bouterline-Young, H. J., and Smith, C. A.: Respiration of full term and premature infants. Am. J. Dis. Child. 80:753, 1950.

Bovet-DuBois, N.: Etude histologique des "membranes hyalines" dans les poumons de nouveau-nés. Thesis. Univ. de Bâle. Ed. S. Karger, S. A., Bâle, 1951.

Bower, B. D., Jones, L. F., and Weeks, M. M.: Cold injury in the newborn. A study of 70 cases. Brit. Med. J. 1:303, 1960.

Boyd, J. D.: The development of the Human Carotid Body. Contrib. Embryol. Carneg. Instit. 26:1, 1937.

Boyd, J. D.: The Inferior aortico-pulmonary glomus. Brit. Med. Bull. 17:79, 1961.

Boyd, R. D. H., Hill, J. R., Humphreys, P. W., Normand, I. C. S., Reynolds, E. O. R., and Strang, L. B.: Permeability of lung capillaries to macromolecules in foetal and newborn lambs and sheep. J. Physiol. 201:567, 1969.

Boyden, E. A., and Tompsett, D. H.: The changing patterns in the developing lungs of infants. Acta Anat. 61:164, 1965.

Boys, C. V.: Soap Bubbles: Their Colours and the Forces Which Mould Them. Dover Public, New York, 1959.

Bozic, C.: Pulmonary hyaline membranes and vascular anomalies of the lung. Description of a case. Pediatrics 32:1094, 1963.

Brady, J., and James, L. S.: Fetal electrocardiographic studies. Tachycardia as a sign of fetal distress. Amer. J. Obstet. Gynec. 86:785, 1963.

Brady, J. P., Cotton, E. C., and Tooley, W. H.: Chemoreflexes in the newborn infant: Effects of 100% oxygen on heart rate and ventilation. J. Physiol. (London) 172:332, 1964.

Brady, J. P., and Rigatto, H.: Pulmonary capillary flow in infants. Circulation (Suppl. III) 40:50, 1969.

Brand, M. M., Durbridge, T. C., Rosan, R. C., and Northway, W. H., Jr.: Neuropathological lesions in respiratory distress syndrome: Acute and chronic changes during hypoxia and oxygen therapy. J. Reprod. Med. 8:267, 1972.

Bratu, M., Brown, M., Carter, M., and Lawson, J. P.: Cystic hygroma of the mediastinum in children. Amer. J. Dis. Child. 119:348, 1970.

Brewis, R. A. L.: Oxygen toxicity during artificial ventilation. Thorax 24:656, 1969.

Briggs, J. N.: Some observations on pulmonary hemorrhage in the newborn period. Abstract. Am. J. Dis. Child. 90:591, 1955.

Briggs, J. N., and Hogg, G.: Perinatal pulmonary pathology. Pediatrics 22:41, 1958.

Brooksaler, F. S., and Graivier, L.: Poland's syndrome. Amer. J. Dis. Child. 121:263, 1971.

Brown, H. W., and Plum, F.: The neurologic basis of Cheyne-Stokes respiration. Am. J. Med. 30:849, 1961.

Brown, R. J. K.: Respiratory difficulties at birth. Brit. Med. J. 1:404, 1959.

Brown, R. S., Nogrady, M. B., Spence, L., and Wiglesworth, F. W.: An outbreak of adenovirus type 7 infection in children in Montreal. C.M.A. Journal. 108:434, 1973.

Brück, K., Parmelee, A. H., and Brück, M.: Neutral temperature range and range of "thermal comfort" in premature infants. Biol. Neonat. 4:32, 1962.

Brumley, G. W., Chernick, V., Hodson, W. A., Normand, C., Fenner, A., and Avery, M. E.: Correlations of mechanical stability, morphology, pulmonary surfactant and phospholipid content in the developing lamb lung. J. Clin. Invest. 46:863, 1967.

Brumley, G. W., Hodson, W. A., and Avery, M. E.: Lung phospholipids and surface tension correlations in infants with and without hyaline membrane disease and in adults. Pediatrics 40:13, 1967.

Brünner, S., Poulsen, P. T., and Vesterdal, J.: Cysts of the lung in infants and children. Acta Paediat. 49:39, 1960.

Bruns, P. D., and Shields, L. V.: High oxygen and hyaline-like membranes. Amer. J. Obstet. Gynec. 67:1224, 1954.

Bruns, P. D., Cooper, W. E., and Drose, V. E.: Maternal-fetal oxygen and acid-base studies and their relationship to hyaline membrane disease in the newborn infant. Amer. J. Obstet. Gynec. 82:1079, 1961.

Bryan, C. S.: Enhancement of bacterial infection by meconium. Johns Hopkins Med. J. 121:9, 1967.

Brzezinski, A., Sadorsky, E., and Shafrir, E.: Electrophoretic distribution of proteins in amniotic fluid and in maternal and fetal serum. Am. J. Obstet. Gynec. 82:800, 1961.

Bucci, G., Iannaccone, G., Scalamandrè, A., Savignoni, P. G., and Mendicini, M.: Observations on the Wilson-Mikity syndrome. Ann. Paediat. 206:135, 1966.

Bucci, G., Scalamandrè, A., Savignoni, P. G., Orzalesi, M., and Mendicini, M.: Cribside sampling of blood from the radial artery. Pediatrics 37:497, 1966.

Bucher, U., and Reid, L.: Development of the intrasegmental bronchial tree: The pattern of branching and development of cartilage at various stages of intrauterine life. Thorax 16:207, 1961.

Bucher, U., and Reid, L.: Development of the mucus-secreting elements in human lung. Thorax 16:219, 1961.

Buckels, L. J., and Usher, R.: Cardiopulmonary effects of placental transfusion. J. Pediat. 67:239, 1965.

Buckingham, S., and Sommers, S. C.: Pulmonary hyaline membranes. Am. J. Dis. Child. 99:216, 1960.

Buckingham, S., and Avery, M. E.: Time of appearance of lung surfactant in the foetal mouse. Nature 193:688, 1962.

Buckingham, S., McNary, W. F., and Sommers, S. C.: Pulmonary alveolar cell inclusions: Their development in the rat. Science 145:1192, 1964.

Buckingham, S., Heinemann, H. O., Sommers, S. C., and McNary, W. F.: Phospholipid synthesis in the large pulmonary alveolar cell. Am. J. Path. 48:1027, 1966.

Buckingham, S., Sommers, S. C., and Sherwin, R. P.: Lesions of the dorsal vagal nucleus in the respiratory distress syndrome. Amer. J. Clin. Path. 48:269, 1967.

Budnick, I. S., Leikin, S., and Hoeck, L. E.: Effect in the newborn infant of reserpine administered ante partum. Am. J. Dis. Child. 90:286, 1955.

Buetow, K. C., Klein, S. W., and Lane, R. B.: Septicemia in premature infants. Am. J. Dis. Child. 110:29, 1965.

Burnard, E. D.: A murmur from the ductus in the newborn baby. Brit. Med. J. 1:806, 1958.

Burnard, E. D.: The cardiac murmur in relation to symptoms in the newborn. Brit. Med. J. 1:134, 1959.

Burnard, E. D.: Changes in the heart size in the dyspnoeic newborn baby. Brit. Med. J. 1:1495, 1959.

Burnard, E. D., and James, L. S.: The cardiac silhouette in newborn infants: A cinematographic study of the normal range. Pediatrics 27:713, 1961.

Burnard, E. D., and James, L. S.: Failure of the heart after undue asphyxia at birth. Pediatrics 28:545, 1961.

Burnard, E. D., and James, L. S.: Atrial pressures and cardiac size in the newborn infant. J. Pediat. 62:815, 1963.

Burnard, E. D., Grattan-Smith, P., Picton-Warlow, C. G., and Grauaug, A.: Pulmonary insufficiency in prematurity. Austr. Paed. J. 1:12, 1965.

Burnell, R. H., Joseph, M. C., and Lees, M. H.: Progressive pulmonary hypertension in newborn infants. Amer. J. Dis. Child. 123:167, 1972.

Burns, B. D.: The central control of respiratory movements. Brit. Med. Bull. 19:7, 1963.

Butler, N., and Claireaux, A. E.: Congenital diaphragmatic hernia as a cause of perinatal mortality. Lancet 1:659, 1962.

Butler, N.: Complications of Birth Asphyxia with Special Reference to Resuscitation. The Obstetrician, Anaesthetist, and the Paediatrician. Pergamon Press, New York, 1963.

Butler, N. R., and Bonham, D. G.: Perinatal Mortality. E & S Livingstone Ltd., London, 1963.

Butterfield, J., and Covey, M. J.: Practical epigram of the Apgar score. Letter. J. A. M. A. 181:353, 1962.

Butterfield, J., Moscovici, C., Berry, C., and Kempe, C. H.: Cystic emphysema in premature infants. A report of an outbreak with isolation of type 19 ECHO virus in one case. N. Eng. J. Med. 268:18, 1963.

Caffey, J.: On the natural regression of pulmonary cysts during early infancy. Pediatrics 11:48, 1953.

Caffey, J.: Pediatric X-Ray Diagnosis, 5th ed., Year Book Publishers Inc., Chicago, 1967.

Caffey, J., and diLiberti, C.: Acute atrophy of the thymus induced by adrenocorticosteroids: Observed roentgenographically in living human infants. Am. J. Roentgen., 82:530, 1959.

Caffey, J., and Silbey, R.: Regrowth of the thymus after atrophy induced by the oral administration of adrenocorticosteroids to human infants. Pediatrics 26:762, 1960.

Camerer, J.: Beiträge zur Frage der Fruchtwasseraspiration. Deutsche Ztschr. ges. gerichtl. Med. 29:333, 1938.

Campbell, A. G. M., Cross, K. W., Dawes, G. S., and Hyman, A. I.: A comparison of air and O_2, in a hyperbaric chamber or by positive pressure ventilation in the resuscitation of newborn rabbits. J. Pediat. 68:153, 1966.

Campbell, A. G. M., Cockburn, F., Dawes, G. S., and Milligan, J. E.: Pulmonary vasoconstriction in asphyxia during cross-circulation between twin foetal lambs. J. Physiol. (London) 192:111, 1967.

Campbell, A. G. M., Dawes, G. S., Fishman, A. P., Hyman, A. I., and Perks, A. M.: The release of a bradykinin-like pulmonary vasodilator substance in foetal and newborn lambs. J. Physiol. 195:83, 1968.

Campbell, J. S., Wiglesworth, F. W., Latorroca, R., and Wilde, H.: Congenital subglottic hemangiomas of the larynx and trachea in infants. Pediatrics 22:727, 1958.

Campbell, K.: Inhalation of excess liquor as a factor in the production of hyaline membrane atelectasis. Med. J. Austr., Nov. 28, 1959, p. 797.

Campbell, R. E.: Roentgenologic features of umbilical vascular catherization in the newborn. Amer. J. Roentgen. 112:68, 1971.

Campbell, R. E.: Intrapulmonary interstitial emphysema: A complication of hyaline membrane disease. Amer. J. Roentgen. 110:449, 1970.

Campiche, M., Prod'hom, S., and Gautier, A.: Etude au microscope électronique du poumon de prématurés morts en destresse respiratoire. Ann. Paediat. 196:81, 1961.

Campiche, M., Jaccottet, M., and Juillard, E.: La pneumonose à membranes hyalines. Ann. Paediat. 199:74, 1962.

Cantrell, J. R., Haller, J. A., and Ravitch, M. M.: A syndrome of congenital defects involving the abdominal wall, sternum, diaphragm, pericardium, and heart. Surg. Gynec. Obstet. 107:602, 1958.

Capers, T. H.: Pulmonary hyaline membrane formation in the adult. Am. J. Med. 31:701, 1961.

Capitanio, M. A., and Kirkpatrick, J. A.: Pneumocystis carinii pneumonia. Am. J. Roentgen., 97:174, 1966.

Capitanio, M. A., Ramos, R., and Kirkpatrick, J. A.: Pulmonary sling. Roentgen observations. Amer. J. Roentgen. Rad. Ther. Nucl. Med. 112:28, 1971.

Capitanio, M. A., and Kirkpatrick, J. A.: Nasopharyngeal lymphoid tissue. Roentgen observations in 257 children two years of age or less. Radiology 96:389, 1970.

Carini, A.: Formas de eschizogonia do Trypanozoma Lewisi. Common. Soc. Med. Sao Paulo, Aug. 16, 1910, p. 204, cited by Gajdusek, Pediat. 19:543, 1957.

Carson, S., Taeusch, H. W., Jr., and Avery, M. E.: The effects of cortisol injection on lung growth in fetal rabbits. J. Appl. Physiol. 34:660, 1973.

Carter, R. W., and Vaughn, H. M.: Congenital pulmonary lymphangiectasis. Am. J. Roentgen. 86:576, 1961.

Cassady, G.: Plasma volume studies in low birth weight infants. Pediatrics 38:1020, 1966.

Cassin, S., Dawes, G. S., Mott, J. C., Ross, B. B., and Strang, L. B.: The vascular resistance of the foetal and newly ventilated lung of the lamb. J. Physiol. 171:61, 1964.

Castilla, P., Irving, I. M., Rees, G. J., and Rickham, P. P.: Posture in the management of esophageal atresia. Variations on a theme by Dr. E. B. D. Neuhauser. J. Pediat. Surg. 6:709, 1971.

Ceballos, R.: Aspiration of maternal blood in the etiology of massive pulmonary hemorrhage in the newborn infant. J. Pediat. 72:390, 1968.

Cederberg, A., Hellstein, S., and Miorner, G.: Oxygen treatment and hyaline pulmonary membranes in adults. Acta path. et Microbiol. Scand. 64:450, 1965.

Celander, O.: In Jonxis, J. H. P., Visser, H. K. A., and Troelstra, J. A. (eds.): The Nutricia Symposium on the Adaptation of the Newborn Infant to Extrauterine Life. Chas. C Thomas, Springfield, 1964.

Ceruti, E.: Chemoreceptor reflexes in the newborn infant: Effect of cooling on the response to hypoxia. Pediatrics 37:556, 1966.

Chagas, C.: Nova tripanozomiaza humana. Estrudos sobre a morfolojia e o ciclo evolutivo do Schizotrypanum cruzi n. gen., n. sp., ajente etiologio de nova entidade morbida de homen. Mem. Insti. Oswaldo Cruz, Rio, 1:159, 1909, cited by Gajdusek, Pediat. 19:543, 1957.

Chang, C. H., and Davis, W. C.: Congenital bifid sternum with partial ectopia cordis. Amer. J. Roentgen. 86:513, 1961.

Chany, C., Lépiue, P., Lelong, M., Le-Tan-Vinh, Satgé, P., Virat, J.: Severe and fatal pneumonia in infants and young children associated with adenovirus infections. Am. J. Hygiene 67:367, 1958.

Chasler, C. N.: Pneumothorax and pneumomediastinum in the newborn. Am. J. Roentgen. 91:550, 1964.

Chatrath, R. R., Shafie, M., and Jones, R. S.: Fate of hypoplastic lungs after repair of congenital diaphragmatic hernia. Arch. Dis. Child. 46:633, 1971.

Cheek, D. B., Malinek, M., and Fraillon, J. M.: Plasma adrenaline and noradrenaline in the neonatal period, and infants with respiratory distress syndrome and placental insufficiency. Pediatrics 31:374, 1963.

Chernick, V., and Avery, M. E.: Spontaneous alveolar rupture in newborn infants. Pediatrics 32:816, 1963.

Chernick, V., Heldrich, F., and Avery, M. E.: Periodic breathing of premature infants. J. Pediat. 64:330, 1964.

Chernick, V., and Reed, M. H.: Pneumothorax and chylothorax in the neonatal period. J. Pediat. 76:624, 1970.

Chernick, V., and Vidyasagar, D.: Continuous negative chest wall pressure in hyaline membrane disease. One year experience. Pediatrics 49:753, 1972.

Chernick, V.: Hyaline membrane disease—therapy with constant lung-distending pressure. New Eng. J. Med. 289:302, 1973.

Ch'In, K. Y., and Tang, M. Y.: Congenital adenomatoid malformation of one lobe of lung with general anasarca. A.M.A. Arch. Path. 48:221, 1949.

Chu, J., Clements, J. A., Cotton, E., Klaus, M. H., Sweet, A. Y., Thomas, M. A., and Tooley, W. H.: The pulmonary hypoperfusion syndrome. Pediatrics 35:733, 1965.

Chu, J., Clements, J. A., Cotton, E. K., Klaus, M. H., Sweet, A. Y., and Tooley, W. H.: Neonatal pulmonary ischemia. Pediatrics (Suppl.) 40:709, 1967.

Chu, J. S., Dawson, P., Klaus, M., and Sweet, A. Y.: Lung compliance and lung volume measured concurrently in normal full-term and premature infants. Pediatrics *34*: 525, 1964.

Claireaux, A. E.: Hyaline membrane in the neonatal lung. Lancet *11*:749, 1953.

Claireaux, A. E.: Neonatal pathology. *In* Holzel, A., and Tizard, J. P. M., (eds.): Modern Trends in Pediatrics, 2nd series. Paul B. Hoeber, Inc., New York, 1958.

Claireaux, A. E., and Ferreira, H. P.: Bilateral pulmonary agenesis. Arch. Dis. Child. *33*:364, 1958.

Clark, D. B.: Werdnig Hoffmann Disease. *In* Nelson, W. E., (ed.): Textbook of Pediatrics, 8th ed., p. 1299. W. B. Saunders Co., Philadelphia, 1969.

Clark, J. M., and Lambertsen, C. J.: Pulmonary oxygen toxicity. A review. Pharmacol. Rev. *23*:37, 1971.

Clark, N. S., Nairn, R. C., and Gowar, F. J. S.: Cystic disease of the lung in the newborn treated by pneumonectomy. Arch. Dis. Child. *31*:358, 1956.

Clarkson, P., Ritter, D. G., Rahimtoola, S. H., Hallermann, F. J., and McGoon, D. C.: Aberrant left pulmonary artery. Am. J. Dis. Child. *113*:373, 1967.

Clement, J. G.: Inhalation bronchography—method and results in the experimental animal. J. Can. Assoc. Radiol. *20*:106, 1969.

Clements, J. A., Platzker, A. C., Tierney, D. F., et al.: Assessment of the risk of the respiratory distress syndrome by a rapid new test for surfactant in amniotic fluid. New Eng. J. Med. *286*:1077, 1972.

Clements, J. A.: Surface tension of lung extracts. Proc. Soc. Exp. Biol. Med. *95*:170, 1957.

Clements, J. A., Brown, E. S., and Johnson, R. P.: Pulmonary surface tension and the mucus lining of the lungs: Some theoretical considerations. J. Appl. Physiol. *12*:262, 1958.

Clements, J. A.: Surface phenomena in relation to pulmonary function (Sixth Bowditch Lecture). Physiologist *5*:11, 1962.

Cochran, W. D., Davis, H. T., and Smith, C. A.: Advantages and complications of umbilical artery catheterization in the newborn. Pediatrics *42*:769, 1968.

Cochran, W. D., Levison, H., Muirhead, D. M., Boston, R. W., Wang, C. C. S., and Smith, C. A.: A clinical trial of high oxygen pressure for the respiratory distress syndrome. New Eng. J. Med. *272*:347, 1965.

Cohen, M. M., Weintraub, D. H., and Lilienfeld, A. M.: The relationship of pulmonary hyaline membrane to certain factors in pregnancy and delivery. Pediatrics *26*:42, 1960.

Cohen, M. M., Jr., Gorlin, R. J., Feingold, M., and ten Bensel, R. W.: The Beckwith-Wiedemann syndrome: seven new cases. Amer. J. Dis. Child. *122*:515, 1971.

Cohn, H. E., Sacks, E. J., Heymann, M. A., and Rudolph, A. M.: Cardiovascular responses to hypoxemia and to acidemia in unanesthetized fetal lambs. Pediat. Res. *6*:342, 1972 (abstract).

Cole, V. A., Normand, I. C. S., Reynolds, E. O. R., and Rivers, R. P. A.: Pathogenesis of hemorrhagic pulmonary edema and massive pulmonary hemorrhage in the newborn. Pediatrics *51*:175, 1973.

Colgan, F. J., Eldrup-Jørgensen, S., and Lawrence, R. M.: Maintenance of Respiration in the Neonatal Respiratory Distress Syndrome. J. A. M. A. *173*:1557, 1960.

Colville, P., Shugg, C., and Ferris, B. G.: Effects of body tilting on respiratory mechanics. J. Appl. Physiol. *9*:19, 1956.

Combes, M. A., Wiggins, K. M., and Fackler, W. R.: Comparison of oral fluid and human fibrinolysin regimens in the management of the respiratory distress syndrome of premature infants. Abstract. Am. Pediat. Soc. p. 60, 1962.

Comer, T. P., and Clagett, O. T.: Surgical treatment of hernia of the foramen of Morgagni. J. Thorac. Cardiovasc. Surg. *52*:461, 1966.

Comline, R. S., and Silver, M.: The release of adrenaline and noradrenaline from the adrenal glands of the foetal sheep. J. Physiol. *156*:424, 1961.

Comline, R. S., Silver, I. A., and Silver, M.: Factors responsible for the stimulation of the adrenal medulla during asphyxia in the foetal lamb. J. Physiol. *178*:211, 1965.

Condorelli, S., and Ungari, C.: The period of functional closure of the foramen ovale and the ductus Botalli in the human newborn. Cardiologia *36*:274, 1960.

Congdon, E. D.: Transformation of the aortic arch system during the development of the human embryo. Contributions to embryology, No. 14, Carnegie Institution of Washington, 1922.

Conway, D. J.: Origin of lung cysts in childhood. Arch. Dis. Child. *26*:504, 1951.

Cook, C. D., Cherry, R. B., O'Brien, D., Karlberg, P., and Smith, C. A.: Studies of respiratory physiology in the newborn infant. I. Observations of normal premature and fullterm infants. J. Clin. Invest. 34:975, 1955.

Cook, C. D., Lucey, J. F., Drorbaugh, J. E., Segal, S., Sutherland, J. M., and Smith, C. A.: Apnea and respiratory distress in the newborn infant. N. Eng. J. Med. 254:562, 604, and 651, 1956.

Cook, C. D., Sutherland, J. M., Segal, S., Cherry, R. B., Mead, J., McIlroy, M. B., and Smith, C. A.: Studies of respiratory physiology in the newborn infant. J. Clin. Invest. 36:440, 1957.

Cook, C. D., Drinker, P. A., Jacobson, H. N., Levison, H., and Strang, L. B.: Control of pulmonary blood flow in the foetal and newly born lamb. J. Physiol. 169:10, 1963.

Cooke, W. D. D.: Prognostic significance of the serum protein content in premature babies and its relation to pulmonary hyaline membrane: Preliminary communication. Med. J. Austr., June 4, 1960, p. 887.

Corbet, A. J. S., and Burnard, E. D.: Oxygen tension measurements on digital blood in the newborn. Pediatrics 46:780, 1970.

Corner, B. D., and Brown, N. J.: Congenital tuberculosis. Thorax 10:99, 1955.

Cotton, B. H., Spaulding, K., and Penido, J. R. F.: An accessory lung. Report of a case. J. Thorac. Surg. 23:508, 1952.

Cotton, E. K., Cogswell, J. J., Cropp, G. J. A., and Losey, R.: Measurements of effective pulmonary blood flow in the normal newborn human infant. Pediatrics 47:520, 1971.

Cournand, A., Motley, H. L., Werkö, L., Richards, D. W.: Physiological studies of the effects of intermittent positive pressure breathing on cardiac output in man. Am. J. Physiol. 152:162, 1948.

Craig, J. M., Kirkpatrick, J., and Neuhauser, E. B. D.: Congenital cystic adenomatoid malformation of the lung in infants. Am. J. Roentgen. 76:516, 1956.

Craig, J. M., Fenton, K., and Gitlin, D.: Obstructive factors in pulmonary hyaline membrane syndrome in asphyxia of newborn. Pediatrics 22:847, 1958.

Cross, K. W.: The respiratory rate and ventilation in the newborn baby. J. Physiol. 109:459, 1949.

Cross, K. W., and Roberts, P. W.: Asphyxia neonatorum treated by electrical stimulation of phrenic nerve. Brit. Med. J. 1:1043, 1951.

Cross, K. W., and Warner, P.: The effect of inhalation of high and low oxygen concentrations on the respiration of the newborn infant. J. Physiol. 114:283, 1951.

Cross, K. W., and Malcolm, J. L.: Evidence of carotid body and sinus activity in newborn and foetal animals. J. Physiol. 118:10P, 1952.

Cross, K. W., and Oppe, T. E.: The effect of inhalation of high and low concentrations of oxygen in the respiration of premature infants. J. Physiol. 117:38, 1952.

Cross, K. W., Hopper, J. M. D., and Oppe, T. E.: The effect of inhalation of carbon dioxide in air on the respiration of the fullterm and premature infant. J. Physiol. 122:264, 1953.

Cross, K. W., Tizard, J. P. M., and Trythall, D. A. H.: The gaseous metabolism of the newborn infant. Acta Paediat. 46:265, 1957.

Cross, K. W., Klaus, M., Tooley, W. H., and Weisser, K.: The response of the newborn baby to inflation of the lungs. J. Physiol. 151:551, 1960.

Cross, K. W., Flynn, D. M., and Hill, J. R.: Oxygen consumption in normal newborn infants during moderate hypoxia in warm and cool environments. Pediatrics 37:565, 1966.

Crosse, V. M.: Atelectasis with hyaline membranes. Ann. Paediat. Fenn. 3:152, 1957.

Cumming, G. R., MacPherson, R. I., and Chernick, V.: Unilateral hyperlucent lung syndrome in children. J. Pediat. 78:250, 1971.

Cumming, W. A., and Reilly, B. J.: Fatigue aspiration. A cause of recurrent pneumonia in infants. Radiology 105:387, 1972.

Daily, W. J. R., Klaus, M., and Meyer, H. B.: Apnea in premature infants: Monitoring, incidence, heart rate changes, and an effect of environmental temperature. Pediatrics 43:510, 1969.

Daily, W. J. R., and Smith, P. C.: Mechanical ventilation of the newborn infant. In Gluck, L. (ed.): Current Problems in Pediatrics, Chicago, Year Book Medical Publishers, 1971.

Daly, W. J., and Bondurant, S.: Direct measurement of respiratory pleural pressure changes in normal man. J. Appl. Physiol. 18:513, 1963.

Daniel, S. S., Adamsons, K., and James, L. S.: Lactate and pyruvate as an index of pre-natal oxygen deprivation. Pediatrics 37:942, 1966.

Daniel, S. S., Dawes, G. S., James, L. S., Ross, B. B., and Windle, W. F.: Hypothermia and the resuscitation of asphyxiated fetal rhesus monkeys. J. Pediat. 68:45, 1966.

Danilowicz, D., Rudolph, A. M., and Hoffman, J. I. E.: Delayed closure of the ductus arteriosus in premature infants. Pediatrics 37:74, 1966.

Danilowicz, D. A., Rudolph, A. M., Hoffman, J. I. E., and Heymann, M. A.: Physiologic pressure difference between main and branch pulmonary arteries in infants. Circulation 45:410, 1972.

Danks, D. M., and Stevens, L. H.: Neonatal respiratory distress associated with a high hematocrit reading. Lancet 11:499, 1964.

Davies, P. A., Robinson, R. J., Scopes, J. W., Tizard, J. P. M., and Wigglesworth, J. S.: Medical Care of Newborn Babies. J. B. Lippincott Co., Philadelphia, 1972.

Davis, C. H., and Stevens, G. W.: Value of routine radiographic examinations of the newborn, based on a study of 702 consecutive babies. Am. J. Obst. Gynec. 20:73, 1930.

Davis, L. A.: Standard roentgen examinations in newborns, infants, and children: Techniques, "portable" films, immobilization devices, and fluoroscopy. Progr. Pediat. Radiol. 1:3, 1967.

Davis, M. E., and Potter, E. L.: Intrauterine respiration of the human fetus. J. A. M. A. 131:1194, 1946.

Davis, W. S., and Allen, P. R.: Accessory diaphragm: duplication of the diaphragm. Radiol. Clin. N. Amer. 6:253, 1968.

Dawes, G. S., Mott, J. C., Widdicombe, J. G., and Wyatt, D. G.: Changes in the lungs of the newborn lamb. J. Physiol. 121:141, 1953.

Dawes, G. S., Mott, J. C., Widdicombe, J. G., and Wyatt, D. G.: Changes in the lungs of the newborn lamb. J. Physiol. 121:141, 1953.

Dawes, G. S., Mott, J. C., and Widdicombe, J. G.: The foetal circulation in the lamb. J. Physiol. 126:563, 1954.

Dawes, G. S.: Foetal and neonatal physiology. Chicago, Year Book Medical Publishers, Inc., 1968.

Dawes, G. S.: Foetal and neonatal physiology. (personal communication from Prichard). Chicago, Year Book Medical Publishers Inc., 1968, p. 165.

Dawes, G. S., Fox, H. E., Leduc, B. M., Liggins, G. C., and Richards, R. T.: Respiratory movements and rapid eye movement sleep in the foetal lamb. J. Physiol. 220:119, 1972.

Dawes, G. S.: Changes in the circulation at birth and the effects of asphyxia. In Gaird-ner, D., (ed.): Recent Advances in Paediatrics. Little Brown & Co., Boston, 1958.

Dawes, G. S., and Mott, J. C.: Reflex respiratory activity in the newborn rabbit. J. Physiol. 145:85, 1959.

Dawes, G. S., and Mott, J. C.: The vascular tone of the foetal lung. J. Physiol. 164:465, 1962.

Dawes, G. S., Hibbard, E., and Windle, W. F.: The effect of alkali and glucose infusion on permanent brain damage in rheus monkeys asphyxiated at birth. J. Pediat. 65:801, 1964.

Dawes, G. S.: Prenatal life: fetal respiratory movements rediscovered. Pediat. 51:965, 1973.

Day, L. R., and Sanford, H. N.: Electrophrenic artificial respiration in newborn. Am. J. Dis. Child. 89:553, 1955.

Day, R., Goodfellow, A. M., Apgar, V., and Beck, G. J.: Pressure-time relations in the safe correction of atelectasis in animal lungs. Pediatrics 10:593, 1952.

De, T.-D., and Anderson, G. W.: Hyaline-like membranes associated with diseases of the newborn lungs: A review of the literature. Obstet. Gynec. Survey 8:1, 1953.

De, T.-D., and Anderson, G. W.: Experimental production of pulmonary hyaline-like membranes with atelectasis. Amer. J. Obstet. Gynec. 68:1557, 1954.

DeBakey, M., Arey, J. B., and Brunazzi, R.: Successful removal of lower accessory lung. J. Thorac. Surg. 19:304, 1950.

DeCarlo, J., Tramer, A., and Startzman, H. H.: Iodized oil aspiration in the newborn. Am. J. Dis. Child. 84:442, 1952.

Dejours, P.: La regulation de la ventilation au cours, de l'exercice musculaire chez l'homme. J. Physiol. (Paris) 51:163, 1959.

deLemos, R., Wolfsdorf, J., Nachman, R., Block, A. J., Leiby, G., Wilkinson, H., Allen, T.,

Haller, J. A., Morgan, W., and Avery, M. E.: Lung injury from oxygen in lambs. Anesthesiology 30:609, 1969.

deLemos, R. A., Shermeta, D. W., Knelson, J. H., Kotas, R., and Avery, M. E.: Acceleration of appearance of pulmonary surfactant in the fetal lamb by administration of corticosteroids. Amer. Rev. Resp. Dis. 102:459, 1970.

Delivoria-Papadopoulos, M., and Swyer, P. R.: Assisted ventilation in terminal hyaline membrane disease. Arch. Dis. Child. 39:481, 1964.

Delivoria-Papadopoulos, M., Roncevic, N. P., and Oski, F. A.: Post-natal changes in oxygen transport of term, premature, and sick infants: the role of red cell 2,3 diphosphoglycerate and adult hemoglobin. Pediat. Res. 5:235, 1971.

deLorimier, A. A., Tierney, D. F., and Parker, H. R.: Hypoplastic lungs in fetal lambs with surgically produced congenital diaphragmatic hernia. Surgery 62:12, 1967.

Deming, J., and Washburn, A. J.: Respiration in infancy. Am. J. Dis. Child. 49:108, 1935.

DeMuth, G. R., and Sloan, H.: Congenital lobar emphysema: Long-term effects and sequelae in treated cases. Surgery 59:601, 1966.

Desmond, M. M., Moore, J., Lindley, J. E., and Brown, C. A.: Meconium staining of the amniotic fluid. A marker of fetal hypoxia. Obstet. Gynec. 9:91, 1957.

Desmond, M. M., Kay, J. L., and Megarity, A. L.: The phases of "transitional distress" occurring in neonates in association with prolonged umbilical cord pulsations. J. Pediat. 55:131, 1959.

Devi, B., and More, J. R. S.: Total tracheopulmonary agenesis. Acta Paed. 55:107, 1965.

Diab, A. E., and Abu-Jaudeh, C. H.: Respiratory distress in infancy. Ann. Otol. 66:198, 1957.

Diamond, E. E., and DeYoung, V. R.: Treatment of neonatal idiopathic respiratory distress syndrome with chlorpromazine. Illinois Med. J. 124:538, 1963.

Dick, F., and Pund, E. R.: Asphyxia neonatorum and the vernix membrane. A.M.A. Arch. Path. (Chicago) 47:307, 1949.

Dietel, K., and Dietel, V.: Intrauterine Atemformen. Ztschr. Kinderh. 79:203, 1957.

DiGeorge, A. M.: Congenital absence of the thymus. J. Pediat. 67:907, 1965.

Dinwiddie, R., and Russell, G.: Relationship of intraesophageal pressure to intrapleural pressure in the newborn. J. Appl. Physiol. 33:415, 1972.

Doershuk, C. F., Downs, T. D., Matthews, L. W., and Lough, M. D.: A method for ventilatory measurements in subjects 1 month – 5 years of age. Normal results and observations in disease. Pediat. Res. 4:165, 1970.

Donald, I., and Steiner, R. E.: Radiography in the diagnosis of hyaline membrane. Lancet 2:846, 1953.

Donald, I.: Augmented respiration: An emergency positive-pressure patient-cycled respirator. Lancet 1:895, 1954.

Doolittle, W. M., Ohmart, D., and Egan, E. A.: Congenital bilateral pleural effusions. Am. J. Dis. Child. 125:435, 1973.

Downes, J. J., Striker, T. W., and Stool, S.: Complications of nasotracheal intubation in children with croup. New Eng. J. Med. 274:226, 1966.

Dripps, R. D., and Comroe, J. H.: The effect of the inhalation of high and low oxygen concentrations on respiration, pulse rate, ballistocardiogram and arterial oxygen saturation (oximeter) of normal individuals. Am. J. Physiol. 149:277, 1947.

Driscoll, S. G., Benirschke, K., and Curtis, G. W.: Neonatal deaths among infants of diabetic mothers. Am. J. Dis. Child. 100:818, 1960.

Driscoll, S. G., Gorbach, A., and Feldman, D.: Congenital listeriosis: Diagnosis from placental studies. Obstet. Gynec. 20:216, 1962.

Driscoll, S. G., and Smith, C. A.: Neonatal pulmonary disorders. Pediat. Clin. N. Amer. 9:325, 1962.

Drorbaugh, J. E., and Fenn, W. O.: A barometric method for measuring ventilation in newborn infants. Pediatrics 16:81, 1955.

Drorbaugh, J. E., Segal, S., Sutherland, J. M., Oppe, T. E., Cherry, R. B., and Smith, C. A.: Compliance of lung during first week of life. Am. J. Dis. Child. 105:63, 1963.

DuBois, A. B., Botelho, S. Y., Bedell, G. N., Marshall, R., and Comroe, J. H., Jr.: A rapid plethysmographic method for measuring thoracic gas volume: A comparison with a nitrogen washout method for measuring functional residual capacity in normal subjects. J. Clin. Invest. 35:322, 1956.

Ducharme, J. C., Bertrand, R., and Debie, J.: Perforation of the pharynx in the newborn: a condition mimicking esophageal atresia. Canad. Med. Assoc. J. 104:785, 1971.

Dunbar, J. S., MacEwen, D. W., and Nogrady, M. B.: Laryngomalacia. Abstract. X International Congress of Radiology, p. 196, 1962.

Dunbar, J. S.: Upper respiratory tract obstruction in infants and children. Amer. J. Roentgen. 109:227, 1970.

Dunbar, J. S., Skinner, G. B., Wortzman, G., and Stuart, J. R.: An investigation of effects of opaque media on the lungs with comparison of barium sulfate, lipiodol and Dionosil. Amer. J. Roentgen. 82:902, 1959.

Dunn, P. M.: Respiratory distress syndrome: Immaturity versus prematurity. Arch. Dis. Child. 40:62, 1965.

Dunnill, M. S.: Postnatal growth of the lung. Thorax 17:329, 1962.

Duran-Jorda, F., Holzel, A., and Patterson, W. H.: A histochemical study of pulmonary hyaline membrane. Arch. Dis. Child. 31:113, 1956.

Dvorak, A. M., and Gavaller, B.: Congenital systemic candidiasis. New Eng. J. Med. 274:540, 1966.

Earle, R., Jr.: Hazards to health. Congenital salicylate intoxication. Report of a case. N. Eng. J. Med. 265:1003, 1961.

Ebel, Kl.-D., and Fendel, H.: The roentgen changes of pneumocystis pneumonia and their anatomic basis. Progr. Pediat. Radiol. 1:177, 1967.

Ebner, H.: Treatment of respiratory distress of the newborn with human fibrinolysin. Rhode Island Med. J. 44:89, 1961.

Edwards, J.: Malformations of the aortic arch system manifested as "vascular rings." Lab. Invest. 2:56, 1953.

Eichenwald, H. F., and Shinefield, H. R.: Viral infections of the fetus and of the premature and newborn infant. Advances Pediat. XII:249, 1962.

Eklof, O., Lohr, G., and Okmian, L.: Submucosal perforation of the esophagus in the neonate. Acta Radiol. 8:187, 1969.

El-Bardeesy, M. W., and Johnson, A. M.: Serum proteinase inhibitors in infants with hyaline membrane disease. J. Pediat. 81:579, 1972.

Eldrige, F. L., Hultgren, H. N., and Wigmore, M. E.: The physiologic closure of the ductus arteriosus in the newborn infant. J. Clin. Invest. 34:987, 1955.

Eliot, M. M.: Deaths around birth—the national score. J. A. M. A. 167:945, 1958.

Elliott, F. M., and Reid, L.: Some new facts about the pulmonary artery and its branching pattern. Clin. Radiol. 16:193, 1965.

Ellis, F. H., Kirklin, J. W., Hodgson, J. R., Woolner, L. B., and Dushane, J. W.: Surgical implications of the mediastinal shadow in thoracic roentgenograms of infants and children. Surg. Gynec. Obstet. 100:532, 1955.

Ellis, K., and Nadelhaft, J.: Roentgenographic findings in hyaline membrane disease in infants weighing 2000 grams and over. Amer. J. Roentgen. 78:444, 1957.

Emerson, C. P.: Pneumothorax, a historical, clinical, and experimental study. Bull. Hopkins Hosp. 11:1, 1903.

Emery, J. L.: Interstitial emphysema, pneumothorax, and "air-block" in the newborn. Lancet 1:405, 1956.

Emmanouilides, G. C., Moss, A. J., Duffie, E. R., and Adams, F. H.: Pulmonary arterial pressure changes in human newborn infants from birth to 3 days of age. J. Pediat. 65:327, 1964.

Emmanouilides, G. C., and Hoy, R. C.: Transumbilical aortography and selective arteriography in newborn infants. Pediatrics 39:337, 1967.

Emmanouilides, G. C., and Moss, A. J.: Respiratory distress in the newborn: effect of cord clamping before and after the onset of respiration. Biol. Neonate 18:363, 1971.

Engel, S.: The Child's Lung. Edward Arnold & Co., London, 1947.

Enhorning, G., and Adams, F. H.: Surface properties of fetal lamb tracheal fluid. Amer. J. Obstet. Gynec. 92:563, 1965.

Eraklis, A. J., Griscom, N. T., and McGovern, J. B.: Bronchogenic cysts of the mediastinum in infancy. New Eng. J. Med. 281:1150, 1969.

Esterly, J. R., and Oppenheimer, E. H.: Massive pulmonary hemorrhage in the newborn. I. Pathologic considerations. J. Pediat. 69:3, 1966.

Evans, H. E., Keller, S., and Mandl, I.: Serum trypsin inhibitory capacity and the idiopathic respiratory distress syndrome. J. Pediat. 81:588, 1972.

Eve, F. C., and Forsyth, N. C.: Asphyxia of the newborn treated by rocking. Brit. Med. J. 2:554, 1948.

Everett, N. B., and Simmons, B. S.: The magnitude of increase in the pulmonary blood volume of the postnatal guinea pig. Anat. Rec. 119:429, 1954.

Farber, S., and Sweet, L. K.: Amniotic sac contents in the lungs of infants. Am. J. Dis. Child. 42:1372, 1931.

Farber, S., and Wilson, J. L.: The hyaline membrane in the lungs. I. A descriptive study. A. M. A. Arch. Path. *14*:437, 1932.

Farber, S., and Wilson, J.: Atelectasis of the new-born. A study and critical review. Am. J. Dis. Child. *46*:572, 1933.

Farber, S.: Studies on pulmonary edema. I. The consequences of bilateral cervical vagotomy in the rabbit. J. Exp. Med. *66*:397, 1937.

Farrell, P. M., and Zachman, R. D.: Enhancement of lecithin synthesis and phosphorylcholine glyceride transferase activity in the fetal rabbit lung after corticosteroid administration (abstract). Pediat. Res. *6*:337, 1972.

Fauré-Fremiet, E., and Dragoiu, J.: Le développement du poumon foetal chez le mouton. Arch. Anat. Microscop. *19*:411, 1923.

Fawcitt, J., Lind, J., and Wegelius, C.: The First Breath. Acta Paediat. (Suppl. 123) *49*:5, 1960.

Fedrick, J.: Comparison of birth weight/gestation distribution in cases of stillbirth and neonatal death according to lesions found at necropsy. Brit. Med. J. *3*:745, 1969.

Fedrick, J., and Butler, N. R.: Hyaline membrane disease. Lancet *II*:768, 1972.

Feinberg, S. B., and Goldberg, M. E.: Hyaline membrane disease: Preclinical roentgen diagnosis; a planned study. Radiology *68*:185, 1957.

Feingold, M. J., Katzew, H., Genieser, N. B., and Becker, M. H.: Lung structure in thoracic dystrophy. Am. J. Dis. Child. *122*:153, 1971.

Feldman, W., Drummond, K. N., and Klein, M.: Hyponatremia following asphyxia neonatorum. Acta Paediat. Scand. *59*:52, 1970.

Felman, A. H., and Talbert, J. L.: Laryngotracheoesophageal cleft. Description of a combined laryngoscopic and roentgenographic diagnostic technique and report of two patients. Radiology *103*:641, 1972.

Felman, A. H., Rhatigan, R. M., and Pierson, K. K.: Pulmonary lymphangectasia observation in 17 patients and proposed classification. Amer. J. Roentgen. Rad. Ther. Nucl. Med. *116*:548, 1972.

Felson, B.: Pulmonary agenesis and related anomalies. Sem. Roentgen. 7:17, 1972.

Felson, B., and Palayew, M. J.: The two types of right aortic arch. Radiology *81*:745, 1963.

Felson, B.: Fundamentals of Chest Roentgenology. W. B. Saunders Co., Philadelphia, 1960.

Felts, J. M.: Carbohydrate and lipid metabolism of lung tissue in vitro. Med. Thorac. *22*:89, 1965.

Fendel, H.: Radiation problems in roentgen examinations of the chest. Progr. Pediat. Radiol. *1*:18, 1967.

Fenton, A. N., and Steer, C. M.: Fetal Distress. Amer. J. Obstet. Gynec. 83:354, 1962.

Ferencz, C.: Congenital abnormalities of pulmonary vessels and their relation to malformations of the lung. Pediatrics 28:993, 1961.

Ferris, B. G., and Pollard, D. S.: Effect of deep and quiet breathing on pulmonary compliance in man. J. Clin. Invest. 39:143, 1960.

Finegold, M. J., Katzew, H., Genieser, N. B., and Becker, M. H.: Lung structure in thoracic dystrophy. Amer. J. Dis. Child. *122*:153, 1971.

Fischer, H. W., Potts, W. J., and Holinger, P. H.: Lobar emphysema in infants and children. J. Pediat. *41*:403, 1952.

Fischer, H. W., Lucido, J. L., and Lynxwiler, C. P.: Lobar emphysema. J. A. M. A. *166*:340, 1958.

Flake, C. G., and Ferguson, C. E.: Congenital choanal atresia in infants and children. Ann. Otol. 73:458, 1964.

Flamm, H.: Die pränatalen Infektionen des Menschen. Georg Thieme Verlag, Stuttgart, 1959.

Fleming, W. H., Szakacs, J. E., Hartney, T. C., and King, E. R.: Hyaline membrane following total body irradiation: relation to lung plasminogen activator. Lancet *II*:1010, 1960.

Fletcher, B. D., Sachs, B. F., and Kotas, R. V.: Radiologic demonstration of post-natal liquid in the lungs of newborn lambs. Pediatrics *46*:252, 1970.

Fletcher, B. D., Outerbridge, E. W., and Dunbar, J. S.: Pulmonary interstitial emphysema in the newborn. J. Canad. Assoc. Radiol. *21*:273, 1970.

Fletcher, B. D., and Taeusch, H. W., Jr.: Radiologic prediction of lung maturity in newborn lambs. Invest. Radiol. 7:378, 1972.

Fletcher, B. D., Outerbridge, E. W., and Stern, L.: Radiologic findings in mechanically ventilated survivors of neonatal respiratory failure. Ann. Radiol. *16*:78, 1973.

Fliegel, C. P., and Kaufmann, H. J.: Problems caused by pneumothorax in congenital diaphragmatic hernia. Ann. Radiol. *15*:159, 1972.

Flowers, C. E., Donnelly, J. F., Creadrick, R. N., Greenberg, B. G., and Wells, H. B.: Spontaneous rupture of the membranes. Amer. J. Obstet. Gynec. 76:761, 1958.

Forbes, G. B.: Chylothorax in infancy. J. Pediat. 25:191, 1944.

Fraillon, J. M. G., and Kitchen, W. H.: The relationship between serum protein levels and hyaline membrane disease in premature babies. Med. J. Austr., Dec. 15, 1962, p. 941.

Frank, J., and Piper, P. G.: Congenital pulmonary cystic lymphangiectasis. J. A. M. A. *171*:1094, 1959.

Frank, M. M., and Gatewood, O. M. B.: Transient pharyngeal incoordination in the newborn. Am. J. Dis. Child. *111*:178, 1966.

Franken, E. A., and Buehl, I.: Infantile lobar emphysema. Report of two cases with unusual roentgenographic manifestation. Am. J. Roent. 98:354, 1966.

Franken, E. A., Jr.: Pneumomediastinum in newborn with associated dextroposition of the heart. Amer. J. Roentgen. *109*:252, 1970.

Fraser, R. G., and Paré, J. A. P.: Roentgenologic signs in the diagnosis of chest disease. An integrated study based on the abnormal roentgenogram. *In* Diagnosis of Diseases of the Chest. Philadelphia, W. B. Saunders Co., 1970.

Freeman, L. C., and Scott, R. B.: Gastric suction in infants delivered by cesarean section: Role in prevention of respiratory complications. Am. J. Dis. Child. 87:570, 1954.

French, J. W., Morgan, B. C., and Guntheroth, W. G.: Infant monkeys—a model for crib death. Amer. J. Dis. Child. *123*:480, 1972.

Friedman, W. F., Pool, P. E., Jacobowitz, D., Seagren, S. C., and Braunwald, E.: Sympathetic innervation of the developing rabbit heart. Circ. Res. 23:25, 1968.

Gairdner, D., (ed.): Respiratory distress syndrome. *In* Recent Advances in Paediatrics, 3rd ed., Little, Brown & Co., Boston, 1965.

Gajdusek, D. C.: Pneumocystic carinii—etiologic agent of plasma cell pneumonia of premature and young infants. Pediatrics *19*:543, 1957.

Galina, M. P., Avnet, M. L., and Einhorn, A.: Iodides during pregnancy. New Eng. J. Med. *267*:1124, 1962.

Gamsu, G., Platzker, A., Gregory, G., Graf, P., and Nadel, J. A.: Powdered tantalum as a contrast agent for tracheobronchography in the pediatric patient. Radiology 107: *151*, 1973.

Gandy, G. M., Adamsons, K., Jr., Cunningham, N., Silverman, W. A., and James, L. S.: Thermal environment and acid-base homeostasis in human infants during the first few hours of life. J. Clin. Invest. *43*:751, 1964.

Gandy, G., Grann, L., Cunningham, N., Adamsons, K., Jr., and James, L. S.: The validity of pH and P_{CO_2} measurements in capillary samples in sick and healthy newborn infants. Pediatrics 34:192, 1964.

Gans, S. L., and Potts, W. J.: Anomalous lobe of lung arising from the esophagus. J. Thorac. Surg. *21*:313, 1951.

Gates, G. F., Dore, E. K., and Kanchanapoom, V.: Thoracic duct leakage in neonatal chylothorax visualized by 198 Au Lymphangiography. Radiology *105*:619, 1972.

Geiger, J. P., O'Connell, T. J., Jr., Carter, S. C., Gomez, A. C., and Aronstam, E. M.: Laryngotracheal-esophageal cleft. J. Thorac. Cardiovasc. Surg. 59:330, 1970.

Gellis, S. S., White, P., and Pfeffer, W.: Gastric suction: A proposed additional technic for the prevention of asphyxia of infants delivered by cesarean section. N. Eng. J. Med. *240*:533, 1949.

Genereux, G. P.: Bronchial atresia: a rare cause of unilateral lung hypertranslucency. J. Canad. Assoc. Radiol. 22:71, 1971.

Gerle, R. D., Jaretzki, A., III, Ashley, C. A., and Berne, A. S.: Congenital bronchopulmonary-foregut malformation: pulmonary sequestration communicating with the gastrointestinal tract. New Eng. J. Med. 278:1413, 1968.

Gershanik, J. J.: Neonatal pneumopericardium. Amer. J. Dis. Child. *121*:438, 1971.

Gersony, W. M.: Persistence of the fetal circulation. A commentary. J. Pediat. 82:1103, 1973.

Geubelle, F., Karlberg, P., Koch, G., Lind, J., Wallgren, G., and Wegelius, C.: L'aeration du poumon chez nouveau-né. Biol. Neonat. *1*:169, 1959.

Giammalvo, J. T.: Congenital lymphangiomatosis of lung: A form of cystic disease; report of case with autopsy findings. Lab. Invest. *4*:450, 1955.

Giannopoulos, G., Mulay, S., and Solomon, S.: Cortisol receptors in rabbit fetal lung. Biochem. Biophys. Res. Commun. 47:411, 1972.

Gil, J., and Weibel, E. R.: Improvements in demonstration of lining layer of lung alveoli by electron microscopy. Resp. Physiol. 8:13, 1969/70.

Girdany, B. R., Sieber, W. K., and Osman, M. Z.: Traumatic pseudodiverticulums of the pharynx in newborn infants. New Eng. J. Med. 280:237, 1969.

Gitlin, D., and Craig, J. M.: Nature of the hyaline membrane in asphyxia of the newborn. Pediatrics 17:64, 1956.

Glasgow, J. F. T., Flynn, D. M., and Swyer, P. R.: A comparison of descending aortic and "arterialized" capillary blood in the sick newborn. Canad. Med. Assoc. J. 106:660, 1972.

Glatt, B. S., and Rowe, R. D.: Cerebral arteriovenous fistula associated with congestive heart failure in the newborn. Pediatrics 26:596, 1960.

Gluck, L., Wood, H. F., and Fousek, M.: Septicemia of the newborn. Pediat. Clin. N. Amer. 13:1131, 1966.

Gluck, L., Kulovich, M. V., Borer, R. C., Brenner, P. H., Anderson, C. G., and Spellacy, W. N.: Diagnosis of the respiratory distress syndrome by amniocentesis. Amer. J. Obstet. Gynec. 109:440, 1971.

Gluck, L., Kulovich, M. V., Eidelman, A. I., Cordero, L., and Khazin, A. F.: Biochemical development of surface activity in mammalian lung. IV. Pulmonary lecithin synthesis in the human fetus, and newborn and etiology of the respiratory distress syndrome. Pediat. Res. 6:81, 1972.

Gluck, L., Motoyama, E. K., Smits, H. L., and Kulovich, M. V.: II. The biochemical development of surface activity in mammalian lung. I. The surface-active phospholipids; the separation and distribution of surface-active lecithin in the lung of the developing rabbit fetus. Pediat. Res. 1:237, 1967.

Gluck, L., Sribney, M., and Kulovich, M.: The biochemical development of surface activity in mammalian lung. II. The biosynthesis of phospholipids in the lung of the developing rabbit fetus and newborn. II. Pediat. Res. 1:247, 1967.

Goetz, O.: Die Ätiologie der interstitiellen sogenannten plasmazellulärem. Pneumonie des Jungen Säuglings. Arch. Kinderh. 163:1, 1960. (Beiherft 41.)

Goldberg, S. J., Levy, R. A., Siassi, B., and Betten, J.: The effects of maternal hypoxia and hyperoxia upon the neonatal pulmonary vasculature. Pediatrics 48:528, 1971.

Goldbloom, R. B., and Dunbar, J. S.: Calcification of cartilage in the trachea and larynx in infancy associated with congenital stridor. Pediatrics 26:669, 1960.

Goldring, D., Behrer, R., Brown, G., and Elliott, G.: Rheumatic pneumonitis. J. Pediat. 53:547, 1958.

Gomez, M. F., and Graven, S. N.: The use of fibrinolysin in the treatment of respiratory distress syndrome. Pediatrics 34:877, 1964.

Gomez, M. R., Whitten, C. F., Nolke, A., Bernstein, J., and Meyer, J. S.: Aneurysmal malformation of the great vein of Galen causing heart failure in early infancy. Pediatrics 31:400, 1963.

Gonzalez-Crussi, F., and Boston, R. W.: The absorptive function of the neonatal lung. Amer. J. Obstet. Gynec. 106:597, 1970.

Gooding, C. A., Gregory, G. A., Taber, P., and Wright, R. R.: An experimental model for the study of meconium aspiration of the newborn. Radiology 100:137, 1971.

Gooding, C. A., and Gregory, G. A.: Roentgenographic analysis of meconium aspiration of the newborn. Radiology 100:131, 1971.

Goodlin, R. C., and Rudolph, A. M.: Tracheal fluid flow and function in fetuses in utero. Lab. Invest. 26:114, 1972.

Goodpasture, E. W., Auerbach, S. H., Swanson, H. S., and Cotter, E. F.: Virus pneumonia of infants secondary to epidemic infections. Am. J. Dis. Child. 57:997, 1939.

Gosselin, O.: Contribution à l'étude de l'invasion des organismes maternal et foetal par les microbes des voies génitales inférierures au cours du travail. Vaillant-Carmanne, S. A., Liège, 1945.

Grady, R. C., and Zuelzer, W. W.: Neonatal tuberculosis. Am. J. Dis. Child. 90:381, 1955.

Graham, B. D., Reardon, H. S., Wilson, J. L., Asao, M. U., and Baumann, M. L.: Physiologic and chemical response of premature infants to oxygen-enriched atmosphere. Pediatrics 6:55, 1950.

Graham, F. K., Caldwell, B. M., Ernhart, C. B., Pennoger, M. M., and Hartmann, A. F.: Anoxia as a significant perinatal experience: A critique. J. Pediat. 50:556, 1957.

Graven, S. N., and Misenheimer, H. R.: Respiratory distress syndrome and the high risk mother. Am. J. Dis. Child. *109*:489, 1965.

Gray, J. S.: Pulmonary ventilation and its physiological regulation. Chas. C Thomas, Springfield, 1950.

Greenspan, R. H., Simon, A. L., Ricketts, H. J., Rojas, R. H., and Watson, J. C.: In vivo magnification angiography. Invest. Radiol. 2:419, 1967.

Greer, M., and Schotland, M.: Myasthenia gravis in the newborn. Pediatrics *26*:101, 1960.

Gregg, R. H., and Bernstein, J.: Pulmonary hyaline membranes and the respiratory distress syndrome. Am. J. Dis. Child. *102*:871, 1961.

Gregory, G. A., Kitterman, J. A., Phibbs, R. H., Tooley, W. H., and Hamilton, W. K.: Treatment of idiopathic respiratory distress syndrome with continuous positive airway pressure. New Eng. J. Med. *284*:1333, 1971.

Gregory, G. A., and Kitterman, J. A.: Pneumotachygraph for use with infants during spontaneous or assisted ventilation. J. Appl. Physiol. *31*:766, 1971.

Gregory, G. A.: Respiratory care of newborn infants. Pediat. Clin. N. Amer. *19*:311, 1972.

Gregory, G. A., and Tooley, W. H.: Gas embolism in hyaline membrane disease. New Eng. J. Med. *282*:1141, 1970.

Gribetz, I., Frank, N. R., and Avery, M. E.: Static volume-pressure relations of excised lungs of infants with hyaline membrane disease, newborn and stillborn infants. J. Clin. Invest. *38*:2168, 1959.

Griscom, N. T.: Harris, G. B. C., Wohl, M. E. B., Vawter, G. F., and Eraklis, A. J.: Fluid-filled lung due to airway obstruction in the newborn. Pediatrics *43*:383, 1969.

Griscom, N. T.: Persistent esophagotrachea: The most severe degree of laryngotracheo-esophageal cleft. Amer. J. Roentgen. 97:211, 1966.

Groll, A.: Anatomische Befunde bei vergifungen mit Phosgen. Virchows Archiv. *231*:48, 1921.

Groniowski, J., and Biczyskowa, W.: The fine structure of the lungs in the course of hyaline membrane disease of the newborn infant. Biol. Neonat. 5:113, 1963.

Grosfeld, J. L., Kilman, J. W., and Frye, T. R.: Spontaneous pneumopericardium in the newborn infant. J. Pediat. 76:614, 1970.

Gross, R. E.: The surgery of infancy and childhood. W. B. Saunders Co., 1953.

Grossman, H., Berdon, W. E., Mizrahi, A., and Baker, D. H.: Neonatal focal hyperaeration of the lungs (Wilson-Mikity syndrome). Radiology 85:409, 1965.

Grossman, H., Winchester, P. H., and Auld, P. A.: Simultaneous frontal and lateral chest roentgenograms on low birth weight infants. Amer. J. Roentgen. *108*:550, 1970.

Grossman, H., Levin, A. R., Winchester, P. H., and Auld, P. A. M.: Pulmonary hypertension in the Wilson-Mikity syndrome. Amer. J. Roentgen. Rad. Ther. Nucl. Med. *114*:293, 1972.

Gruber, H. S., and Klaus, M. H.: Intermittent mask and bag therapy: An alternative approach to respiration therapy for infants with severe respiratory distress. J. Pediat. 76:194, 1970.

Gruenwald, P.: Surface tension as a factor in the resistance of neonatal lungs to aeration. Amer. J. Obstet. Gynec. *53*:996, 1947.

Gruenwald, P.: Degenerative changes in the right half of the liver resulting from intrauterine anoxia. Amer. J. Clin. Path. *19*:801, 1949.

Gruenwald, P.: In Conference on Hyaline Membranes. Fourth M & R Pediatric Research Conf., Ross Laboratories, Columbus, Ohio, 1952.

Gruenwald, P.: Prenatal origin of the respiratory distress (hyaline-membrane) syndrome of premature infants. Letter. Lancet, Jan. 23, 1960, p. 230.

Gruenwald, P., Johnson, R. P., Hustead, R. F., and Clements, J. A.: Correlation of mechanical properties of infants' lungs with surface activity of extracts. Proc. Soc. Exp. Biol. Med. *109*:369, 1962.

Gruenwald, P.: Normal and abnormal expansion of the lungs of newborn infants obtained at autopsy. II. Opening pressure, maximal volume, and stability of expansion. Lab. Invest. *12*:563, 1963.

Gruenwald, P., Nitowsky, H. M., and Siegel, I. A.: Respiratory distress syndrome. N.Y. State J. Med. 63:277, 1963.

Gruenwald, P.: Effect of age on surface properties of excised lungs. Proc. Soc. Exp. Biol. Med. *122*:388, 1966.

Gruenwald, P.: Pulmonary surfactant and stability of aeration in young human fetuses. Pediatrics 38:912, 1966.

Gunther, M.: The transfer of blood between baby and placenta in the minutes after birth. Lancet 1:1277, 1957.

Gupta, J. M.: The effect of THAM on the oxygen tension of arterial blood in neonatal respiratory-distress syndrome. Lancet 1:734, 1965.

Gupta, J. M., Dahlenburg, G. W., and Davis, J. A.: Changes in blood gas tensions following administration of amine buffer (THAM) to infants with respiratory distress syndrome. Arch. Dis. Child. 42:416, 1967.

Guyton, A. C., Crowell, J. W., and Moore, J. W.: Basic oscillating mechanism of Cheyne-Stokes breathing. Am. J. Physiol. 187:395, 1956.

Haight, C.: Congenital tracheoesophageal fistula without esophageal atresia. J. Thorac. Surg. 17:600, 1948.

Haldane, J. S., and Priestley, J. G.: The regulation of lung ventilation. J. Physiol. 32:225, 1905.

Hall, R. J., Nelson, W. P., Blake, H. A., and Geiger, J. P.: Massive pulmonary arteriovenous fistula in the newborn. Circulation 31:762, 1965.

Ham, A. W., and Baldwin, K. W.: Histological study of the development of the lung with particular reference to the nature of alveoli. Anat. Rec. 81:363, 1941.

Han, S. Y., Rudolph, A. J., and Teng, C. T.: Pneumomediastinum in infancy. J. Pediat. 62:754, 1963.

Hanson, J. S., and Shinozaki, T.: Hybrid computer studies of ventilatory distribution and lung volume. I. Normal newborn infants. Pediatrics 46:900, 1970.

Hardy, J. B., Hardy, P. H., Oppenheimer, E. H., Ryan, S. H., Jr., and Sheff, R. N.: Failure of penicillin in a newborn with congenital syphilis. J. Amer. Med. Assoc. 212:1345, 1970.

Harell, G. S., Friedland, G. W., Daily, W. J., and Cohn, R. B.: Neonatal Boerhaave's syndrome. Radiology 95:665, 1970.

Harned, H., MacKinney, L., Rowshan, G., Wolkoff, A., and Sugioka, K.: Relationships of PO_2, PCO_2, and pH to onset of breathing as studied by a cuvette electrode assembly. Abstract. Am. J. Dis. Child. 104:517, 1962.

Harned, H. S., MacKinney, L. G., Berryhill, W. S., and Holmes, C. K.: Effects of hypoxia and acidity on the initiation of breathing in the fetal lamb at term. Am. J. Dis. Child. 112:334, 1966.

Harned, H. S., Griffin, C. A., Berryhill, W. S., MacKinney, L. G., and Sugioka, K.: Role of carotid chemoreceptors in the initiation of effective breathing of the lamb at term. Pediatrics 39:329, 1967.

Harned, H. S., Jr., Herrington, R. T., and Ferreiro, J. I.: The effects of immersion and temperature on respiration in newborn lambs. Pediatrics 45:598, 1970.

Harris, G. B. C.: The newborn with respiratory distress: Some roentgenographic features. Radiol. Clin. N. Amer. 1:497, 1963.

Harris, G. B. C.: Comments to the special treatment article. In Progress in Pediatric Radiology, Vol. I. H. Kaufmann (ed.) Chicago, Year Book, 1967.

Harris, L. E., and Steinberg, A. G.: Abnormalities observed during the first 6 days of life in 8,716 liveborn infants. Pediatrics 14:314, 1954.

Harris, P. D., Neuhauser, E. B. D., and Gerth, R.: The osmotic effect of water soluble contrast media on circulating plasma volume. Amer. J. Roentgen. 91:694, 1964.

Harrison, V. C., Heese, H. de V., and Klein, M.: The significance of grunting in hyaline membrane disease. Pediatrics 41:549, 1968.

Harrison, V. C., Heese, H. de V., and Klein, M.: Intracranial hemorrhage associated with hyaline membrane disease. Arch. Dis. Child. 43:116, 1968.

Hashida, Y., and Sherman, F. E.: Accessory diaphragm associated with neonatal respiratory distress. J. Pediat. 59:529, 1961.

Hatasa, K., and Nakamura, T.: Electron microscopic observations of lung alveolar epithelial cells of normal young mice, with special reference to formation and secretion of osmiophilic lamella bodies. Z. Zellforschung 68:266, 1965.

Hays, D. M., Wooley, M. M., and Snyder, W. H.: Esophageal atresia and tracheoesophageal fistula: management of the uncommon types. J. Pediat. Surg. 1:240, 1966.

Heese, H. deV., Witmann, W., and Malan, A. F.: The management of the respiratory distress syndrome of the newborn with positive-pressure respiration. S. Afr. Med. J. 37:123, 1963.

Heird, W. C., Driscoll, J. M., Schullinger, J. N., Grebin, B., and Winters, R. W.: Intravenous alimentation in pediatric patients. J. Pediat. 80:351, 1972.

Heitzman, E. R., Ziter, F. M., Markarian, B., McClennan, B. L., and Sherry, H. S.: Kerley's interlobular septal lines: Roentgen pathologic correlation. Amer. J. Roentgen. 80:578, 1967.

Heitzman, E. R., and Ziter, F. M., Jr.: Acute interstitial pulmonary edema. Amer. J. Roentgen. 98:291, 1966.

Helmrath, T. A., Hodson, W. A., and Oliver, T. K.: Positive pressure ventilation in the newborn infant: the use of a face mask. J. Pediat. 76:202, 1970.

Helwig, H., Pullmann, H.: Effects of orciprenaline (Alupent) in newborn infants of low birth weight. Z. Kinderheilk. 109:76, 1970.

Hendry, W. S., and Patrick, R. L.: Observations on thirteen cases of pneumocystis carinii pneumonia. Amer. J. Clin. Path. 38:401, 1962.

Hermann, L.: Uber den atelectatischen Zustand der Lungen und dessen Aufhoren bei der Geburt. Arch. ges. Physiol. 20:365, 1879-1880.

Herrington, R. T., Harned, H. S., Jr., Ferreiro, J. I., Griffin, C. A.: The role of the central nervous system in perinatal respiration: studies of chemoregulatory mechanisms in the term lamb. Pediatrics 47:857, 1971.

Hers, J. F. P., Mulder, J., Masurel, N., and Kuip, L. V. D.: Studies on the pathogenesis of influenza virus pneumonia in mice. J. Path. Bact. 83:207, 1962.

Hess, O. W.: Factors influencing perinatal mortality in cesarean section. Amer. J. Obstet. Gynec. 75:376, 1958.

Heymann, M. A., Rudolph, A. M., Nies, A. S., and Melmon, K. L.: Bradykinin production associated with oxygenation of the fetal lamb. Circ. Res. 25:521, 1969.

Heymann, M. A., and Rudolph, A. M.: Effect of exteriorization of the sheep fetus on its cardiovascular function. Circ. Res. 21:741, 1967.

Heymann, M. A., and Rudolph, A. M.: Effects of congenital heart disease on fetal and neonatal circulations. Prog. Cardiovasc. Dis. 15:115, 1972.

Heymans, C.: Chemoreceptors and regulation of respiration. Acta Physiol. Scand. 22:4, 1950.

Himwich, H. E., Bernstein, A. O., Herrlich, H., Chesler, A., and Fazekas, J. F.: Mechanisms for the maintenance of life in the newborn during anoxia. Amer. J. Physiol. 134:387, 1942.

Hobolth, N., Buchmann, G., and Sandberg, L. E.: Congenital choanal atresia. Acta Paediat. Scand. 56:286, 1967.

Hochheim, K.: Ueber einige Befunde in den Lungen von Neugeborenen und die Beziehung derselben zur Aspiration von Fruchtwasser. Centralblatt fur Path. 14:537, 1903.

Hodgman, J. E., Mikity, V. G., Tatter, D., and Cleland, R. S.: Chronic respiratory distress and the premature infant. Wilson-Mikity syndrome. Pediatrics 44:179, 1969.

Hodson, W. A., Chernick, V., and Avery, M. E.: A rebreathing method for measurement of arterial carbon dioxide tension in newborn infants and children. Lancet 1:515, 1966.

Hodson, W. A., Fenner, A., Brumley, G., Chernick, V., and Avery, M. E.: Cerebrospinal fluid and blood acid-base relationships in fetal and neonatal lambs and in pregnant ewes. Resp. Physiol. 5:241, 1968.

Hoffman, J. I. E., Rudolph, A. M., and Danilowicz, D.: Left to right atrial shunts in infancy. Amer. J. Cardiol. 30:868, 1972.

Hoffman, L. E., and Van Mierop, L. H. S.: Effect of epinephrine on heart rate and arterial blood pressure of the developing chick embryo. Pediat. Res. 5:472, 1971.

Hogg, J. C., Williams, J., Richardson, J. B., Macklem, P. T., and Thurlbeck, W. M.: Age as a factor in the distribution of lower airway conductance and in the pathologic anatomy of obstructive lung disease. N. Eng. J. Med. 282:1283, 1970.

Holden, A. M., Fyler, D. C., Shillito, J., Jr., and Nadas, A. S.: Congestive heart failure from intracranial arteriovenous fistula in infancy. Clinical and physiologic considerations in eight patients. Pediatrics 49:30, 1972.

Holden, K. R., and Alexander, F.: Diffuse neonatal hemangiomatosis. Pediatrics 46:411, 1970.

Holder, T. M., and Christy, M. G.: Cystic adenomatoid malformation of the lung. J. Thorac. Cardiov. Surg. 47:590, 1964.

Holinger, P. H., Johnston, K. C., and Zoss, A. R.: Tracheal and bronchial obstruction due to congenital cardio-vascular anomalies. Ann. Otol. 57:808, 1948.

Holinger, P. H., Johnston, K. C., and Schiller, F.: Congenital anomalies of the larynx. Ann. Otol. 63:581, 1954.

Holinger, P. H.: Congenital anomalies of the tracheobronchial tree. Postgrad. Med. 36:454, 1954.

Holzel, A., Bennet, E., and Vaughan, B. F.: Congenital lobar emphysema. Arch. Dis. Child. 31:216, 1956.

Hooper, J. M. D., Evans, I. W. J., and Stapleton, T.: Resting pulmonary water loss in the newborn infant. Pediatrics 13:206, 1954.

Hottinger, A., Kaufmann, H. J., Weisser, K., and Wertheman, A.: Uber eine seltene Lungenerkrankung Fruhgeborener. Ann. Paediat. (Basal) 201:13, 1963.

Howard, P. J., and Bauer, A. R.: Respiration of the Newborn infant. Variation in respiratory minute volume with change in per cent of oxygen in respired mixture. Am. J. Dis. Child. 79:611, 1950.

Howatt, W. F., Avery, M. E., Humphreys, P. W., Normand, I. C. S., Reid, L., and Strang, L. B.: Factors affecting pulmonary surface properties in the foetal lamb. Clin. Sci. 29:239, 1965.

Howatt, W. F., Humphreys, P. W., Normand, I. C. S., and Strang, L. B.: Ventilation of liquid by the fetal lamb during asphyxia. J. Appl. Physiol. 20:496, 1965.

Howie, V. M., and Weed, A. S.: Spontaneous pneumothorax in the first ten days of life. J. Pediat. 50:6, 1957.

Howland, J., and Marriott, W. McK.: Acidosis occurring with diarrhea. Am. J. Dis. Child. 11:309, 1916.

Hudson, P.: Congenital Web of Larynx. Am. J. Dis. Child. 81:545, 1951.

Huggett, A. St. G.: Foetal blood-gas tensions and gas transfusion through the placenta of the goat. J. Physiol. 62:373, 1927.

Humphreys, G. H., Hogg, B. M., and Ferrer, J.: Congenital atresia of esophagus. J. Thorac. Surg. 32:332, 1956.

Humphreys, P. W., Normand, I. C. S., Reynolds, E. O. R., an Strang, L. B.: Pulmonary lymph flow and the uptake of liquid from the lungs of the lamb at the start of breathing. J. Physiol. 193:1, 1967.

Huneycutt, H. C., Anderson, W. R., and Hendry, W. S.: Pneumocystis carinii pneumonia. Case studies with electron microscopy. Am. J. Clin. Path. 41:411, 1964.

Hung, K. S., Hertweck, M. S., Hardy, J. D., and Loosli, C. G.: Innervation of pulmonary alveoli of the mouse lung. An electron microscopic study. Amer. J. Anat. 135:477, 1972.

Hustead, R. F., and Avery, M. E.: Observations of mask pressure achieved with the Kreiselman infant resuscitator. New Eng. J. Med. 265:939, 1961.

Hutchinson, D. L., Hunter, C. B., Neslen, E. B., and Plentl. A. A.: The exchange of water and electrolytes in the mechanism of amniotic fluid formation and the relationship to hydramnios. Surg. Gynec. Obstet. 100:391, 1955.

Hutchison, J. H., Kerr, M. M., McPhail, M. F. M., Douglas, T. A., Smith, G., Norman, J. N., and Bates, E. H.: Studies in the treatment of the pulmonary syndrome of the newborn. Lancet II:465, 1962.

Hutchison, J. H., Kerr, M. M., Williams, K. G., and Hopkinson, W. I.: Hyperbaric oxygen in the resuscitation of the newborn. Lancet II:1019, 1963.

Hryniuk, W., Foerster, J., Shojania, M., and Chow, A.: Cytarabine for herpesvirus infections. J. Amer. Med. Assoc. 219:715, 1972.

Iannaccone, G., Bucci, G., and Savignoni, P. G.: Diagnostic and prognostic value of x-ray findings in respiratory distress syndrome of newborn premature infants. Ann. Radiol. (Paris) 8:237, 1965.

Illingworth, R. S.: Cyanotic attacks in newborn infants. Arch. Dis. Child. 32:328, 1957.

Inall, J. A., Bluhm, M. M., Kerr, M. M., Douglas, T. A., Hope, C. S., and Hutchison, J. H.: Blood volume and hematocrit studies in respiratory distress syndrome of the newborn. Arch. Dis. Child. 40:480, 1965.

Ingalls, T. H.: Epidemiology of retrolental fibroplasia in etiologic relation to pulmonary hyaline membrane. New Eng. J. Med. 251:1017, 1954.

Ingram, D. R., and Poznanski, A. K.: Nasopharyngeal dermoid. Radiology 92:297, 1969.

Jacobson, H. N., Strang, L. B., Cook, C. D., Drinker, P. A., and Levison, H.: Pulmonary blood flow in the fetal and neonatal lamb. Physiologist 5:161, 1962.

James, L. S., Burnard, E. D., and Rowe, R. D.: Abnormal shunting through the foramen ovale after birth. Amer. J. Dis. Child. 102:550, 1961 (abstract).

James, L. S.: Changes in the heart and lungs at birth. J. Pediat. 51:95, 1957.

James, L. S., and Rowe, R. D.: The pattern of response of pulmonary and systemic arterial pressures in newborn and older infants to short periods of hypoxia. J. Pediat. 51:5, 1957.

James, L. S., Weisbort, I. M., Price, C. E., Holaday, D. A., and Apgar, V.: The acid-base status of human infants in relation to birth asphyxia and the onset of respiration. J. Pediat. 52:379, 1958.

James, L. S.: Physiology of respiration in newborn infants and in the respiratory distress syndrome. Pediatrics 24:1069, 1959.

James, L. S., Moya, F., Burnard, E. D., and Apgar, V.: Intragastric administration of oxygen. Lancet 1:737, 1959.

James, L. S., Apgar, V. A., Burnard, E. D., and Moya, F.: Intragastric oxygen and resuscitation of the newborn. Acta Paediat. 52:245, 1963.

James, L. S.: Onset of breathing and resuscitation. Pediat. Clin. N. Amer. 13:621, 1966.

Javett, S. N., Webster, I., and Braudo, J. L.: Congenital dilatation of the pulmonary lymphatics. Pediatrics 31:416, 1963.

Jäykkä, S.: Capillary erection and lung expansion. Acta Paediat. 46: (Suppl. 112) 1957.

Jefft, M.: The radiotherapeutic management of subglottic hemangioma in children. Radiology, 86:207, 1966.

Jeiger, W., Blankenship, W., Lind, J., and Kitchin, A.: The changing circulatory pattern of the newborn infant studied by the indicator dilution technique. Acta. Pediat. 53:541, 1964.

Jeresaty, R. M., Huszar, R. J., and Basu, S.: Pierre Robin syndrome. Cause of respiratory obstruction, cor pulmonale, and pulmonary edema. Amer. J. Dis. Child. 117:710, 1969.

Jeune, M., Carron, R., Berand, C., and Loaec, Y.: Polychondrodystrophie avec blocage thoracique d'evolution fatale. Pediatrie 9:390, 1954.

Johnson, A. L., Wiglesworth, F. W., Dunbar, J. S., Siddoo, S., and Grajo, M.: Infradiaphragmatic total anomalous pulmonary venous connection. Circulation 17:340, 1958.

Johnson, G. H., Brinkman, C. R., and Assali, N. S.: Response of the hypoxic fetal and neonatal lamb to administration of base solution. Amer. J. Obstet. Gynec. 114:914, 1972.

Johnson, J. W. C., and Fariday, E. E.: Respiratory distress in the newborn. Pulmonary mechanics following fluid installation in the lungs of neonatal lambs. Amer. J. Obstet. Gynec. 92:253, 1965.

Johnson, W. C., and Meyer, J. R.: A study of pneumonia in the stillborn and newborn. Amer. J. Obstet. Gynec. 9:151, 1925.

Jones, C. J.: Unusual hamartoma of the lung in a newborn infant. Arch. Path. (Chicago) 48:150, 1949.

Joshi, V. V., Mandavia, S. G., Stern, L., and Wiglesworth, F. W.: Acute lesions induced by endotracheal intubation. Occurrence in the upper respiratory tract of newborn infants with respiratory distress syndrome. Amer. J. Dis. Child. 124:646, 1972.

Jost, A., and Policard, A.: Contribution expérimentale à l'étude du dévelopment du poumon chez le lapin. Arch. Anat. Microsc. 37:323, 1948.

Jue, K. L., Amplatz, K., Adams, P., Jr., and Anderson, R. C.: Anomalies of great vessels associated with lung hypoplasia. The Scimitar syndrome. Am. J. Dis. Child. 111:35, 1966.

Kafer, E. R.: Pulmonary oxygen toxicity. A review of the evidence for acute and chronic oxygen toxicity in man. Brit. J. Anesth. 43:687, 1971.

Kafka, V., Padorcova, H., Kabelka, M., and Kleint, Z.: A congenital arteriovenous pulmonary aneurysm in a two-and-a-half-year-old boy. (Case report and review of the literature). J. Cardiov. Surg. 2:396, 1961.

Kampmeier, O. F.: On the lymph flow of the human heart with reference to the development of the channels and the first appearance, distribution, and physiology of their valves. Am. Heart J. 4:210, 1928.

Kappelman, M. M., Dorst, J., Haller, A., and Stambler, A.: H-type tracheo-esophageal fistula. Amer. J. Dis. Child. 118:568, 1969.

Kapteyn, J. L. T. O., Wolvius, G. G., and Wagenvoort, C. A.: The pulmonary arteries and arterioles in hyaline membrane disease. Arch. Dis. Child. 38:468, 1963.

Karlberg, P., Cook, C. D., O'Brien, D., Cherry, R. B., and Smith, C. A.: Studies of respiratory physiology in the newborn infant: Observations during and after respiratory distress. Acta Paediat. 43:397, 1954.

Karlberg, P.: Physiology of prematurity. *In* Lanman, J. T. (ed.): Trans. 2nd Macy Conference. The Josiah Macy Jr. Foundation, New York, 1957.

Karlberg, P.: The adaptive changes in the immediate postnatal period, with particular reference to respiration. J. Pediat. *56*:585, 1960.

Karlberg, P., Cherry, R. B., Escardó, F., and Köch, G.: Respiratory studies in newborn infants. Acta Paediat. *49*:345, 1960.

Karlberg, P., Cherry, R. B., Escardó, F. E., and Köch, G.: Respiratory studies in newborn infants. II. Pulmonary ventilation and mechanics of breathing in the first minutes of life, including the onset of respiration. Acta Paediat. *51*:121, 1962.

Karlberg, P., Adams, F. H., Geubelle, F., and Wallgren, G.: Alteration of the infant's thorax during vaginal delivery. Acta Obstet. Gynec. Scand. *41*:223, 1962.

Karlberg, P., Moore, R. E., and Oliver, T. K.: The thermogenic response of the newborn infant to noradrenaline. Acta Paediat. *51*:284, 1962.

Karrer, H. E.: The ultrastructure of mouse lung. General architecture of capillary and alveolar walls. J. Biophys. Biochem. Cty. *2*:241, 1956.

Kattwinkel, J., Fleming, D., Cha, C. C., Fanaroff, A. A., and Klaus, M. H.: A device for administration of continuous positive airway pressure by the nasal route. Pediatrics 52:131, 170, 1973.

Kauffman, S. L., and Stout, A. P.: Hemangiopericytoma in children. Cancer *13*:695, 1960.

Kaufman, O. Ya.: Intrauterine development of pulmonary vessels in man. Arkh. Anat. *46*:58, 1964. Fed. Proc. (Transl. Suppl.) *24*:T584, 1965.

Keidan, S. E.: Transient diabetes in infancy. Arch. Dis. Child. *30*:291, 1955.

Keith, J. D.: Congestive heart failure. Pediatrics *18*:491, 1956.

Keith, J. D., Rose, V., Braudo, M., and Rowe, R. D.: The electrocardiogram in the respiratory distress syndrome and related cardiovascular dynamics. J. Pediat. *59*:167, 1961.

Kergin, F. G.: Congenital cystic disease of lung associated with anomalous arteries. J. Thorac. Surg. *23*:55, 1952.

Kesson, C. W.: Asphyxia neonatorum due to a nasopharyngeal teratoma. Arch. Dis. Child. *29*:254, 1954.

Keuth, U.: Das Membransyndrom der Früh-und Neugeborenen. Springer-verlag, Berlin, 1965.

Keuth, U., Razeghi, H., Frisch, H. J., and Bockemuhl, J.: Ungunstiger Effekt von orciprenalin bei Fruh- und Neugeborenen. Mschr. Kinderheilk. *120*:257, 1972.

Kibrick, S.: Myasthenia gravis in the newborn. Pediatrics *14*:365, 1954.

Kidd, L., Levison, H., Gemmel, P., Aharon, A., and Swyer, P. R.: Limb blood flow in the normal and sick newborn. A plethysmographic study. Am. J. Dis. Child. *112*:402, 1966.

Kikkawa, Y., Motoyama, E. K., and Cook, C. D.: The ultrastructure of the lungs of lambs. Am. J. Path. *47*:877, 1965.

Kikkawa, Y., Motoyama, E. K., and Gluck, L.: Study of the lungs of fetal and newborn rabbits, Morphologic, biochemical, and surface physical development. Amer. J. Path. *52*:177, 1968.

Kirkpatrick, J. A., Jr., and DiGeorge, A. M.: Congenital absence of the thymus. Amer. J. Roentgen. *103*:32, 1968.

Kirkpatrick, J. A., Jr., and Capitanio, M. A.: Pulmonary manifestations of systemic diseases in infants. Sem. Roentgen. 7:149, 1972.

Kirkpatrick, J. A., Cresson, S. L., and Pilling, G. P.: The motor activity of the esophagus in association with esophageal atresia and tracheoesophageal fistula. Amer. J. Roentgen. 86:884, 1961.

Kitterman, J. A., Edmunds, L. H., Gregory, G. A., Heymann, M. A., Tooley, W. H., and Rudolph, A. M.: Patent ductus arteriosus in premature infants. New Eng. J. Med. *287*:473, 1972.

Kjellberg, S. R., Rudhe, U., and Zetterstrom, R.: Heart volume variations in the neonatal period. Acta Radiol. *42*:173, 1954.

Klaus, M., Reiss, O. K., Tooley, W. H., Piel, C., and Clements, J. A.: Alveolar epithelial cell mitochondria as a source of the surface-active lung lining. Science *137*:750, 1962.

Klaus, M., Tooley, W. H., Weaver, K. H., and Clements, J. A.: Lung volume in the newborn infant. Pediat. *30*:111, 1962.

Klein, Z. L.: An accessory lobe of lung in a newborn. Pediatrics *45*:118, 1970.

Kleinman, L. I., Sell, J. E., and Petering, H. G.: Carbonic anhydrase isoenzymes in infants with respiratory distress syndrome. Amer. J. Dis. Child. 124:696, 1972.

Knelson, J. H., Howatt, W. F., and deMuth, G. R.: The physiologic significance of grunting respiration. Pediatrics 44:393, 1969.

Kohler, E., and Babbitt, D. P.: Dystrophic thoraces and infantile asphyxia. Radiology 94:55, 1970.

Korngold, H. W., and Baker, J. M.: Nonsurgical treatment of unilobar obstructive emphysema of the newborn. Pediatrics 14:296, 1954.

Kotas, R. V.: Accelerated pulmonary surfactant after intrauterine infection in the fetal rabbit. Pediat. 51:655, 1973.

Kotas, R. V., Fazen, L. E., and Moore, T. E.: Umbilical cord and serum trypsin inhibitor capacity and the idiopathic respiratory distress syndrome. J. Pediat. 81:593, 1972.

Kotas, R. V., and Avery, M. E.: Accelerated appearance of pulmonary surfactant in the fetal rabbit. J. Appl. Physiol. 30:358, 1971.

Kovalcík, V.: The response of the isolated ductus arteriosus to oxygen and anoxia. J. Physiol. 164:185, 1963.

Krauss, A. N., and Auld, P. A. M.: Measurement of mixed venous oxygen tension in premature infants by a rebreathing method. Pediat. Res. 6:158, 1972.

Krauss, A. N., Soodalter, J. A., and Auld, P. A. M.: Adjustment of ventilation and perfusion in the full term normal and distressed neonate as determined by urinary alveolar nitrogen gradients. Pediatrics 47:865, 1971.

Krauss, A. N., Tori, C. A., Brown, J., Soodalter, J., and Auld, P. A. M.: Oxygen chemoreceptors in low birth weight infants. Pediat. Res. 7:569, 1973.

Krieger, I.: Studies on mechanics of respiration in infancy. Am. J. Dis. Child. 105:439, 1963.

Krogh, A.: The Anatomy and Physiology of Capillaries. p. 340, Yale Univ. Press, New Haven, Conn. 1936.

Kuhn, J. P., Fletcher, B. D., and deLemos, R. A.: Roentgen findings in transient tachypnea of the newborn. Radiology 92:751, 1969.

Kuhns, L. R., Poznanski, A. K.: Endotracheal tube position in the infant. J. Pediat. 78: 991, 1971.

Kumode, S.: On pulmonary surface tension of fetal lung in various gestational ages. Acta. Pediat. Jap. 10:51, 1968.

Kuroya, M., and Ishida, N.: Newborn virus pneumonitis (type Sedai). II. Report: The isolation of a new virus possessing hemagglutinin activity. Yokohama Med. Bull. 4:217, 1953.

Kwitten, J., and Reiner, L.: Congenital cystic adenomatoid malformation of the lung. Pediatrics 30:759, 1962.

Landing, B. H.: Pathologic features of the respiratory distress syndromes in newborn infants. Am. J. Roentgen. 74:796, 1955.

Landing, B. H.: Pulmonary lesions of newborn infants. A statistical study. Pediatrics 19:217, 1957.

Lane, S. D., Burko, H., and Scott, H. W.: Congenital bronchopulmonary-foregut malformation. Radiology 101:291, 1971.

Lange, R. L., and Hecht, H. H.: The mechanism of Cheyne-Stokes respiration, J. Clin. Invest. 41:42, 1962.

Langer, L. O., Jr., Spranger, J. W., Greinacher, I., and Herdman, R. C.: Thanatophoric dwarfism. A condition confused with achondroplasia in the neonate, with brief comments on achondrogenesis and homozygous achondroplasia. Radiology 92: 285, 1969.

Langer, L. O., Jr.: Thoracic-pelvic-phalangeal dystrophy. Radiology 91:447, 1968.

Lanman, J. H., Schaffer, A., Herod, L., Ogawa, Y., and Castellanos, R.: Distensibility of the fetal lung with fluid in sheep. Pediat. Res. 5:586, 1971.

Larroche, J. C., Nodot, A., and Minkowski, A.: Développement des artères et artérioles pulmonaries de la période foetale à la période néonatale. Biol. Neonat. 1:37, 1959.

Latham, E. F., Nesbitt, R. E. L., and Anderson, G. W.: A clinical pathological study of newborn lung with hyaline-like membranes. Bull. Hopkins Hosp. 96:173, 1955.

Laumonier, R.: Remarques sur la structure pulmonaire des prématurés. Sem. Hôp. Paris 28:2047, 1952.

Laurence, K. M.: Congenital pulmonary lymphangiectasis. J. Clin. Path. 12:62, 1959.

Lauweryns, J., Bonte, J., and van derSchueren, G.: A haemodynamic study of the syndrome of secondary pulmonary atelectasis. Acta Anat. (Basel). 46:142, 1961.

Lauweryns, J. M., Claessens, S., and Boussauw, L.: The pulmonary lymphatics in neonatal hyaline membrane disease. Pediatrics 41:917, 1968.

Lauweryns, J. M., Eggermont, E., van den Driessche, A., and Denys, P.: L'atelectasie pulmonaire neonatale secondaire avec membranes hyalines. Arch. Franç. Pédiat. 22:5, 1965.

Lauweryns, J. M.: "Hyaline membrane disease" in newborn infants. Macroscopic, radiographic, and light and electron microscopic studies. Human Path. 1:175, 1970.

Laxdal, O. E., McDougall, H., and Mellin, G. W.: Congenital eventration of the diaphragm. N. Eng. J. Med. 250:401, 1954.

Leape, L. L., and Longino, L. A.: Infantile lobar emphysema. Pediatrics 34:246, 1964.

Leape, L. L., Ching, N., and Holder, T. M.: Lobar emphysema and patent ductus arteriosus. Development of emphysema while under observation. Pediatrics 46: 97, 1970.

Ledbetter, M. K., Homma, T., and Farhi, L. E.: Readjustment in distribution of alveolar ventilation and lung perfusion in the newborn. Pediat. 40:940, 1967.

Ledesma, J., and Girdany, B. R.: Congenital lobar emphysema: A case report with a thirty-two year follow-up. Ann. Radiol. 15:181, 1972.

Lee, S. B., and Kuhn, J. P.: Pneumatosis intestinalis following pneumomediastinum in a newborn infant. J. Pediat. 79:813, 1971.

Lendrum, F. C.: The "Pulmonary Hyaline Membrane" as a manifestation of heart failure in the newborn infant. J. Pediat. 47:149, 1955.

Lertzman, M., and Ciner, E.: A rebreathing technique for the estimation of arterial carbon dioxide tension in infants and children with details for use in a routine hospital laboratory. J. Pediat. 67:291, 1965.

Le Tan-Vinh, Cochard, A., and Vu Trieu Dong: Lymphangiectasies pulmonaires congénitales et lymphangite pleuro-pulmonaire cancéreuse métastique de l'enfant. Arch. Franç. Pédiat. 21:165, 1964.

Le Tan-Vinh, G. G.: La pneumonie à pneumocystis: ses rapports avec la pneumonic interstitielle à plasmocytes. Arch. Franç. Pédiat. 11:1035, 1954.

Levine, O. R., Jameson, A. G., Nellhaus, G., and Gold, A. P.: Cardiac complications of cerebral arteriovenous fistula in infancy. Pediatrics 30:563, 1962.

Levine, O. R., and Blumenthal, S.: Digoxin dosage in premature infants. Pediatrics 29:18, 1962.

Levy, J. L., Jr., Guynes, W. A., Jr., Louis, J. E., and Linder, L. H.: Bilateral congenital diaphragmatic hernias through the foramina of Bochdalek. J. Pediat. Surg. 4:557, 1969.

Lewis, A. J., and Besant, D. F.: Muscular dystrophy in infancy. J. Pediat. 60:376, 1962.

Lewis, M. R.: Persistence of the thymus in the cervical area. J. Pediat. 61:887, 1962.

Lewis, S.: A follow-up study of the respiratory distress syndrome. Proc. Roy. Soc. Med. 61:771, 1968.

Lieberman, J.: Clinical syndromes associated with deficient lung fibrinolytic activity. I. New concept of hyaline membrane disease. N. Eng. J. Med. 260:619, 1959.

Lieberman, J.: Clinical syndromes associated with deficient fibrinolytic activity of lung. II. Cystic fibrosis of pancreas. Pediatrics. 25:419, 1960.

Liberman, J.: The nature of the fibrinolytic enzyme defect in hyaline membrane disease. N. Eng. J. Med. 265:363, 1961.

Liggins, G. C.: Premature delivery of foetal lambs infused with glucocorticoids. J. Endocrinal. 45:515, 1969.

Lincoln, J. C. R., Stark, J., Subramanian, S., Aberdeen, E., Bonham-Carter, R. E., Berry, C. L., and Waterston, D. J.: Congenital lobar emphysema. Ann. Surg. 173:55, 1971.

Lind, J., and Wegelius, C.: Human fetal circulation: Changes in the cardiovascular system at birth and disturbances in the post-natal closure of the foramen ovale and ductus arteriosus. Cold Spr. Harb. Symp. Quant. Biol. 19:109, 1954.

Lind, J., and Wegelius, C.: Atrial septal defects in children. Circulation 7:819, 1953.

Lind, J., Stern, L., and Wegelius, C.: The Human Foetal and Neonatal Circulation. Charles C Thomas, Springfield, 1964.

Lind, J., Tähti, E., and Hirvensalo, M.: Roentgenologic studies of the size of the lungs of the newborn baby before and after aeration. Ann. Paediat. Fenn. 12:20, 1966.

Lind, T., Billewicz, W. Z., and Cheyne, G. A.: Composition of amniotic fluid and maternal blood through pregnancy. J. Obstet. Gynaec. Brit. Commonw. 78:505, 1971.

Lind, T., Parkin, F. M., and Cheyne, G. A.: Biochemical and cytological changes in liquor amnii with advancing gestation. J. Obstet. Gynaec. Brit. Commun. 76:673, 1969.

Lipp, J. A. M., and Rudolph, A. M.: Sympathetic nervous development in the rate of guinea pig heart. Biol. Neonate, 21:76, 1972.

Litt, R. E., Mencia, F., and Altman, D. H.: Congenital stenosis of the right mainstem bronchus. Am. J. Roentgen. 89:1017, 1963.

Little, W. J.: The influence of abnormal parturition, difficult labours, premature birth, and asphyxia neonatorum, on the mental and physical condition of the child, especially in relation to deformities. Trans. Obst. Soc. London 3:293, 1861.

Lloyd, B. B., Jukes, M. G. M., and Cunningham, D. J. C.: The relation between alveolar oxygen pressure and the respiratory response to carbon dioxide in man. Quart. J. Exp. Physiol. 43:214, 1958.

Lloyd, J. R., and Clatworthy, H. W.: Hydramnios as an aid to early diagnosis of congenital obstruction of the alimentary tract: A study of the maternal and fetal factors. Pediatrics 21:903, 1958.

Lloyd, T. C., Jr.: Hypoxic pulmonary vasoconstriction: Role of perivascular tissue. J. Appl. Physiol. 25:560, 1968.

Loeb, W. J., and Smith, E. E.: Airway obstruction in a newborn by pedunculated pharyngeal dermoid. Pediatrics 40:20, 1967.

Lofgren, R. H.: Respiratory distress from congenital lingual cysts. Am. J. Dis. Child. 106:610, 1963.

Long, E. C., and Hull, W. E.: Respiratory volume-flow in the crying newborn infant. Pediatrics 27:373, 1961.

Longino, L. A., and Jewett, T. C.: Congenital bifid sternum. Surg. 38:610, 1955.

Loosli, C. G., and Potter, E. L.: Pre- and postnatal development of the respiratory portion of the human lung. Amer. Rev. Resp. Dis. 80:5, 1959.

Love, W. G., and Tillery, B.: New treatment for atelectasis of the newborn. Am. J. Dis. Child. 86:423, 1953.

Low, F. N.: Pulmonary alveolar epithelium of laboratory mammals and man. Anat. Rec. 117:241, 1953.

Low, F. N., and Sampaio, M. M.: The pulmonary alveolar epithelium as an entodermal derivative. Anat. Rec. 127:51, 1957.

Lubchenco, L. O.: Recognition of spontaneous pneumothorax in premature infants. Pediatrics 24:996, 1959.

Lynch, M. J. G., and Mellor, L. D.: Hyaline membrane disease of lungs. J. Pediat. 48:165, 1956.

MacEwan, D. W., Dunbar, J. S., Smith, R. D., and Brown, B. St. J.: Pneumothorax in young infants — recognition and evaluation. J. Can. Assoc. Radiol. 22:264, 1971.

MacKay, R. B.: Observations on the oxygenation of the foetus in normal and abnormal pregnancy. J. Obstet. Gynec. Brit. Emp. 44:185, 1957.

Macklin, C. C.: Pulmonic alveolar epithelium. J. Thorac. Surg. 6:82, 1936.

Macklin, C. C.: Transport of air along sheaths of pulmonic blood vessels from alveoli to mediastinum. A.M.A. Arch. Intern. Med. 64:913, 1939.

Macklin, C. C.: The pulmonary alveolar mucoid film and the pneumonocytes. Lancet I:1099, 1954.

Maguire, G. H.: The larynx: Simplified radiological examination using heavy filtration and high voltage. Radiology 87:102, 1966.

Maier, H. C., and Bortone, F.: Complete failure of sternal fusion with herniation of pericardium. J. Thorac. Surg. 18:851, 1949.

Makepeace, A. W., Fremont-Smith, F., Dailey, M. E., and Carroll, M. D.: The nature of the amniotic fluid. Surg. Gynec. Obst. 53:635, 1931.

Malan, A. F., and Hesse, H. deV.: Spontaneous pneumothorax in the newborn. Acta Paediat. Scand. 55:224, 1966.

Maloney, J. V., and Whittenberger, J. L.: The direct effects of pressure breathing on the pulmonary circulation. Ann. N. Y. Acad. Sci. 66:931, 1957.

Mandelbaum, B., and Evans, T.: Life in the amniotic fluid. Amer. J. Obstet. Gynec. 104:365, 1969.

Mann, T. P., and Elliott, R. I. K.: Neonatal cold injury due to accidental exposure to cold. Lancet I:229, 1957.

Margolis, C. Z., Orzalesi, M. M., and Schwartz, A. D.: Disseminated intravascular coagulation in the respiratory distress syndrome. Am. J. Dis. Child. 125:324, 1973.

Margulies, S. I., Brunt, P. W., Donner, M. W., and Silbiger, M. L.: Familial dysautonomia: A cineradiographic study of the swallowing mechanism. Radiology 90:107, 1968.

Markarian, M., Githens, J. H., Jackson, J. J., Bannon, A. E., Lindley, A., Rosenblut, E., Martorell, R., and Lubchenco, L.: Fibrinolytic activity in premature infants. Relationship of the enzyme system to the respiratory distress syndrome. Am. J. Dis. Child. 113:312, 1967.

Martin, C. M., Kunin, C. M., Gottlieb, L. S., Barnes, M. W., Liu, C., and Finland, M.: Asian Influenza A in Boston 1957-58. I. Observations in thirty-two influenza-associated fatal cases. A. M. A. Arch. Int. Med. 103:515, 1959.

Martin, J. F., and Friedell, H. L.: The roentgen findings in atelectasis of the newborn. Amer. J. Roentgen. 67:905, 1952.

Martin, J. K.: A controlled trial of digoxin in the prevention of the respiratory distress syndrome. Canad. Med. Ass. J. 89:995, 1963.

Mathews, D. H., Avery, M. E., and Jude, J. R.: Closed-chest cardiac massage in the newborn infant. J. A. M. A. 183:964, 1963.

Matsaniotis, N., Karpouzas, J., Tzortzatou-Vallianou, M., and Tsagournis, E.: Aspiration due to difficulty in swallowing. Arch. Dis. Child. 46:788, 1971.

Matthes, F. T., Kirschner, R., Yow, M. D., and Brennan, J. C.: Acute poisoning associated with inhalation of mercury vapor. Pediatrics 22:675, 1958.

Mathis, R. K., Freier, E. F., Hunt, C. E., Krivit, W., and Sharp, H. L.: Alpha-1-antitrypsin in the respiratory distress syndrome. New Eng. J. Med. 288:59, 1973.

McAdams, A. J.: Pulmonary hemorrhage in the newborn. Am. J. Dis. Child. 113:255, 1967.

McAdams, A. J., Coen, R., Kleinman, L. L., Tsang, R., and Sutherland, J.: The experimental production of hyaline membranes in premature rhesus monkeys. Amer. J. Path. 70:277, 1973.

McCracken, G. H., and Jones, L. G.: Gentamicin in the neonatal period. Amer. J. Dis. Child. 120:524, 1970.

McCracken, G. H.: Changing pattern of the antimicrobial susceptibilities of Escherichia Coli in neonatal infections. J. Pediat. 78:942, 1971.

McCue, C. M., Robertson, L. W., Lester, R. G., and Mauck, H. P., Jr.: Pulmonary artery coarctations. J. Pediat. 67:222, 1965.

McDonald, I. H., and Stocks, J. G.: Prolonged nastotracheal intubation. Brit. J. Anaesth. 37:161, 1965.

McHugh, H. E., and Loch, W. E.: Congenital webs of the larynx. Laryngoscope 52:43, 1942.

McKay, E., and Richardson, J.: Pneumocystis carinii pneumonia associated with hypogammaglobulinemia. Lancet II:713, 1959.

McKendry, J. B. J., Lindsay, W. K., and Gerstein, M. C.: Congenital defects of the lymphatics in infancy. Pediatrics 19:22, 1957.

McLain, C. R.: Amniography: A versatile diagnostic procedure in obstetrics. Obstet. Gynec. 23:45, 1964.

McNamara, T. O., Gooding, C. A., Kaplan, S. L., and Clark, R. E.: Exomphalos-macroglossia-gigantism (visceromegaly) syndrome (the Beckwith-Wiedemann syndrome). Amer. J. Roentgen. 114:264, 1972.

Mead, J., Whittenberger, J. L., and Radford, E. P.: Surface tension as a factor in pulmonary volume-pressure hysteresis. J. Appl. Physiol. 10:191, 1957.

Mead, J., and Gaensler, E. A.: Esophageal and pleural pressures in man, upright and supine. J. Appl. Physiol. 14:81, 1959.

Mead, J., and Collier, C.: Relation of volume history of lungs to respiratory mechanics in anesthetized dogs. J. Appl. Physiol. 14:669, 1959.

Medovy, H., and Beckman, J. H.: Asphyxial attacks in the newborn infant due to congenital occlusion of the posterior nares. Report of five cases. Pediatrics 8:678, 1951.

Mentesti, P.: The protein pattern of the amniotic fluid; determination with free microelectrophoresis. II. In pathological obstetrics. Minerva Ginec. 11:552, 1959.

Meschan, I., Marvin, H. N., Gordon, V. H., and Regnier, G.: The radiographic appearances of hyaline disease of the lungs in the newborn. Radiology 60:383, 1953.

Meschia, G., Cotter, J. R., Barron, D. H., and Breathnach, C. S.: Haemoglobin, oxygen, carbon dioxide and hydrogen ion concentrations in the umbilical bloods of sheep and goats as sampled via indwelling plastic catheters. Quart. J. Exp. Physiol. 50:185, 1965.

Mikity, V., Hodgman, J. E., and Tatter, D.: The radiological findings in delayed pulmonary maturation in premature infants. Progr. Pediat. Radiol. 1:149, 1967.

Millen, R. S., and Davies, J.: See-saw resuscitation for the treatment of asphyxia in the newborn. Amer. J. Obstet. Gynec. 52:508, 1946.

Millen, R. S., Rowsom, A. F., Mayberger, H. W.: Prevention of neonatal asphyxia with the use of a rocking resuscitator. Amer. J. Obstet. Gynec. 70:1087, 1955.

Miller, C. A., and Reed, H. R.: The relation of serum concentrations of bilirubin to respiratory function of premature infants. Pediatrics 21:362, 1958.

Miller, H. C., and Hamilton, T. R.: The pathogenesis of the "vernix Membrane." Relation to aspiration pneumonia in stillborn and newborn infants. Pediatrics 3:735, 1949.

Miller, H. C., and Jennison, M. H.: Study of pulmonary hyaline-like material in 4117 consecutive births. Incidence, pathogenesis, diagnosis. Pediatrics 5:7, 1950.

Miller, H. C., Behrle, F. C., and Gibson, D. M.: Comparison of pulmonary hyaline membranes in vagotomized rabbits with those in newborn infants. Pediatrics 7:611, 1951.

Miller, H. C.: Effect of high concentration of carbon dioxide and oxygen on the respiration of full term infants. Pediatrics 14:104, 1954.

Miller, H. C., and Behrle, F. C.: The effect of hypoxia on the respiration of newborn infants. Pediatrics 14:93, 1954.

Miller, H. C., and Conklin, E. V.: Clinical evaluation of respiratory insufficiency in newborn infants. Pediatrics 16:427, 1955.

Miller, H. C., and Behrle, F. C.: Changing patterns of respiration in newborn infants. Pediatrics 22:665, 1958.

Miller, H. C., Behrle, F. C., and Smull, N. W.: Apnea and irregular respiratory rhythms among premature infants. Pediatrics 23:676, 1959.

Miller, H. C.: Respiratory distress syndrome of newborn infants. II. Clinical study of pathogenesis. J. Pediat. 61:9, 1962.

Miller, J. A.: In Windle, W. F. (ed.): Neurological and Psychological Deficits of Asphyxia Neonatorum, p. 105. Chas. C Thomas, Springfield, 1958.

Miller, J. A., and Miller, F. S.: Factors in neonatal resistance to anoxia. III. Potentiation by narcosis of the effects of hypothermia in the newborn guinea pig. Amer. J. Obstet. Gynec. 84:44, 1962.

Miller, J. A., Zakhary, R., and Miller, F. S.: Hypothermia, asphyxia and cardiac glycogen in guinea pigs. Science 144:1226, 1964.

Miller, K. E., Allen, R. P., and Davis, W. S.: Rib gap defects with micrognathia: The cerebro-costo-mandibular syndrome—A Pierre Robin-like syndrome with rib dysplasia. Amer. J. Roentgen. 114:253, 1972.

Miller, W. S.: The Lung. 2nd ed. Chas. C Thomas, Springfield, 1950.

Mitchell, S.: Ductus arteriosus in the neonatal period. J. Pediat. 51:12, 1957.

Mithal, A., and Emery, J. L.: Postnatal development of alveoli in premature infants. Arch. Dis. Child. 36:449, 1961.

Moffat, A. D.: Congenital cystic disease of the lungs and its classification. J. Path. Bact. 79:361, 1960.

Moog, F.: The influence of the pituitary-adrenal system on the differentiation of phosphatase in the duodenum of the suckling mouse. J. Exp. Zool. 124:329, 1953.

Morgan, J.: Neuromuscular incoordination of swallowing in the newborn. J. Laryng. 70:294, 1956.

Morris, E. D., and Beard, R. W.: The rationale and technique of foetal blood sampling and amnioscopy. J. Obstet. Gynaec. Brit. Common. 72:489, 1965.

Morrow, G., Hope, J. W., and Boggs, T. R.: Pneumomediastinum, a silent lesion in the newborn. J. Pediat. 70:554, 1967.

Mortensson, W., and Lundstrom, N. R.: Bronchopulmonary vascular malformation syndrome causing left heart failure during infancy. Acta Radiol. 11:449, 1971.

Moscovici, C., LaPlaca, M., and Amer, J.: Respiratory illness in prematures and children. Illness caused by parainfluenza type 3 virus. Am. J. Dis. Child. 102:91, 1961.

Moseley, J. E.: Loculated pneumomediastinum in the newborn. A thymic "Spinnaker sail" Sign. Radiology 75:788, 1960.

Moss, A. J., Duffie, E. R., and Fagan, L. M.: Respiratory distress syndrome in the newborn. J. A. M. A. 184:48, 1963.

Moss, A. J., Emmanouilides, G., and Duffie, E. R.: Closure of the ductus arteriosus in the newborn infant. Pediatrics 32:25, 1963.

Moss, A. J., Rettori, O., and Simmons, N. S.: The relationship of amniotic fluid viscosity to respiratory distress in lambs. Pediatrics 38:858, 1966.

Motoyama, E. K., Orzalesi, M. M., Kikkawa, Y., Kaibara, M., Wu, B., Zigas, C. J., and Cook, C. D.: Effect of cortisol on the maturation of fetal rabbit lungs. Pediatrics 48:547, 1971.

Mott, J. C.: The ability of young mammals to withstand total oxygen lack. Brit. Med. Bull. 17:144, 1961.

Moya, F., James, L. S., Burnard, E. D., and Hanks, E. C.: Cardiac massage in the newborn infant through the intact chest. Amer. J. Obstet. Gynec. 84:798, 1962.

Moya, F., Morishima, H. O., Shnider, S. M., and James, L. S.: Influence of maternal hyperventilation on the newborn infant. Am. J. Obstet. Gynec. 91:76, 1965.

Mueller-Heubach, E., Myers, R. E., and Adamsons, K.: Effects of adrenalectomy on pregnancy length in rhesus monkey. Amer. J. Obstet. Gynec. 112:221, 1972.

Mulvey, R. B.: The thymic "wave" sign. Radiology 81:834, 1963.

Murdock, A. I., Corey, P., and Swyer, P. R.: An objective multifactorial linear discriminant scoring system for neonates with the respiratory distress syndrome. Biol. Neonate 18:263, 1971.

Murdock, A., Kidd, B. S. L., Llewellyn, M. A., McReid, M., and Swyer, P. R.: Intrapulmonary venous admixture in the respiratory distress syndrome. Biol. Neonat. 15:1, 1970.

Murphy, D. P., and Thorpe, E. S.: Breathing measurements on normal newborn infants. J. Clin. Invest. 10:545, 1931.

Nabarro, S.: Calcification of the laryngeal and tracheal cartilages associated with congenital stridor in an infant. Arch. Dis. Child. 27:185, 1952.

Nadel, J. A., Wolfe, W. G., Graf, P. D., Youker, J. E., Zamel, N., Austin, J. H. M., Hinchcliffe, W. A., Greenspan, R. H., and Wright, R. R.: Powdered tantalum. A new contrast medium for roentgenographic examination of human airways. New Eng. J. Med. 283:281, 1970.

Nadelhaft, J., and Ellis, K.: Roentgen appearances of the lungs in 1,000 apparently normal full term newborn infants. Amer. J. Roentgen. 78:440, 1957.

Naeye, R. L.: Arterial changes during the perinatal period. Arch. Path (Chicago) 71:121, 1961.

Naeye, R. L.: Human intrauterine parabiotic syndrome and its complications. N. Eng. J. Med. 268:804, 1963.

Naeye, R. L.: Pulmonary arterial abnormalities associated with hyaline membrane disease. Amer. J. Path. 48:869, 1966.

Naeye, R. L., and Letts, H. W.: The effects of prolonged neonatal hypoxemia on the pulmonary vascular bed and heart. Pediatrics 30:902, 1962.

Naeye, R. L., and Blanc, W. A.: Relation of poverty and race to antenatal infection. New Eng. J. Med. 283:555, 1970.

Naeye, R. L., Dellinger, W. S., and Blanc, W. A.: Fetal and maternal features of antenatal bacterial infections. J. Pediat. 69:733, 1971.

Naeye, R. L.: The epidemiology of perinatal mortality. The power of the autopsy. Pediat. Clin. N. Amer. 19:295, 1972.

Nahmias, A. J., Alford, C. A., and Korones, S. B.: Infection of the newborn with herpesvirus homonis. Adv. Pediat. 17:185, 1970.

Nash, G., Blennerhassett, J. B., and Pontoppidan, H.: Pulmonary lesions associated with oxygen therapy and artificial ventilation. New Eng. J. Med. 276:357, 1967.

Neal, W. A., Reynolds, J. W., Jarvis, C. W., and Williams, H. J.: Umbilical artery catheterization: demonstration of arterial thrombosis by aortography. Pediatrics 50:6, 1972.

Neches, W. H., Williams, R. L., and McNamara, D. G.: Pulmonary angiographic findings in infantile lobar emphysema. Amer. J. Dis. Child. 123:171, 1972.

Needham, J.: Chemical Embryology. Vol. 3, p. 1547, Cambridge Univ. Press, Oxford. 1931.

Neill, C. A.: Development of the pulmonary veins. Pediatrics 18:880, 1956.

Neill, C. A., Ferencz, C., Sabiston, D. C., and Sheldon, H.: The familial occurrence of hypoplastic right lung with systemic arterial supply and venous drainage "Scimitar Syndrome." Bull. Hopkins Hosp. 107:1, 1960.

Neligan, G., and Smith, C. A.: The blood pressure of newborn infants in asphyxial states and in hyaline membrane disease. Pediatrics 26:735, 1960.

Nelson, N. M., Prod'hom, L. S., Cherry, R. B., Lipsitz, P. J., and Smith, C. A.: Pulmonary function in the newborn infant. II. Perfusion-estimation by analysis of the arterial-alveolar carbon dioxide differences. Pediatrics 30:975, 1962.

Nelson, N. M., Prod'hom, L. S., Cherry, R. B., Lipsitz, P. J., and Smith, C. A.: Pulmonary function in the newborn infant: The alveolar-arterial oxygen gradient. J. Appl. Physiol. 18:534, 1963.

Nelson, N. M., Prod'hom, L. S., Cherry, R. B., and Smith, C. A.: A further extension of the in vitro oxygen-dissociation curve for the blood of the newborn infant. J. Clin. Invest. 43:606, 1964.

Nelson, N. M.: On the etiology of hyaline membrane disease. Pediat. Clin. N. Amer. 17:943, 1970.

Nelson, N. M., Prod'hom, L. S., Cherry, R. B., Lipsitz, P. J., and Smith, C. A.: Pulmonary function in the newborn infant. V. Trapped gas in the normal infant's lung. J. Clin. Invest. 42:1850, 1963.

Nelson, T. Y.: Tension emphysema in infants. Arch. Dis. Child. 32:38, 1957.

Neuhauser, E. B. D., and Harris, G. B. C.: Familial dysautonomia of Riley-Day roentgenographic features. Abstract X International Congr. Radiol. p. 194, 1962.

Neuhauser, E. B. D., and Wittenborg, M. H.: Medical progress: Pediatric radiology. New Eng. J. Med. 249:62, 1953.

Newman, D. E., and Poznanski, A. K.: A simple device for infant warming during radiography. Radiology 97:439, 1970.

Newman, W., McKinnon, L., Phillips, L., Paterson, P., and Wood, C.: Oxygen transfer from mother to fetus during labor. Amer. J. Obstet. Gynec. 99:61, 1967.

Nicolopoulos, D. A., and Smith, C. A.: Metabolic aspects of idiopathic respiratory distress (hyaline membrane syndrome) in newborn infants. Pediatrics 28:206, 1961.

Niemoeller, H., and Schaefer, K. E.: Development of hyaline membranes and atelectasis in experimental chronic respiratory acidosis. Proc. Soc. Exp. Biol. Med. 110:804, 1962.

Noonan, J. A., Walters, L. R., and Reeves, J. T.: Congenital pulmonary lymphangiectasis. Amer. J. Dis. Child. 120:314, 1970.

Normand, I. C. S., Reynolds, E. O. R., and Strang, L. B.: Passage of macromolecules between alveolar and interstitial spaces in foetal and newly ventilated lungs of the lamb. J. Physiol. 210:151, 1970.

Normand, I. C. S., Oliver, R. E., Reynolds, E. O., and Strang, L. B.: Permeability of lung capillaries and alveoli to non-electrolytes in the foetal lamb. J. Physiol. 219:303, 1971.

Northway, W. H., Jr., Rosan, R. C., and Porter, D. Y.: Pulmonary disease following respirator therapy. New Eng. J. Med. 276:357, 1967.

Northway, W. H., Jr., Daily, W. J. R., Parker, B. R., Hackel, A., Bensch, K. G., Vosti, K. L., and Sunshine, P.: Perinatal pulmonary study. Invest. Radiol. 6:354, 1971.

Nourse, C. H., and Nelson, N. M.: Uniformity of ventilation in the newborn infant: direct assessment of the arterial-alveolar N_2 difference. Pediatrics 43:226, 1969.

Oberhansli-Wiess, I., Heymann, M. A., Rudolph, A. M., and Melmon, K. L.: The pattern and mechanisms of response to oxygen by the ductus arteriosus and umbilical artery. Pediat. Res. 6:693, 1972.

O'Brien, D., Hansen, J. D. L., and Smith, C. A.: Effect of supersaturated atmospheres on insensible water loss in the newborn infant. Pediatrics 13:126, 1954.

Oh, W., Lind, J., and Gessner, I. H.: The circulatory and respiratory adaptation to early and late cord clamping in newborn infants. Acta Paediat. Scand. 55:17, 1966.

Oh, W., Wallgren, G., Hanson, J. S., and Lind, J.: The effects of placental transfusion on respiratory mechanics of normal term infants. Pediatrics 40:6, 1967.

O'Hara, A. E., Wallace, J. D., and Nerlinger, R. E.: Controlled pulmonary roentgenographic exposures in newborn infants. Am. J. Roentgen. 95:99, 1965.

Olding, L.: Bacterial infection in cases of perinatal death. Acta Paediat. Scand. 171:1, 1966.

Oliver, T. K., Demis, J. A., and Bates, G. D.: Serial blood-gas tensions and acid-base balance during the first hour of life in human infants. Acta Paediat. 50:346, 1961.

Oliver, T. K., Jr., and Karlberg, P.: Gaseous metabolism in newly born human infants. Am. J. Dis. Child. 105:427, 1963.

O'Neal, R. M., Ahlvin, R. C., Bauer, W. C., and Thomas, W. A.: Development of fetal pulmonary arterioles. A. M. A. Arch. Path. 63:309, 1957.

Opie, E. L.: The pathologic anatomy of influenza; based chiefly on American and British sources. Arch. Path. Lab. Med. 5:285, 1928.

Oppenheimer, E. H., and Hardy, J. B.: Congenital syphilis in the newborn infant: clinical and pathological observations in recent cases. Johns Hopkins Med. J. 129:63, 1971.

Oppenheimer, E. M.: Congenital varicella with disseminated visceral lesions. Bull. Hopkins Hosp. 74:240, 1944.

Opsahl, T., and Berman, E. J.: Bronchiogenic mediastinal cysts in infants. Case report and review of the literature. Pediatrics 30:372, 1962.

Orazalesi, M. M., Motoyama, E. K., Jacobson, H. N., Kikkawa, Y., Reynolds, E. O. R., and Cook, C. D.: The development of the lungs of lambs. Pediatrics 35:373, 1965.

Orzalesi, M. M., and Hay, W. W.: The regulation of oxygen affinity of fetal blood. I. In vitro experiments and results in newborn infants. Pediatrics 48:857, 1971.

Outerbridge, E. W., Nogrady, M. B., Beaudry, P. H., and Stern. L.: Idiopathic respiratory distress syndrome. Recurrent respiratory illness in survivors. Amer. J. Dis. Child. 123:99, 1972.

Outerbridge, E. W., Roloff, D. W., and Stern, L.: Continuous negative pressure in the management of severe respiratory distress syndrome. J. Pediat. 81:384, 1972.

Oyamada, A., Gasul, B. M., and Holinger, P. H.: Agenesis of the lung: Report of a case with a review of all previously reported cases. Am. J. Dis. Child. 85:182, 1953.

Pagtakhan, R. D., Fariday, E. E., and Chernick, V.: Interaction between arterial PO_2 and PCO_2 in the initiation of respiration in sheep. J. Appl. Physiol. 30:382, 1971.

Pagtakhan, R. D., Faridy, E. E., and Chernick, V.: Role of the carotid body in the interaction between arterial PO_2 and PCO_2 in the initiation of breathing. Physiologist 12:321, 1969.

Park, E. A.: Defective development of the right lung due to anomalous development of the right pulmonary artery and vein, accompanied by dislocation of the heart simulating dextrocardia. Proc. N.Y. Path. Soc. 12:88, 1912.

Parmentier, R.: L'aération néonatale du poumon. Contribution expérimentale et anatomo-clinique. Revue Belge Path. Méd. Expèr. 29:123, 1962.

Partlow, W. F., and Taybi, H.: Teratomas in infants and children. Amer. J. Roentgen. 112:155, 1971.

Pasamanick, B., and Lilienfeld, A. M.: Association of maternal and fetal factors with development of mental deficiency. I. Abnormalities in the prenatal and paranatal periods. J. A. M. A. 159:155, 1955.

Patten, B. M.: Human Embryology. p. 684, The Blakiston Co., Philadelphia, 1947.

Patterson, J. H., Lindsey, I. L., Edwards, E. S., and Logan, W. D.: Pneumocystic carinii pneumonia and altered host resistance: Treatment of one patient with pentamidine isethionate. Pediatrics 38:388, 1966.

Pattle, R. E.: Properties, function, and origin of the alveolar lining layer. Proc. Roy. Soc. B. 148:217, 1958.

Pattle, R. E., Claireaux, A. E., Davies, P. A., and Cameron, A. H.: Inability to form a lung-lining film as a cause of the respiratory-distress syndrome in the newborn. Lancet II:469, 1962.

Paul, W. M., Enns, T., Reynolds, S. R. M., and Chinard, F. P.: Sites of water exchange between the maternal system and the amniotic fluid of rabbits. J. Clin. Invest. 35:634, 1956.

Pavlica, F.: The first observation of congenital pneumocystic pneumonia in a fully developed stillborn child. Ann. Paediat. 198:177, 1962.

Pearl, M.: Sequestration of the lung. Amer. J. Dis. Child. 124:706, 1972.

Pennoyer, M. M., Graham, F. K., and Hartmann, A. F.: The relationship of paranatal experience to oxygen saturation in newborn infants. J. Pediat. 49:685, 1956.

Perlstein, P. H., Edwards, N. K., and Sutherland, J. M.: Apnea in premature infants and incubator air temperature changes. New Eng. J. Med. 282:461, 1970.

Perry, R. E., Hodgman, J., and Cass, A. B.: Pleural effusion in the neonatal period. J. Pediat. 62:838, 1963.

Peterson, H. G., Jr., and Pendleton, M. E.: Contrasting roentgenographic pulmonary patterns of the hyaline membrane and fetal aspiration syndromes. Am. J. Roentgen. 74:800, 1955.

Pettay, O., Leinikki, P., Donner, M., and Lapinleimu, K.: Herpes simplex virus infection in the newborn. Arch. Dis. Child. 47:97, 1972.

Pettersson, G.: Inhibited separation of larynx and the upper part of the trachea from the esophagus in a newborn; report of a case successfully operated upon. Acta. Chir. Scand. 110:250, 1955.

Phelan, P., and Campbell, P.: Pulmonary complications of rubella embryopathy. J. Pediat. 75:202, 1969.

Phelps, D. L., Lachman, R. S., Leake, R. D., and Oh, W.: The radiologic localization of the major aortic tributaries in the newborn infant. J. Pediat. 81:336, 1972.

Phillips, L. L., and Skrodelis, V.: A comparison of the fibrinolytic enzyme system in maternal and umbilical cord blood. Pediatrics 22:715, 1958.

Pirnar, T., and Neuhauser, E. B. D.: Asphyxiating thoracic dystrophy of the newborn. Am. J. Roentgen. 98:358, 1966.

Pitkin, R. M., Reynolds, W. A., and Burchell, R. C.: Fetal contribution to amniotic fluid. Amer. J. Obstet. Gynec. 100:834, 1968.

Platzker, A. C. G., Kitterman, J. A., Clements, J. A., and Tooley, W. H.: Surfactant appearance and secretion in fetal lamb lung in response to dexamethasone (abstract). Pediat. Res. 6:406, 1972.

Pleasure, J., and Geller, S. A.: Neurofibromatosis in infancy presenting with congenital stridor. Am. J. Dis. Child. 113:390, 1967.

Plentl, A. A.: The dynamics of the amniotic fluid. Ann. N. Y. Acad. Sci. 75:746, 1959.

Plott, D.: Congenital laryngeal abductor paralysis due to anucleus ambiguous dysgenesis in three brothers. New Eng. J. Med. 271:593, 1964.

Pochaczevsky, R., Ratner, H., Perles, D., Kassner, G., and Naysan, P.: Spondylothoracic dysplasia. Radiology 98:53, 1971.

Polgar, G.: Airway resistance in the newborn infant. J. Pediat. 59:915, 1961.

Polgar, G., and Kong, G. P.: The nasal resistance of newborn infants. J. Pediat. 67:557, 1965.

Polgar, G., and Lacourt, G.: A method for measuring respiratory mechanics in small newborn (premature) infants. J. Appl. Physiol. 32:555, 1972.

Polgar, G., and String, S. T.: The viscous resistance of the lung tissues in newborn infants. J. Pediat. 69:787, 1966.

Potter, E. L., and Bohlender, G. P.: Intra-uterine respiration in relation to development of the fetal lung. Amer. J. Obstet. Gynec. 42:14, 1941.

Potter, E. L.: Bilateral renal agenesis. J. Pediat. 29:68, 1946.

Potter, E. L.: Pulmonary pathology in the newborn. In Levine, S. Z. (ed.): Adv. Pediat. VI:157, 1953.

Potter, E. L.: Pathology of the fetus and infant. Year Book Medical Publishers, Inc., Chicago, 1961.

Prec, K. J., and Cassels, D. E.: Dye dilution curves and cardiac output in newborn infants. Circulation 11:789, 1955.

Prec, K. J., and Cassels, D. E.: Oximeter studies in newborn infants during crying. Pediatrics 9:756, 1952.

Prechtl, H. F. R., and Dijkstra, J.: Neurologic diagnosis of cerebral injury in the newborn. In Birge, B. S. (ed.): Proc. Symposium on Prenatal Care. P. Noordhoff, Ltd., Groningen, 1959.

Presberg, H. J., and Singleton, E. B.: Combined immune deficiency disease. Its radiographic expression. Radiology 91:959, 1968.

Pritchard, J. A.: Fetal swallowing and amniotic fluid volume. Obstet. Gynec. 28:606, 1966.

Pritchard, J. A.: Deglutition by normal and anencephalic fetuses. Obstet. Gynec. 25:289, 1965.

Prod'hom, L. S., Levison, H., Cherry, R. B., Drorbaugh, J. E., Hubbell, J. P., and Smith, C. A.: Evolution of right to left shunt and acid base balance in newborn infants with respiratory distress. Abstract. Am. Pediat. Soc. p. 20, 1962.

Prod'hom, L. S., Levison, H., Cherry, R. B., Drorbaugh, J. E., Hubbell, J. P., and Smith, C. A.: Adjustment of ventilation, intrapulmonary gas exchange and acid-base balance during the first day of life. Pediatrics 33:632, 1964.

Prod'hom, L. S., Levison, H., Cherry, R. B., and Smith, C. A.: Adjustment of ventilation, intrapulmonary gas exchange, and acid base balance during the first day of life. Infants with early respiratory distress. Pediatrics 35:662, 1965.

Pryce, D. M.: Lining of healed but persistent abscess cavities in lung with epithelium of ciliated columnar type. J. Path. Bact. 60:259, 1948.

Pryles, C. V., Steg, N. L., Nair, S., Gellis, S. S., and Tenney, B.: A controlled study of the influence on the newborn of prolonged premature rupture of the amniotic membranes and/or infection in the mother. Pediatrics 31:608, 1963.

Pryse-Davies, J.: The pathology of the lung. Proc. Roy. Soc. Med. 65:823, 1972.

Prystowsky, H.: Fetal blood studies. VII. The oxygen pressure gradient between the maternal and fetal blood of the human in normal and abnormal pregnancy. Bull. Hopkins Hosp. *101*:48, 1957.

Purves, M. J.: Fluctuations of arterial oxygen tension which have the same period as respiration. Resp. Physiol. *1*:281, 1966.

Purves, M. J., and Biscoe, T. J.: Development of chemoreceptor activity. Brit. Med. Bull. *22*:56, 1966.

Purves, M. J.: The effect of a single breath of oxygen on respiration in the newborn lamb. Resp. Physiol. *1*:297, 1966.

Purves, M. J.: The respiratory response of the newborn lamb to inhaled CO_2 with and without accompanying hypoxia. J. Physiol. (London.) *185*:78, 1966.

Purves, M. J.: The effects of hypoxia in the newborn lamb before and after denervation of the carotid chemoreceptors. J. Physiol. *185*:60, 1966.

Quie, P. G., and Wannamaker, L. W.: The plasminogen-plasmin system of newborn infants. Am. J. Dis. Child. *100*:836, 1960.

Radford, E. P., Jr., Ferris, B. G., and Kriete, B. C.: Clinical use of a nomogram to estimate proper ventilation during artificial respiration. N. Eng. J. Med. *251*:877, 1954.

Radford, E. P., Jr.: Ventilation standards for use in artificial respiration. J. Appl. Physiol. *7*:451, 1954-1955.

Randolph, J. G., and Gross, R. E.: Congenital chylothorax, A. M. A. Arch. Surg. *74*:405, 1957.

Rankin, N. E., and Mendelson, I. R.: A case of atresia of the larynx. A. M. A. Arch. Dis. Child. *31*:324, 1956.

Rasche, R. F. H., and Kuhns, L. R.: Histopathologic changes in airway mucosa of infants after endotracheal intubation. Pediatrics *50*:632, 1972.

Rasche, R. F. H., and Kuhns, L. R.: Airway changes and intubation in infants. Pediatrics *50*:513, 1972.

Ravitch, M. M., and Hardy, J. B.: Congenital cystic disease of the lung in infants and children. A. M. A. Arch. Surg. *59*:1, 1949.

Ravitch, M. M.: Atypical deformities of the chest wall—absence and deformities of the ribs and costal cartilages. Surgery *59*:438, 1966.

Ravitch, M. M.: *In* Benson, C. D., et al. (eds.): Pediatric Surgery. Year Book Medical Publishers, Inc., Chicago, 1962.

Reardon, H. S.: Treatment of acute respiratory distress in newborn infants of diabetic and "prediabetic" mothers. Am. J. Dis. Child. *94*:558, 1957.

Reardon, H. S., Baumann, M. L., and Haddad, E. J.: Chemical stimuli of respiration in the early neonatal period. J. Pediat. *57*:151, 1960.

Recavarren, S., Benton, C., and Gall, E. A.: The pathology of acute alveolar diseases of the lung. Seminars Roentgen. *2*:22, 1967.

Redding, R. A., Douglas, W. H. J., and Stein, M.: Thyroid hormone influence upon lung surfactant metabolism. Science *175*:994, 1972.

Redmond, A., Isana, S., and Ingall, D.: Relation of onset of respiration to placental transfusion. Lancet *1*:283, 1965.

Reich, S. B.: Production of pulmonary edema by aspiration of water-soluble nonabsorable contrast media. Radiology *92*:367, 1969.

Reid, L., and Rubino, M.: The connective tissue septa in the foetal human lung. Thorax *14*:3, 1959.

Reid, L.: The embryology of the lung, p. 109. *In* De Reuck, A. V. S., and Porter, R. (eds.): Ciba Foundation Symposium: Development of the lung. J. & A. Churchill, Ltd., London, 1967.

Reid, L.: The Pathology of emphysema. Chicago, Year Book Medical Publishers, 1967.

Reifferscheid, W., and Schmiemann, R.: Räntgenographischer nachweis der intrauterinen Atenbewegung des Foetus. Zentralbl. Gynäk. *63*:146, 1939.

Reinstorff, D., and Fenner, A.: Ventilatory response to hyperoxia in premature and newborn infants during the first three days of life. Resp. Physiol. *15*:159, 1972.

Rémy, J., Ponté, C., Bonte, C., and Flinois, C.: Le stade I de la détresse respiratoire idiopathique du prématuré. Valeur diagnostique et prognostique. Ann. Radiol. *13*:645, 1970.

Renert, W. A., Berdon, W. E., Baker, D. H., and Rose, J. S.: Obstructive urologic malformations of the fetus and infant—relation to neonatal pneumomediastinum and pneumothorax (air block). Radiology *105*:97, 1972.

Reynolds, E. O. R., Jacobson, H. N., Motoyama, E. K., Kikkawa, Y., Craig, J. M., Orzalesi, M. M., and Cook, C. D.: The effect of immaturity and prenatal asphyxia on the lungs and pulmonary function of newborn lambs: The experimental production of respiratory distress. Pediatrics 35:382, 1965.

Reynolds, E. O. R., Orzalesi, M. M., Motoyama, E. K., Craig, J. M., and Cook, C. D.: Surface properties of saline extracts from lungs of newborn infants. Acta Paediat. Scand. 54:511, 1965.

Reynolds, E. O. R.: Hyaline membrane disease. Amer. J. Obstet. Gynec. 106:780, 1970.

Reynolds, E. O. R., Roberton, N. R. C., and Wigglesworth, J. S.: Hyaline membrane disease, respiratory distress and surfactant deficiency. Pediatrics 42:758, 1968.

Reynolds, R. N., and Etsten, B. E.: Mechanics of respiration of apneic anesthetized infants. Anesthesiology 27:13, 1966.

Reynolds, S. R. M.: A source of amniotic fluid in the lamb. The naso-pharyngeal and buccal cavities. Nature 172:307, 1953.

Reynolds, S. R. M.: Homeostatic regulation of resting heart rate in fetal lambs. Amer. J. Physiol. 176:162, 1954.

Reynolds, S. R. M.: The fetal and neonatal pulmonary vasculature in the guinea pig in relation to hemodynamic changes at birth. Am. J. Anat. 98:97, 1956.

Reynolds, S. R. M.: Regulation of the fetal circulation. Its relation to fetal distress. Clin. Obstet. Gynec. 3:834, 1960.

Reynolds, S. R. M., and Mackie, J. D.: Development of chemoreceptor response sensitivity: Studies in fetuses, lambs, and ewes. Amer. J. Physiol. 201:239, 1961.

Reynolds, W. A.: Fetal sources of amniotic fluid: An enigma. In Hodari, A. A., and Mariona, F. G. (eds.): In Physiological Biochemistry of the Fetus. Charles C Thomas, Publisher, Springfield, Ill., 1972.

Rhodes, P. G., and Hall, R. T.: Continuous positive airway pressure delivered by face mask in infants with the idiopathic respiratory distress syndrome. A controlled study. Pediatrics 52:17, 1973.

Richard, J., Chevalier, V., Capelle, R., Cavrot, E., Content, J., and Delforge, J.: Diaphragmatic obstetric paralysis. Report of 10 cases. Arch. Franç. Pédiat. 14:563, 1957.

Richards, C. C., and Bachman, L.: Lung and chest wall compliance of apneic paralyzed infants. J. Clin. Invest. 40:273, 1961.

Rigatto, H., and Brady, J. P.: Periodic breathing and apnea in preterm infants. I. Evidence for hypoventilation possibly due to central respiratory depression. Pediatrics 50:202, 1972.

Rigatto, H., and Brady, J. P.: Periodic breathing and apnea in preterm infants. II. Hypoxia as a primary event. Pediatrics 50:219, 1972.

Rimoin, D. L., Fletcher, B. D., and McKusick, V. A.: Spondylocostal dysplasia. Amer. J. Med. 45:948, 1968.

Robbins, J. B.: Pneumocystis carinii pneumonitis: A review. Pediat. Res. 1:131, 1967.

Robertson, A. M., and Crichton, J. U.: Neurological sequelae in children with neonatal respiratory distress. Amer. J. Dis. Child. 117:271, 1969.

Robertson, B., and Ivemark, B.: Abnormalities of the costochondral junction in cases of perinatal death, with special reference to hyaline membrane disease. Acta Path. Microbiol. Scand. 77:172, 1969.

Robertson, B.: The normal intrapulmonary arterial pattern of the human late fetal and neonatal lung. A microangiographic and histologic study. Acta Paediat. Scand. 56:249, 1967.

Robillard, E., Alarie, Y., Dagenais-Perusse, P., Baril, E., and Guilbeault, A.: Microaerosol administration of synthetic β-γ-dipalmitoyl-L-α-lecithin in the respiratory distress syndrome. A preliminary report. Canad. Med. Ass. J. 90:55, 1964.

Robinson, F. R., Harper, D. T., Thomas, A. S., and Kaplan, H. P.: Proliferative pulmonary lesions in monkeys exposed to high concentrations of oxygen. Aerosp. Med. 38:481, 1967.

Roe, B. B., and Stephens, H. B.: Congenital diaphragmatic hernia and hypoplastic lung. J. Thorac. Surg. 32:279, 1956.

Roghair, G. D.: Non-operative management of lobar emphysema. Long-term follow-up. Radiology 102:125, 1972.

Rokos, J., Vaeusorn, O., Nachman, R., and Avery, M. E.: Hyaline membrane disease in twins. Pediatrics 42:204, 1968.

Rosen, M. S., and Reich, S. B.: Umbilical venous catheterization in the newborn: Identification of correct positioning. Radiology 95:335, 1970.

Rosenfeld, M., and Snyder, F. F.: Stages of development of respiratory regulation and the changes occurring at birth. Amer. J. Physiol. 121:242, 1938.

Ross, B. B.: Comparison of foetal pulmonary fluid with foetal plasma and amniotic fluid. Nature 199:1100, 1963.

Rowe, M. I., Furst, A. J., Altman, D. H., and Poole, C. A.: The neonatal response to gastrografin enema. Pediatrics 48:29, 1971.

Rowe, R. D., and James, L. S.: The normal pulmonary arterial pressure during the first year of life. J. Pediat. 51:1, 1957.

Rowe, R. D.: Maternal rubella and pulmonary artery stenosis. Pediatrics 32:180, 1963.

Rowe, S., and Avery, M. E.: Massive pulmonary hemorrhage in the newborn. II. Clinical considerations. J. Pediat. 69:12, 1966.

Rudhe, U., Margolin, F. R., and Robertson, B.: Atypical roentgen appearances of the lung in hyaline membrane disease of the newborn. Acta Radiol. 10:57, 1970.

Rudnick, D.: Developmental capacities of the chick lung in chorioallantoic grafts. J. Exptl. Zool. 66:125, 1933.

Rudolph, A. J., and Smith, C. A.: Idiopathic respiratory distress syndrome of the newborn. J. Pediat. 57:905, 1960.

Rudolph, A. J., Vallbona, C., and Desmond, M. M.: Patterns of cardiac activity in premature infants with and without distress. Abstract. Soc. Pediat. Res., p. 140, 1962.

Rudolph, A. J., Vallbona, C., and Desmond, M. M.: Cardiodynamic studies in the newborn. III. Heart rate patterns in infants with idiopathic respiratory distress syndrome. Pediatrics 36:551, 1965.

Rudolph, A. J., Desmond, M. M., and Pineda, R. G.: Clinical diagnosis of respiratory difficulty in the newborn. Pediat. Clin. N. Amer. 13:669, 1966.

Rudolph, A. M.: The fourth Edgar Mannheimer memorial lecture: The foetal circulation and changes in the circulation after birth. Proc. Ass. Europ. Paediat. Cardiol. 6:2, 1970.

Rudolph, A. M., Drorbaugh, J. E., Auld, P. A. M., Rudolph, A. J., Nadas, A. S., Smith, C. A., and Hubbell, J. P.: Studies on the circulation in the neonatal period. The circulation in the respiratory distress syndrome. Pediatrics 27:551, 1961.

Rudolph, A. M., Mesel, E., and Levy, J.: Epinephrine in the treatment of cardiac failure due to shunts. Circulation 28:3, 1963.

Rudolph, A. M., Heymann, M. A., Teramo, K. A. W., Barrett, C. T., and Raiha, N. C. R.: Studies on the circulation of the previable human fetus. Paediat. Res. 5:452, 1971.

Rudolph, A. M., and Heymann, M. A.: Pulmonary circulation in fetal lambs. Paediat. Res. 6:341, 1972 (abstract).

Rudolph, A. M., and Yuan, S.: Response of the pulmonary vasculature to hypoxia and H ion concentration changes. J. Clin. Invest. 45:399, 1966.

Rudolph, A. M., and Heymann, M. A.: The circulation of the fetus in utero. Circ. Res. 21:163, 1967.

Rudolph, A. M., and Heymann, M. A.: Circulatory changes during growth in the fetal lamb. Circ. Res. 26:289, 1970.

Ruge, C.: Pneumothorax bei Einem Neugebornem. Zeitsch. Geburtsch Gyn. 2:31, 1878.

Russo, P. E., and Coin, C. G.: Calcification of the hyoid, thyroid, and tracheal cartilages in infancy. Amer. J. Roentgen. 80:440, 1958.

Sabga, G. A., Neville, W. E., and DelGuercio, L. R. M.: Anomalies of the lungs associated with congenital diaphragmatic hernia. Surg. 50:547, 1961.

Sabiston, D. C.: The surgical management of congenital bifid sternum with partial ectopia cordis. J. Thorac. Surg. 35:118, 1958.

Safar, P., Escarraga, L. A., and Elam, J. O.: A comparison of the mouth-to-mouth and mouth-to-airway methods of artificial respiration with the chest-pressure arm-lift methods. New Eng. J. Med. 258:671, 1958.

Saldino, R. M.: Lethal short-limbed dwarfism: achondrogenesis and thanatophoric dwarfism. Amer. J. Roentgen. 112:185, 1971.

Saling, E.: Neues Vorgehen zur Untersuching des Kindes unter der Geburt Arch. f. Gynäk 197:108, 1962.

Saling, E.: The endoscopic technique of obtaining foetal blood for microanalysis. German Med. Monthly 9:449, 1964.

Samartzis, E. A., Cook, C. D., and Rudolph, A. J.: Fibrinolytic activity in the serum of infants with and without the hyaline membrane syndrome. Acta Paediat. *49*:727, 1960.

Sampaolo, G., and Sampaolo, C. L.: La trachea di feti di cavia in coltura organotipica. Indagini sugli aspetti istologici, sugli atteggiamenti morfogenetici e sulla differenziazione in vitro deel'epitelio e della cartilagine. Quaderni Anat. Prat. *14*:149, 1958.

Sandison, A. T.: Partial absence of the trachea with live birth. Arch. Dis. Child. *30*:475, 1955.

Sano, T., Niitsu, I., and Nakagawa, I.: Newborn virus pneumonitis (Type Sendai). I. Report: Clinical observation of a new virus pneumonitis of the newborn. Yokohama Med. Bull. *4*:199, 1953.

Sapin, S. O., Donoso, E., and Blumenthal, S.: Digoxin dosage in infants. Pediatrics *18*:730, 1956.

Sarnoff, S. J., Maloney, J. V., Sarnoff, L. C., Ferris, B. G., and Whittenberger, J. L.: Electrophrenic respiration in acute bulbar poliomyelitis. J. A. M. A. *143*:1383, 1950.

Schachter, F. F., and Apgar, V.: Perinatal asphyxia and psychologic signs of brain damage in childhood. Pediatrics *24*:1006, 1959.

Schaefer, K. E., Avery, M. E., and Bensch, K.: Time course of changes in surface tension and morphology of alveolar epithelial cells in CO_2-induced hyaline membrane disease. J. Clin. Invest. *43*:2080, 1964.

Schaeffer, M.: Fox, M. J., and Li, C. P.: Intrauterine poliomyelitis infection: Report of a case. J. A. M. A. *155*:248, 1954.

Schaffer, A. J., Markowitz, M., and Perlman, A.: Pneumonia in newborn infants. J. A. M. A. *159*:663, 1955.

Schaffer, A. J.: The pathogenesis of intrauterine pneumonia. I. A critical review of the evidence concerning intrauterine respiratory-like movements. Pediatrics *17*:747, 1956.

Schaffer, A. J., and Avery, M. E.: Diseases of the Newborn. W. B. Saunders Co., Philadelphia, 1971.

Schapiro, R. L., and Evans, E. T.: Surgical disorders causing neonatal respiratory distress. Amer. J. Roentgen. *114*:305, 1972.

Scheidegger, S.: Lungenmisbildungen. (Beitragzur Entstehung der Nebenlunge.) Frankfurt Z. Path. *49*:362, 1936.

Schenck, S. G.: Congenital cystic disease of the lungs. Am. J. Roentgen. *35*:608, 1936.

Schifrin, N.: Unilateral paralysis of the diaphragm in the newborn infant due to phrenic nerve injury with and without associated brachial palsy. Pediatrics 9:69, 1952.

Schmidt, A. G.: Portal vein gas due to administration of fluids via the umbilical vein. Radiology *88*:293, 1967.

Schmidt, C. F., and Comroe, J. H.: Functions of the carotid and aortic bodies. Physiol. Rev. *20*:115, 1940.

Schulman, J. D., Queenan, J. T., Scarpelli, E. M., Church, E., and Auld, P. A. M.: Lecithin-sphingomyelin ratios in amniotic fluid. Relation to neonatal condition and gestational age. Obstet. Gynec. *40*:697, 1972.

Schulz, H.: The Submicroscopic Anatomy and Pathology of the Lung. Springer, Berlin, 1959.

Scopes, J. W.: Metabolic rate and temperature control in the human baby. Brit. Med. Bull. *22*:88. 1966.

Secher, O., and Karlberg, P.: Placental blood transfusion. Lancet *I*:1203, 1962.

Seeds, A. E.: Water metabolism of the fetus. Amer. J. Obstet. Gynec. 92:727, 1965.

Sehlkopf, K. L., and von Werz, R.: Über die Rolle der Kohlensäure bei der Sauerstoffvergiftung. Arch. exper. Path. Pharmakol. *205*:351, 1948.

Setnikar, I., Agostoni, E., and Taglietti, A.: The fetal lung, a source of amniotic fluid. Proc. Soc. Exp. Biol. Med. *101*:842, 1959.

Shackelford, G. D., and McAlister, W. H.: Congenital laryngeal cyst. Amer. J. Roentgen. Rad. Ther. Nucl. Med. *114*:289, 1972.

Shanklin, D. R.: Cardiovascular factors in the development of pulmonary hyaline membrane. A.M.A. Arch. Path. *68*:49, 1959.

Shanklin, D. R.: The influence of fixation on the histologic features of hyaline membrane disease. Am. J. Path. *44*:823, 1964.

Shawker, T. H., Nilprabhassorn, P., and Dennis, J. M.: Benign intrathoracic lipoma with rib erosion in an infant. Radiology *104*:111, 1972.

Shearer, W. T., Biller, H. F., Ogura, J. H., and Goldring, D.: Congenital laryngeal web and interventricular septal defect. Amer. J. Dis. Child. *123*:605, 1972.

Sheldon, W. H.: Pulmonary pneumocystis carinii infection. J. Pediat. *61*:780, 1962.

Shepard, F. M., Johnston, R. B., Jr., Klatte, E. C., Burko, H., and Stahlman, M.: Residual pulmonary findings in clinical hyaline membrane disease. New Eng. J. Med. *279*: 1063, 1968.

Sherrick, D. W., Kincaid, O. W., and DuShane, J. W.: Agenesis of a main branch of the pulmonary artery. Amer. J. Roentgen. *87*:917, 1962.

Shinebourne, E. A., Vapaavuori, E. K., Williams, R. L., Heymann, M. A., and Rudolph, A. M.: Development of baroreflex activity in unanesthetized fetal and neonatal lambs. Circ. Res., *31*:710, 1972.

Siassi, B., Goldberg, S. J., Emmanouilides, G. C., Higashino, S. M., and Lewis, E.: Persistent pulmonary vascular obstruction in newborn infants. J. Pediat. *78*:610, 1971.

Sidaway, M. E.: Duplication of oesophagus. Ann. Radiol. *7*:400, 1964.

Sieber, O. F., Fulginiti, V. A., Brazie, J., and Umlauf, H. J.: In utero infection of the fetus by herpes simplex virus. J. Pediat. *69*:30, 1966.

Siggaard-Andersen, O.: The Acid-Base Status of the Blood. Williams and Wilkins, Baltimore, 1964.

Silverman, B. K., Breckx, T., Craig, J., and Nadas, A. S.: Congestive heart failure in the newborn caused by cerebral A-V fistula. Am. J. Dis. Child. *89*:539, 1955.

Silverman, W. A., and Anderson, D. H.: A controlled clinical trial of effects of water mist on obstructive respiratory signs, death rate and necropsy findings among premature infants. Pediatrics *17*:1, 1956.

Silverman, W. A., and Silverman, R. H.: "Incidence" of hyaline membrane in premature infants. Letter. Lancet *II*:588, 1958.

Silverman, W. A.: Dunham's Premature Infants, 3rd ed., p. 144, Paul B. Hoeber, Inc., New York, 1961.

Silverman, W. A., Sinclair, J. C., and Agate, F. J.: The oxygen cost of minor changes in heat balance of small newborn infants. Acta Paediat. Scand. *55*:294, 1966.

Silverman, W. A., Sinclair, J. C., and Buck, J. B.: A valved mask for respiratory studies in the neonate. J. Pediat. *68*:468, 1966.

Silverman, W. A., Sinclair, J. C., Gandy, G. M., Finster, M., Bauman, W. A., and Agate, F. J.: A controlled trial of management of respiratory distress syndrome in a body-enclosing respirator. I. Evaluation of safety. Pediatrics *39*:740, 1967.

Sime, F., Banchero, N., Penaloza, D., Gamoa, R., Cruz, J., and Marticoerena, E.: Pulmonary hypertension in children born and living at high altitudes. Amer. J. Cardiol. *11*:143, 1963.

Simon, H.: Die Sogenaunte Pneumocystis Carinii, eine besondere Vegatationsform des Soor. Naturwissenschaften *40*:625, 1953.

Sinclair, J. C.: Prevention and treatment of the respiratory distress syndrome. Pediat. Clin. N. Amer. *13*:711, 1966.

Singleton, E. B.: Respiratory distress syndrome. *In* Kaufman, H. J. (ed.): Progress in Pediatric Radiology. Chicago, Year Book Medical Publishers, Inc., 1967.

Sinniah, D., and Somasundaram, K.: Lateral cervical cyst. A cause of respiratory distress in the newborn. Amer. J. Dis. Child. *124*:582, 1972.

Sivanesan, S.: Neonatal pulmonary pathology in Singapore. J. Pediat. *59*:600, 1961.

Sjöstedt, S., and Rooth, G.: Low oxygen tension in the management of newborn infants. Arch. Dis. Child. *32*:397, 1957.

Sladen, A., Laver, M. B., and Pontoppidan, H.: Pulmonary complications and water retention in prolonged mechanical ventilation. New Eng. J. Med. *279*:448, 1968.

Sloan, H.: Lobar obstructive emphysema in infancy treated by lobectomy. J. Thorac. Surg. *26*:1, 1953.

Smart, J.: Complete congenital agenesis of a lung. Quart. J. Med. *15*:125, 1946.

Smith, B. T.: Isolated phrenic nerve palsy in the newborn. Pediatrics *49*:449, 1972.

Smith, C. A., and Barker, R. H.: Ether in the blood of the newborn infant: A quantitative study. Amer. J. Obstet. Gynec. *43*:763, 1942.

Smith, C. A.: The Physiology of the Newborn Infant. Chas. C Thomas, Springfield, 1959.

Smith, C. A.: Circulatory factors in relation to idiopathic respiratory distress (hyaline membrane disease) in the newborn. J. Pediat. *56*:605, 1960.

Smith, P. C., Schach, E., and Daily, W. J. R.: Mechanical ventilation of newborn infants: II. Effects of independent variation of rate and pressure on arterial oxygenation of infants with respiratory distress syndrome. Anesthesiology 37:498, 1972.

Smith, R. A.: A theory of the origin of intralobar sequestration of lung. Thorax 11:10, 1956.

Smith, R. M.: Diagnosis and treatment: Nasotracheal intubation as a substitute for tracheostomy. Pediatrics 38:652, 1966.

Snyder, F. F., and Rosenfeld, M.: Direct observation and intrauterine respiratory movements of the fetus and the role of carbon dioxide and oxygen in their regulation. Am. J. Physiol. 119:153, 1937.

Snyder, F. F.: Pulmonary hyaline membrane disease. Origin in premature infants delivered by cesarean section during labor or after placenta previa or abruptio placentae. Obst. Gynec. 18:677, 1961.

Solis-Cohen, L., and Bruck, S.: A roentgen examination of the chest of 500 newborn infants for pathology other than enlarged thymus. Radiology 23:173, 1934.

Sorokin, S., Padykula, H. A., and Herman, E.: Comparative histochemical patterns in developing mammalian lungs. Develop. Biol. 1:125, 1959.

Sorokin, S.: Histochemical events in developing human lungs. Acta Anat. 40:105, 1960.

Sorokin, S.: A study of development in origin cultures of mammalian lungs. Develop. Biol. 3:60, 1961.

Sorokin, S. P.: A morphologic and cytochemical study of the great alveolar cell. J. Histochem. Cytochem. 14:884, 1967.

Spear, G. S., Vaeusorn, O., Avery, M. E., Nachman, R., Wolfsdorf, J., and Bergman, R. A.: Inclusions in terminal air spaces of fetal and neonatal human lung. Biol. Neonate 14:344, 1969.

Spector, R. G., Claireaux, A. E., and Williams, E. R.: Congenital adenomatoid malformation of lung with pneumothorax. Arch. Dis. Child. 35:475, 1960.

Spencer, H.: Pathology of the Lung. The Macmillan Co., New York, 1962.

Spencer, R. P., Spackman, T. J., and Pearson, H. A.: Diagnosis of right diaphragmatic eventration by means of liver scan. Radiology 99:375, 1971.

Spock, A., Schneider, S., and Baylin, G. J.: Mediastinal gastric cysts: A case report and review of English literature. Am. Rev. Resp. Dis. 94:97, 1966.

Spock, A., Hinton, M. L., and Albertson, T. H.: A microtechnique for measurement of oxygen tension in capillary blood. J. Pediat. 68:987, 1966.

Stafford, A., and Weatherall, J. A. C.: The survival of young rats in nitrogen. J. Physiol. 153:457, 1960.

Stahlman, M.: The use of carbon monoxide diffusion capacity in the evaluation of pulmonary function in infants and children. Abstract. Am. J. Dis. Child. 100:527, 1960.

Stahlman, M., and Sexton, C.: Ventilation control in the newborn. Am. J. Dis. Child. 101:216, 1961.

Stahlman, M. T.: Pulmonary ventilation and diffusion in the human newborn infant. J. Clin. Invest. 36:1081, 1957.

Stahlman, M., Young, W., and Payne, G.: Studies of ventilatory aids in hyaline membrane disease. Abstract. Am. J. Dis. Child. 104:126, 1962.

Stahlman, M. T., Merrill, R. E., and LeQuire, V. S.: Cardiovascular adjustments in normal newborn lambs. Am. J. Dis. Child. 104:360, 1962.

Stahlman, M., LeQuire, V. S., Young, W. C., Merrill, R. E., Birmingham, R. T., Payne, G. A., and Gray, J.: Pathophysiology of respiratory distress in newborn lambs. Am. J. Dis. Child. 108:375, 1964.

Stahlman, M. T., Young, W. C., and Payne, G.: Prognostic significance of blood lactic acid levels in hyaline membrane disease. Abstract. South. Med. J. 55:1320, 1962.

Stahlman, M.: Assessment of the cardiovascular status of infants with hyaline membrane disease. In Cassels, D. (ed.): Proceedings: Fetal and Newborn Circulation. Grune and Stratton, New York, 1966.

Stahlman, M. T., Young, W. C., Gray, J., and Shepard, F. M.: The management of respiratory failure in the idiopathic respiratory distress syndrome of prematurity. Ann. N. Y. Acad. Sci. 121:930, 1965.

Stahlman, M. T.: Perinatal circulation. Pediat. Clin. N. Amer. 13:753, 1966.

Stahlman, M. T., Battersby, E. J., Shepard, F. M., and Blankenship, W. J.: Prognosis in hyaline-membrane disease. Use of a linear discriminant. New Eng. J. Med. 276:303, 1967.

Stahlman, M., Blankenship, W. J., Shepard, F. M., Gray, J., Young, W. C., and Malan, A. F.: Circulatory studies in clinical hyaline membrane disease. Biol. Neonate 20:300, 1972.

Staple, T. W., Hudson, H. H., Hartmann, A. F., Jr.: The angiographic findings in four cases of infantile lobar emphysema. Amer. J. Roentgen. 97:195, 1966.

Staub, N. C.: Site of action of hypoxia on the pulmonary vasculature. Fed. Proc. 22:453, 1963 (abstract).

Steele, R. W., Metz, J. R., Bass, J. W., and DuBois, J. J.: Pneumothorax and pneumomediastinum in the newborn. Radiology 98:629, 1971.

Steele, R. W., and Copeland, G. A.: Delayed resorption of pulmonary alveolar fluid in the neonate. Radiology 103:637, 1972.

Steiner, R. E.: The radiology of respiratory distress in the newborn. Brit. J. Radiol. 27:491, 1954.

Steinschneider, A.: Prolonged apnea and the sudden infant death syndrome. Clinical and laboratory observations. Pediatrics 50:646, 1972.

Stephenson, J. M., Du, J. N., and Oliver, T. K.: The effect of cooling on blood gas tensions in newborn infants. J. Pediat. 76:848, 1970.

Stern, L., Fletcher, B. D., Dunbar, J. S., Levant, M. N., and Fawcett, J. S.: Pneumothorax and pneumomediastinum associated with renal malformations in newborn infants. Amer. J. Roentgen. 116:785, 1972.

Stern, L., and Lind, J.: Cardiovascular disease: Perinatal circulation. Ann. Rev. Med. 11:113, 1960.

Stern, L., Ramos, A. D., Outerbridge, E. W., and Beaudry, P. H.: Negative pressure artificial respiration. Use in treatment of respiratory failure of the newborn. Canad. Med. Assoc. J. 102:595, 1970.

Stern. L.: Therapy of the respiratory distress syndrome. Pediat. Clin. N. Amer. 19:221, 1972.

Stern, L., Ramos, A., and Wiglesworth, F.: Congestive heart failure secondary to cerebral arteriovenous aneurysm in the newborn infant. Amer. J. Dis. Child. 115:581, 1968.

Stern, L. M., Fonkalsrud, E. W., Hassakis,P., and Jones, M. H.: Management of Pierre Robin Syndrome in infancy by prolonged nasoesophageal intubation. Amer. J. Dis. Child. 124:78, 1972.

Stoerk, O.: Ueber augeborene blasige Missbildung der Lunge. Wien. Klin. Wschr. 10:25, 1897.

Stool, S. E., Johnson, D., Rosenfeld, P. A.: Unintentional esophageal intubation in the newborn. Pediatrics 48:299, 1971.

Stone, H. H., Henderson, D., and Guidio, F. A.: Teratomas of the neck. Amer. J. Dis. Child. 113:222, 1967.

Storey, C. F., and Marrangoni, A. G.: Lobar agenesis of the lung. J. Thorac. Surg. 28:536, 1954.

Strang, L. B., Anderson, G. S., and Platt, J. W.: Neonatal death and elective cesarean section. Lancet 1:954, 1957.

Strang, L. B.: Alveolar gas and anatomical dead-space measurements in normal newborn infants. Clin. Sci., 21:107, 1961.

Strang, L. B., and MacLeish, M. H.: Ventilatory failure and right-to-left shunt in newborn infants with respiratory distress. Pediatrics 28:17, 1961.

Strang, L. B., and McGrath, M. W.: Alveolar ventilation in normal newborn infants studied by air wash-in after oxygen breathing. Clin. Sci. 23:129, 1962.

Strang, L. B.: Uptake of liquid from the lungs at the start of breathing, p. 348. In De Reuck, A. V. S., and Porter, R. (eds.): Ciba Foundation Symposium: Development of the Lung. J. & A. Churchill, Ltd., London, 1967.

Strauss, J., Beran, A. V., and Baker, R.: Continuous O_2 monitoring of newborn and older infants and of children. J. Appl. Physiol. 33:238, 1972.

Strickroot, F. L., Schaeffer, R. L., and Bergo, H. L.: Myasthenia gravis occurring in an infant born of a myasthenic mother. J. A. M. A. 120:1207, 1942.

Strunge, P.: Infantile lobar emphysema with lobar agenesia and congenital heart disease. Acta Paediat. Scand. 61:209, 1972.

Sundell, H., Garrott, J., Blankenship, W. J., Shepard, F. M., and Stahlman, M. T.: Studies on infants with type II respiratory distress syndrome. J. Pediat. 78:754, 1971.

Sunderland, C. O., Morgan, C. L., and Lees, M. H.: Cerebral arteriovenous fistula producing temporary heart failure in a newborn infant. Clin. Pediat. 10:309, 1971.

Sutherland, J. M., Oppé, T. E., Lucey, J. F., and Smith, C. A.: Leg volume changes observed in hyaline membrane disease. Am. J. Dis. Child. 98:24, 1959.

Sutherland, J. M., and Epple, H. H.: Cardiac massage of stillborn infants. Obst. Gynec. 18:182, 1961.

Sutherland, J. M., and Ratcliff, J. W.: Crying vital capacity. Am. J. Dis. Child. 101:67, 1961.

Swischuk, L. E.: Transient respiratory distress of the newborn (TRDN): A temporary disturbance of a normal phenomenon. Amer. J. Roentgen. 108:557, 1970.

Swyer, P. R., Reiman, R. C., and Wright, J. J.: Ventilation and ventilatory mechanics in the newborn. J. Pediat. 56:612, 1960.

Swyer, P. R., Delivoria-Papadopoulos, M., Levison, H., Reilly, B. J., and Balis, J. U.: The pulmonary syndrome of Wilson and Mikity. Pediatrics 36:374, 1965.

Taeusch, H. W., Jr., Heitner, M., and Avery, M. E.: Accelerated lung maturation and increased survival in premature rabbits treated with hydrocortisone. Amer. Rev. Resp. Dis. 105:972, 1972.

Tausend, M. E., and Stern, W. Z.: Thymic patterns in the newborn. Amer. J. Roentgen. 95:125, 1965.

Taussig, F. J.: The amniotic fluid and its quantitative variability. Amer. J. Obstet. Gynec. 14:505, 1927.

Taylor, F. B., and Abrams, M. E.: Effect of surface active lipoprotein on clotting and fibrinolysis, and of fibrinogen on surface tension of surface active lipoprotein. Amer. J. Med. 40:346, 1966.

Tchou, C.-S., Fletcher, B. D., Franke, P., Outerbridge, E. W., and Dunbar, J. S.: Asymmetric distribution of the roentgen pattern in hyaline membrane disease. J. Can. Assoc. Radiol. 23:85, 1972.

Tefft, M.: The radiotherapeutic management of subglottic hemangioma in children. Radiology 86:207, 1966.

Teng, P., and Osserman, K. E.: Studies in myasthenia gravis: Neonatal and juvenile types. J. Mt. Sinai Hosp. N. Y. 23:711, 1956.

Thaler, M. M., and Stobie, H. C.: An improved technic of external cardiac compression in infants and young children. New Eng. J. Med. 269:606, 1963.

Theros, E. G.: An exercise in radiologic-pathologic correlation. Radiology 89:524, 1967.

Thibeault, D. W., Clutario, B., and Auld, P. A. M.: Arterial oxygen tension in premature infants. J. Pediat. 69:449, 1966.

Thomas, D. V., Fletcher, G., Sunshine, P., Schafer, I. A., and Klaus, M. H.: Prolonged respirator use in pulmonary insufficiency of the newborn. J. A. M. A. 193:183, 1965.

Thomas, M. R.: A cystic hamartoma of the lung in a new-born infant. J. Path. Bact. 61:599, 1949.

Thomson, J., and Forfar, J. O.: Regional obstructive emphysema in infancy. Arch. Dis. Child. 33:97, 1958.

Thorburn, M. J.: Neonatal death and massive pulmonary haemorrhage in Jamaica. Arch. Dis. Child. 38:589, 1963.

Thunberg, T.: The barospirator: A new machine for producing artificial respiration. Scand. Arch. Physiol. 48:80, 1926.

Thurlbeck, W. M., Benjamin, B., and Reid, L.: A sampling method for estimating the number of mucous glands in the foetal human trachea. Brit. J. Dis. Chest 55:49, 1961.

Tierney, D. F., Clements, J. A., and Trahan, H. J.: Rates of replacement of lecithins and alveolar stability in rat lungs. Amer. J. Physiol. 213:671, 1967.

Tobin, C. E.: Human pulmonic lymphatics. Anat. Rec. 127:611, 1957.

Tolstedt, G. E., and Tudor, R. B.: Esophagopleural fistula in a newborn infant. Arch. Surg. 97:780, 1968.

Tombropoulos, E. G.: Fatty acid synthesis by subcellular fractions of lung tissue. Science 146:1180, 1964.

Tooley, W. H., Klaus, M., Weaver, K. H., and Clements, J. A.: The distribution of ventilation in normal newborn infants. Am. J. Dis. Child. 100:731, 1960.

Tooley, W. H., Gardner, R., Thung, N., and Finley, T.: Factors affecting the surface tension of lung extracts. Fed. Proc. 20:428, 1961.

Tooley, W. H., Klaus, M., Costley, C., Way, W., and Rock, R.: The lung and acid-base balance in the newborn. Abstract. Am. J. Dis. Child. 104:120, 1962.

Townsend, E. H., and Squire, L.: Treatment of atelectasis by thoracic traction. Pediatrics 17:250, 1956.

Toyama, W. M.: Combined congenital defects of the anterior abdominal wall, sternum, diaphragm, pericardium, and heart: A case report and review of the syndrome. Pediatrics 50:778, 1972.

Turner, L. B., and Bakst, A. A.: Phrenic nerve paralysis associated with Erb's palsy in the newborn. A clinical and anatomicrophathologic study. J. Mt. Sinai Hosp., N. Y. 15:374, 1948-1949.

Usdin, G. L., and Weil, M. L.: Effect of apnea neonatorum on intellectual development. Pediatrics 9:387, 1952.

Usher, R.: The respiratory distress syndrome of prematurity. I. Changes in potassium in the serum and the electrocardiogram and effects of therapy. Pediatrics 24:562, 1959.

Usher, R.: The respiratory distress syndrome of prematurity. Pediat. Clin. N. Am. 8:525, 1961.

Usher, R.: Reduction of mortality from respiratory distress syndrome of prematurity with early administration of intravenous glucose and sodium bicarbonate. Pediatrics 32:966, 1963.

Usher, R., Shephard, M., and Lind, J.: The blood volume of the newborn infant and placental transfusion. Acta Paed. 52:497, 1963.

Usher, R., McLean, F., and Maughan, G. B.: Respiratory distress syndrome in infants delivered by cesarean section. Amer. J. Obstet. Gynec. 88:806, 1964.

Utian, H. L., and Thomas, R. G.: Cricopharyngeal incoordination in infancy. Pediatrics 43:402, 1969.

V. Hesse, H. de, and Wittman, W.: Respiratory distress syndrome in the newborn. Letter. Lancet II:1058, 1962.

Van Breeman, V. L., Neustein, H. B., and Bruns, P. D.: Pulmonary hyaline membranes studied with the electron microscope. Am. J. Path. 33:769, 1961.

Vapaavuori, E. K., Shinebourne, E. A., Williams, R. L., Heymann, M. A., and Rudolph, A. M.: Cardiovascular responses to autonomic blockade in intact fetal and newborn lambs. Pediat. Res. 5:425, 1971 (abstract).

Vidyasagar, D., and Chernick, V.: Continuous positive transpulmonary pressure in hyaline membrane disease. Pediatrics 48:296, 1971.

Villavicencio, J. L., Jurado, E., Sagaon, J., and Alvarez de los Cobos, J.: The use of human fibrinolysin by aerosol in the treatment of pulmonary hyaline membrane syndrome. Studies on the fibrinolytic system of normal premature infants and older children. Surg. Forum 11:8, 1960.

Villee, C. A.: Physiology of Prematurity. Trans. 2nd Conference, Josiah Macy Jr. Foundation, New York, 1958.

Vivel, O.: Die Serologie der interstitiellen Pneumonie. Monatsschr. Kinderh. 108:146, 1960.

von Hottinger, A., Kaufmann, H. J., Weisser, K., and Werthemann, A.: Über eine seltene Lungenerkrankung Frühgeborener. Ann. Paediat. 201:13, 1963.

von Neergaard, K.: Neue Auffassungen uber einen Grundbegriff der Atemmechanik die Retraktion-Skraft der Lunge abhängig von der Oberflackenspannung in den Alveolen. Z. Ges. Exp. Med. 66:373, 1929.

Voyce, M. A., and Hunt, A. C.: Congenital tuberculosis. Arch. Dis. Child. 41:299, 1966.

Wade-Evans, T.: Thrombi in the hepatic sinusoids of the newborn and their relation to pulmonary hyaline membrane formation. Arch. Dis. Child. 36:286, 1961.

Wagenvoort, C. A., Losekoot, G., and Mulder, E.: Pulmonary veno-occlusive disease of presumably intrauterine origin. Thorax 26:429, 1971.

Wagenvoort, C. A., and Wagenvoort, N.: Arterial anastomoses, bronchopulmonary arteries, and pulmobronchial arteries in perinatal lungs. Lab. Invest. 16:13, 1967.

Walker, J. S.: Transpalative surgery for congenital bilateral choanal atresia. J. A. M. A. 154:753, 1954.

Wallgren, G., Hanson, J. S., Tabakin, B. S., Raiha, N., and Vapaavuori, E.: Qualitative studies of the human neonatal circulation. V. Hemodynamic findings in premature infants with and without respiratory distress. Acta Paediat. Scand. (Suppl.) 179:69, 1967.

Wang, N. S., Kotas, R. V., Avery, M. E., and Thurlbeck, W. M.: Accelerated appearance of osmiophilic bodies in fetal lungs following steroid injection. J. Appl. Physiol. 30:362, 1971.

Warley, M. A., and Gairdner, D.: Respiratory distress syndrome of the newborn— principles in treatment. Arch. Dis. Child. 37:455, 1962.

Warren, S., and Gates, O.: Radiation pneumonitis; experimental and pathologic observations. A.M.A. Arch. Path. 30:440, 1940.

Waterston, D. J., Bonham-Carter, R. E., and Aberdeen, E.: Congenital tracheo-oesophageal fistula in association with oesophageal atresia. Lancet 11:55, 1963.

Weaver, R. L., and Ahlgren, E. W.: Umbilical artery catheterization in neonates. Amer. J. Dis. Child. 122:499, 1971.

Webb, J. K. S., John, T. J., Jadhav, M., Graham, M. D., and Walter, A.: The incidence of hyaline membrane syndrome in South India. J. Indian Pediat. Soc. 1:193, 1962.

Weibel, E. R., and Gomez, D. M.: Architecture of the human lung. Science 137:577, 1962.

Weisbrot, I. M., James, L. S., Price, C. E., Holaday, D. A., and Apgar, V.: Acid-base homeostasis of the newborn infant during the first 24 hours of life. J. Pediat. 52:395, 1958.

Werkö, L.: The influence of positive pressure breathing on the circulation in man. Acta Med. Scand. (Suppl. 193) 1, 1947.

Weseman, C. M.: Tracheotomy in the newborn. Am. J. Dis. Child. 100:881, 1960.

Wesenberg, R. L., Graven, S. N., and McCabe, E. B.: Radiological findings in wet-lung disease. Radiology 98:69, 1971.

Wessel, M. A.: Chylothorax in a two-week-old infant with spontaneous recovery. J. Pediat. 25:201, 1944.

Westin, B., Miller, J. A., Jr., Nyberg, R., and Wedenberg, E.: Neonatal asphyxia pallida treated with hypothermia alone or with hypothermia and transfusion of oxygenated blood. Surgery 45:868, 1959.

Wexels, P.: Agenesis of the lung. Thorax 6:171, 1951.

Whitehead, W. H., Windle, W. F., and Becker, R. F.: Changes in lung structure during aspiration of amniotic fluid and during air breathing at birth. Anat. Rec. 83:255, 1942.

Whitfield, C. R., Chan, W. H., Sproule, W. B., and Stewart, A. D.: Amniotic fluid lecithin sphingomyelin ratio and fetal lung development. Brit. Med. J. 2:85, 1972.

Whittenberger, J. L.: Artificial respiration. Physiol. Rev. 35:611, 1955.

Whittenberger, J. L. (ed.): Artificial Respiration. Theory and Applications. Hoeber Med. Div., Harper and Row, 1962.

Wigger, H. J., Bransilver, B. R., and Blanc, W. A.: Thromboses due to catheterization in infants and children. J. Pediat. 76:1, 1970.

Williams, H., and Campbell, P.: Generalized bronchiectasis associated with deficiency of cartilage in the bronchial tree. Arch. Dis. Child. 35:182, 1960.

Williams, H. J., and Carey, L. S.: Rubella embryopathy. Roentgenologic lesions. Amer. J. Roentgen. 97:92, 1966.

Williams, R. L., Hof, R. P., Heymann, M. A., and Rudolph, A. M.: Cardiovascular effects of hypothalamic stimulation in the chronic fetal lamb preparation. Abstract presented at the American Heart Association Meeting, Dallas, Texas, November 1972.

Wilson, J. L., Long, S. B., and Howard, P. J.: Respiration of premature infants — respone to variations of oxygen and to increased carbon dioxide in inspired air. Am. J. Dis. Child. 63:1080, 1942.

Wilson, M. G., and Mikity, V. G.: A new form of respiratory disease in premature infants. Am. J. Dis. Child. 99:489, 1960.

Wilson, T. G.: Discussion on stridor in infants. Proc. Roy. Soc. Med. 45:355, 1952.

Windle, W. F., Becker, R. F., Barth, E. E., and Schulz, M. D.: Aspiration of amniotic fluid by fetus. (An experimental roentgenological study in the guinea pig.) Surg. Gynec. Obstet. 69:705, 1939.

Windle, W. F.: Neuropathology of certain forms of mental retardation. Science 140:1186, 1963.

Wittenborg, M. H., Gyepes, M. T., and Crocker, D.: Tracheal dynamics in infants with respiratory distress, stridor, and collapsing trachea. Radiology 88:653, 1967.

Witzleben, C. L.: Aplasia of the trachea. Pediatrics 32:31, 1963.

Witzleben, C. L., and Driscoll, S. G.: Possible transplacental transmission of Herpes simplex infection. Pediatrics 36:192, 1965.

Wolfson, S. L., Frech, R., Hewitt, C., and Shanklin, D. R.: Radiographic diagnosis of hyaline membrane disease. Radiology 93:339, 1969.

Woodrum, D. E., Oliver, T. K., Jr., and Hodson, W. A.: The effect of prematurity and hyaline membrane disease on oxygen exchange in the lung. Pediatrics 50:380, 1972.

Woodrum, D. E., Parer, J. T., Wennberg, R. P., and Hodson, W. A.: Chemoreceptor response in initiation of breathing in the fetal lamb. J. Appl. Physiol. 33:120, 1972.

Woodside, G. L., and Dalton, A. J.: The ultrastructure of lung tissue from newborn and embryo mice. J. Ultrastructure Res. 2:28, 1958.

Wright, R. C.: Prevention of hyalin-membrane disease in the term cesarean-section infant. Obstet. Gynec. 18:695, 1961.

Wu, B., Kikkawa, Y., Orzalesi, M. M., Motoyama, E. K., Kaibara, M., Zigas, C. J., and Cook, C. D.: Accelerated maturation of fetal rabbit lungs by thyroxine. Physiologist 14:253, 1971.

Wunderlich, B., and Reynolds, R. N.: Arterial blood sampling in babies. Amer. J. Dis. Child. 123:446, 1972.

Yancy, W. S., and Spock, A.: Spontaneous neonatal pleural effusion. J. Pediat. Surg. 2:313, 1967.

Yates, P. O.: Birth trauma to the vertebral arteries. Arch. Dis. Child. 34:436, 1959.

Young, L. W., Rubin, P., and Hanson, R. E.: The extra-adrenal neuroblastoma: High radiocurability and diagnostic accuracy. Amer. J. Roentgen. 108:75, 1970.

Younozai, M. K.: Hyaline membranes in Lebanon. Pediatrics 29:332, 1962.

Yow, M., Teng, N. E., Bangs, J., Bangs, T., and Stephenson, W.: The ototoxic effects of Kanamycin Sulfate in infants and children. Abstract. Am. J. Dis. Child. 102:546, 1961.

Yow, M. D., and Tengg, N. E.: The Use of Kanamycin Sulfate as a therapeutic agent for infants and children. J. Pediat. 58:538, 1961.

Zachman, R. D.: The enzymes of lecithin biosynthesis in human newborn lungs. I. Choline Kinase. Biol. Neonate 19:211, 1971.

Index